Marine Natural Products with Antifouling Activity

Marine Natural Products with Antifouling Activity

Editors

Tom Turk
Joana Reis Almeida

MDPI • Basel • Beijing • Wuhan • Barcelona • Belgrade • Manchester • Tokyo • Cluj • Tianjin

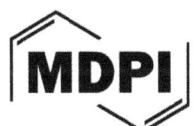

Editors
Tom Turk
University of Ljubljana
Slovenia

Joana Reis Almeida
University of Porto
Portugal

Editorial Office
MDPI
St. Alban-Anlage 66
4052 Basel, Switzerland

This is a reprint of articles from the Special Issue published online in the open access journal *Marine Drugs* (ISSN 1660-3397) (available at: https://www.mdpi.com/journal/marinedrugs/special_issues/Marine_Natural_Products_Antifouling_Activity).

For citation purposes, cite each article independently as indicated on the article page online and as indicated below:

LastName, A.A.; LastName, B.B.; LastName, C.C. Article Title. *Journal Name* **Year**, *Volume Number*, Page Range.

ISBN 978-3-0365-2145-9 (Hbk)
ISBN 978-3-0365-2146-6 (PDF)

© 2021 by the authors. Articles in this book are Open Access and distributed under the Creative Commons Attribution (CC BY) license, which allows users to download, copy and build upon published articles, as long as the author and publisher are properly credited, which ensures maximum dissemination and a wider impact of our publications.

The book as a whole is distributed by MDPI under the terms and conditions of the Creative Commons license CC BY-NC-ND.

Contents

About the Editors vii

Preface to "Marine Natural Products with Antifouling Activity" ix

Ho Yin Chiang, Jinping Cheng, Xuan Liu, Chunfeng Ma and Pei-Yuan Qian
Synthetic Analogue of Butenolide as an Antifouling Agent
Reprinted from: *Marine Drugs* **2021**, *19*, 481, doi:10.3390/md19090481 1

Lexin Long, Ruojun Wang, Ho Yin Chiang, Wei Ding, Yong-Xin Li, Feng Chen and Pei-Yuan Qian
Discovery of Antibiofilm Activity of Elasnin against Marine Biofilms and Its Application in the Marine Antifouling Coatings
Reprinted from: *Marine Drugs* **2021**, *19*, 19, doi:10.3390/md19010019 13

Daniela Pereira, Catarina Gonçalves, Beatriz T. Martins, Andreia Palmeira, Vitor Vasconcelos, Madalena Pinto, Joana R. Almeida, Marta Correia-da-Silva and Honorina Cidade
Flavonoid Glycosides with a Triazole Moiety for Marine Antifouling Applications: Synthesis and Biological Activity Evaluation
Reprinted from: *Marine Drugs* **2020**, *19*, 5, doi:10.3390/md19010005 25

Bruna Costa, Rita Mota, Paula Tamagnini, M. Cristina L. Martins and Fabíola Costa
Natural Cyanobacterial Polymer-Based Coating as a Preventive Strategy to Avoid Catheter-Associated Urinary Tract Infections
Reprinted from: *Marine Drugs* **2020**, *18*, 279, doi:10.3390/md18060279 47

Luciana C. Gomes, Sara I. Faria, Jesus Valcarcel, José A. Vázquez, Miguel A. Cerqueira, Lorenzo Pastrana, Ana I. Bourbon and Filipe J. Mergulhão
The Effect of Molecular Weight on the Antimicrobial Activity of Chitosan from *Loligo opalescens* for Food Packaging Applications
Reprinted from: *Marine Drugs* **2021**, *19*, 384, doi:10.3390/md19070384 63

Guoyong Yan, Jin Sun, Zishuai Wang, Pei-Yuan Qian and Lisheng He
Insights into the Synthesis, Secretion and Curing of Barnacle Cyprid Adhesive via Transcriptomic and Proteomic Analyses of the Cement Gland
Reprinted from: *Marine Drugs* **2020**, *18*, 186, doi:10.3390/md18040186 83

Shuai Zhang, Xinjin Liang, Geoffrey Michael Gadd and Qi Zhao
Marine Microbial-Derived Antibiotics and Biosurfactants as Potential New Agents against Catheter-Associated Urinary Tract Infections
Reprinted from: *Marine Drugs* **2021**, *19*, 255, doi:10.3390/md19050255 103

Yunqing Gu, Lingzhi Yu, Jiegang Mou, Denghao Wu, Maosen Xu, Peijian Zhou and Yun Ren
Research Strategies to Develop Environmentally Friendly Marine Antifouling Coatings
Reprinted from: *Marine Drugs* **2020**, *18*, 371, doi:10.3390/md18070371 125

About the Editors

Tom Turk Ph. D., 1959. He obtained his Ph. D. 1992 at the University of Ljubljana. His Ph.D. thesis was on microbial enzymology in denitrification. Most of his research was conducted at the Graduate Department of Biochemistry, Brandeis University, Waltham, Ma., USA. His later research was dedicated to cytolytic toxins from sea anemones and other organisms, predominantly fungi which harbor cytolytic compounds. In the following years, he studied different aspects of marine natural compounds, mainly those isolated from sponges, among them the biological activity of alkylpyridnium polymers from marine sponge Reniera sarai. Currently, his main focus and the core of his interest is in the possible application of these compounds as antifouling agents and in the development of anticancer drugs for the treatment of certain types of lung cancer. He was a visiting professor at University of Florida, Gainesville, Fl. USA. Currently, he holds a position as a full-time professor of Biochemisty at the University of Ljubljana, Slovenia.

Joana Reis Almeida Biomedical Sciences Ph. D. (2012, ICBAS—University of Porto), is Assistant Researcher at the Interdisciplinary Center of Marine and Environmental Research, University of Porto (CIIMAR-UP), and Invited Assistant Professor at the Faculty of Sciences, University of Porto (FCUP-UP). She works in the areas of natural sciences, environmental sciences, marine biology, and blue biotechnology, and her current research interests focus on marine biofouling and the search for eco-efficient antifouling strategies based on new alternative environmentally compatible products. She currently leads a research team focusing on new bio-inspired antifouling strategies and related environmental aspects. She has published over 20 papers in ISI journals and has two patents on antifouling bioactivity of new compounds. She is the Principal Investigator of the project NASCEM (FCT-PT) on the bioprospection of alternative and sustainable antifouling compounds, and has been part of several national and European research projects on biotechnological applications of natural products, and also in cooperation with sustainable aquaculture industry for antifouling infrastructure improvement.

Preface to "Marine Natural Products with Antifouling Activity"

In a highly competitive marine benthic environment, competition for available space is an important survival strategy for many species. Therefore, antifouling compounds are important components of an arsenal used by many benthic sessile organisms in order to prevent fouling by other organisms. Additionally, among marine microorganisms, a huge diversity of secondary metabolites are produced and have been disclosed to be bioactive against different components of biofouling communities. This Special Issue covers different aspects of the chemistry of marine-based antifouling compounds and their use in various antifouling applications. This collection of articles includes research publications on the discovery of new agents against marine biofouling, namely a butenolide analogue (Boc-butenolide) (1), elasnin (2), and polymethoxylated flavones and chalcones (3); a cyanobacterial polymer-based coating as an antibiotic-free alternative strategy to fight catheter-associated urinary tract infections (4); antimicrobial poly(lactic acid) (PLA) surfaces coated with β-chitosan and β-chitooligosaccharides for food packaging apllicatins (5); insights into the molecular mechanisms underlying the synthesis, secretion, and curing of barnacle cyprid adhesive as potential molecular targets for the development of environmentally friendly antifouling compounds (6); and two review articles focusing on new potential marine microbial-derived antibiotics and biosurfactants against catheter-associated urinary tract infections (7) and recent strategies for the development of marine ecofriendly coatings (8).

This compilation of selected scientific publications highlights the interdisciplinarity underlying the theme of antifouling strategies, and their wide biotechnological applicability.

Tom Turk, Joana Reis Almeida
Editors

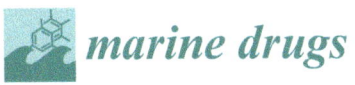

Article

Synthetic Analogue of Butenolide as an Antifouling Agent

Ho Yin Chiang [1], Jinping Cheng [1], Xuan Liu [1], Chunfeng Ma [2] and Pei-Yuan Qian [1,3,*]

[1] Department of Ocean Science, Division of Life Science and Hong Kong Branch of the Southern Marine Science and Engineering Guangdong Laboratory (Guangzhou), The Hong Kong University of Science and Technology, Hong Kong, China; hoyinchiang@ust.hk (H.Y.C.); jincheng@ust.hk (J.C.); ocesxliu@ust.hk (X.L.)
[2] Faculty of Materials Science and Engineering, South China University of Technology, Guangzhou 510000, China; msmcf@scut.edu.cn
[3] Southern Marine Science and Engineering Guangdong Laboratory (Guangzhou), Nansha 510000, China
* Correspondence: boqianpy@ust.hk

Abstract: Butenolide derivatives have the potential to be effective and environmentally friendly antifouling agents. In the present study, a butenolide derivative was structurally modified into Boc-butenolide to increase its melting point and remove its foul smell. The structurally modified Boc-butenolide demonstrated similar antifouling capabilities to butenolide in larval settlement bioassays but with significantly lower toxicity at high concentrations. Release-rate measurements demonstrated that the antifouling compound Boc-butenolide could be released from polycaprolactone-polyurethane (PCL-PU)-based coatings to inhibit the attachment of foulers. The coating matrix was easily degraded in the marine environment. The performance of the Boc-butenolide antifouling coatings was further examined through a marine field test. The coverage of biofouler on the Boc-butenolide coatings was low after 2 months, indicating the antifouling potential of Boc-butenolide.

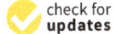

Citation: Chiang, H.Y.; Cheng, J.; Liu, X.; Ma, C.; Qian, P.-Y. Synthetic Analogue of Butenolide as an Antifouling Agent. *Mar. Drugs* **2021**, *19*, 481. https://doi.org/10.3390/md19090481

Academic Editors: Orazio Taglialatela-Scafati, Tom Turk and Joana Reis Almeida

Received: 21 June 2021
Accepted: 21 August 2021
Published: 25 August 2021

Publisher's Note: MDPI stays neutral with regard to jurisdictional claims in published maps and institutional affiliations.

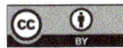

Copyright: © 2021 by the authors. Licensee MDPI, Basel, Switzerland. This article is an open access article distributed under the terms and conditions of the Creative Commons Attribution (CC BY) license (https://creativecommons.org/licenses/by/4.0/).

Keywords: antifouling compounds; structural optimisation; butenolide; larval attachment assay

1. Introduction

Since the prohibition of tributyltin in 2008, many studies have attempted to discover novel antifouling compounds from marine natural products [1]. Many bioactive marine natural products have been screened and tested in recent decades, and several reviews on marine natural products and their synthetic analogues as antifouling compounds have been published [2–5]. Although many potent antifouling compounds have been discovered, those compounds are rarely commercialised. The low supply of antifouling compounds has hindered the development of antifouling paints based on the marine natural products [2,3,6,7]. Two solutions to the problem exist. The first solution is to explore marine natural products from microorganisms, as microorganisms can produce a wide range of bioactive secondary metabolites [8–10]. The convenience of bacterial cultivation and the mass production of metabolites in a short period of time have benefits over the extraction of compounds from the microorganism [6,7,10]. The second solution involves structural optimisation using organic synthesis [6,11]. Secondary metabolites extracted from organisms are often complex in structure; thus, they can be difficult to synthesise effectively in large quantities for commercial-scale usage [6,11]. By studying the structure–activity relationship of bioactive compounds isolated from organisms, pharmacophores that are responsible for antifouling abilities can be identified [11]. Optimisation of the compound's structure is performed with the goal of increasing its potency, decreasing the toxicity of the original compound [12], improving other physical or chemical properties of the compound and simplifying the chemical structure for chemical synthesis.

The antifouling compound 5-octylfuran-2(5H)-one (butenolide) has a melting point at 23 °C, which causes it to change from solid form to liquid at high ambient temperatures. In the present study, a butenolide derivative was modified with a Boc-protecting-group at the terminal of the alkyl side chain, *tert*-butyl (5-(5-oxo-2,5-dihydrofuran-2-yl)pentyl)carbamate

(Boc-butenolide) (Figure 1). This modification aims to improve its environmental stability and to remove its foul smell by increasing its melting point from 23 °C to 132 °C. A higher melting temperature above ambient temperature could lead to a more precise control of the proportion of antifoulant added during coating formulation. The modified Boc-butenolide (Figure 1) was further characterized for its melting point, stability and antifouling bioactivity using anti-larval settlement bioassays with larvae of barnacles (*Amphibalanus amphitrite*) and tubeworms (*Hydroides elegans*) in the laboratory. The modified Boc-butenolide was further formulated into an antifouling paint using polymer matrix poly(ε-caprolactone) based polyurethane (PCL-PU). Release-rate measurements of Boc-butenolide and a marine field antifouling test were conducted to evaluate the feasibility of using Boc-butenolide as an active ingredient in antifouling coatings.

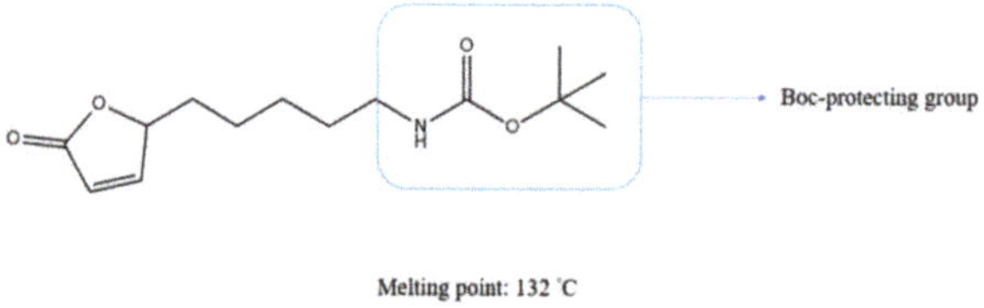

Figure 1. Chemical structure of *tert*-butyl (5-(5-oxo-2,5-dihydrofuran-2yl)pentyl)carbamate (Boc-butenolide).

2. Results and Discussion

2.1. Stability and Solubility of Boc-Butenolide and Butenolide

Figure 2a illustrates the measured concentrations of Boc-butenolide in ASW for 3 months. The concentration of Boc-butenolide measured at day 0 is around 64 ppm and dropped to approximately 50 ppm after 3 months in ASW. In the following anti-larval settlement bioassay experiments, the same nominal concentrations for each condition were used to compare their bioactivity. To understand the relationship between nominal concentration and soluble or working concentrations of the two compounds, the working concentrations for all nominal concentrations used in the experiments were tested using HPLC. Figure 2b shows that the measured working concentrations of Boc-butenolide are higher than all tested working concentrations for butenolide under all tested nominal concentrations (3.125, 6.25, 12.5, 25, 50, and 100 ppm). The average dissolution rate of Boc-butenolide is approximately 40%, while the average dissolution rate of butenolide is only around 10%.

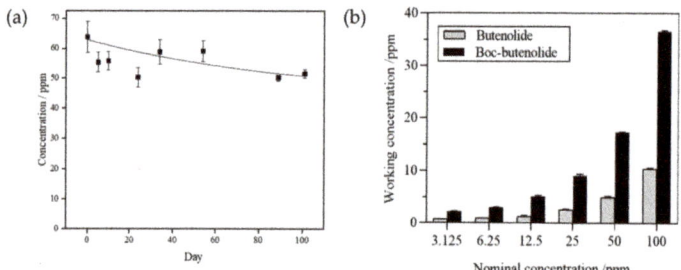

Figure 2. Measured concentrations of Boc-butenolide in ASW for 3 months (**a**), and working concentrations of butenolide and Boc-butenolide (**b**) used in Figures 3 to 6.

2.2. Antifouling Performance of Boc-Butenolide

Figure 3 shows the settlement rate of *A. amphitrite* larvae treated with Boc-butenolide and butenolide. At nominal concentrations of 50 ppm to 100 ppm, both compounds inhibited the settlement of barnacle cyprids. Settlement rates between the two compounds began to differ at 25 ppm. For Boc-butenolide, the cyprids showed some settlement at a rate of approximately 3%. The settlement rate continuously increased, reaching approximately 70% at a concentration of 3.125 ppm. For butenolide, the attachment of cyprids was inhibited between the concentrations of 6.25 ppm and 100 ppm, and approximately only 10% of the larvae settled in the treatment of 3.125 ppm.

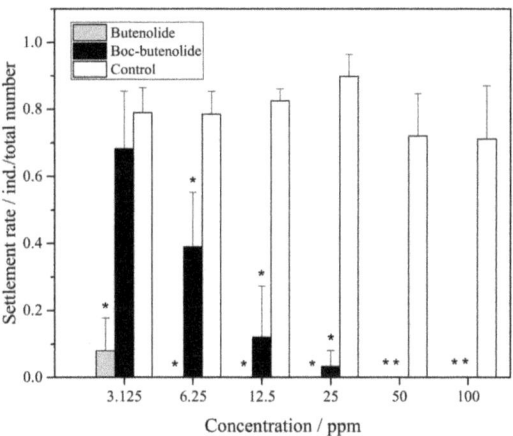

Figure 3. *A. amphitrite* larval settlement rate after Boc-butenolide and butenolide treatments. Asterisks indicate a significant difference from the control with $p < 0.05$.

Figure 4 shows the mortality rate of *A. amphitrite* larvae treated with Boc-butenolide and butenolide. For both compounds, there was no significant difference in toxic effects compared with the control group between the nominal concentrations of 3.125 ppm and 12.5 ppm. A pronounced difference in toxic effects was observed at 25 ppm. A very low toxicity was observed for Boc-butenolide-treated larvae, i.e., the mortality rate was approximately 8%, compared with the obvious toxic effect observed for the butenolide-treated larvae, in which mortality rate was over 90% among the individuals at high concentrations. All cyprids died in both treatments with higher antifoulant concentrations (50 and 100 ppm), indicating the toxic effects of the antifouling compounds at high concentrations.

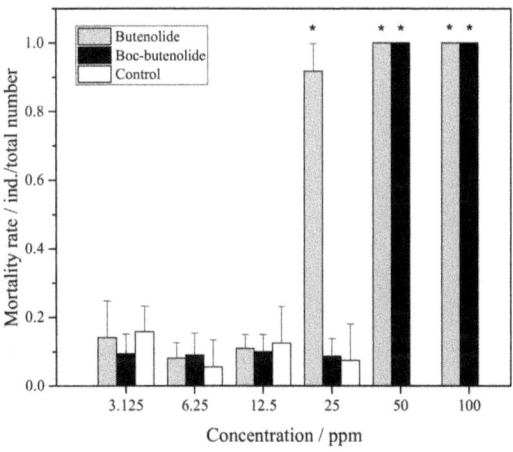

Figure 4. *A. amphitrite* larval mortality rate after Boc-butenolide and butenolide treatments. Asterisks indicate a significant difference from the control with $p < 0.05$.

The *H. elegans* larval settlement bioassay results were similar to those of the *A. amphitrite* larval settlement bioassay. No settlement of larvae was observed after treatments with Boc-butenolide at 50 and 100 ppm (Figure 5), whereas for butenolide treatments, effective inhibition of larval settlement was found even at a low concentration of 12.5 ppm. For Boc-butenolide treatments, a significant difference from the control group was still observed at 25 ppm, with a settlement rate of approximately 20%. An increase in settlement inhibition was observed from 3.125 ppm to 25 ppm. For butenolide treatments, a significant difference was found between treatment and control groups across all concentrations, with a settlement rate of approximately 50% at low concentrations of 3.125 and 6.25 ppm.

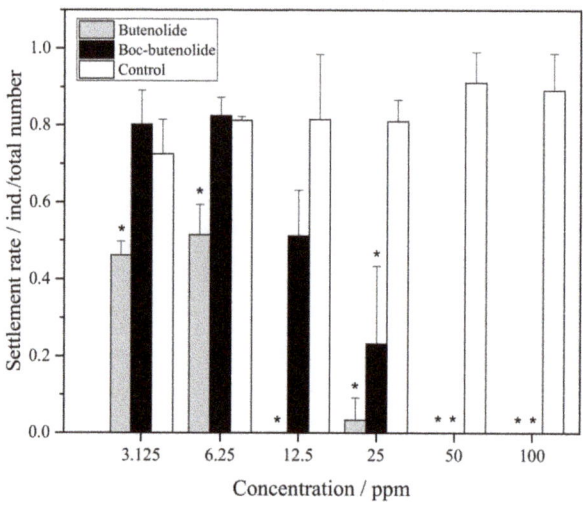

Figure 5. *H. elegans* larval settlement rate after Boc-butenolide and butenolide treatments. Asterisks indicate a significant difference from the control with $p < 0.05$.

In terms of the toxicity of the compounds (Figure 6), only Boc-butenolide treatments at 50 and 100 ppm showed significant toxicity on the *H. elegans* larvae. However, for butenolide treatments, toxic effects started to appear at 12.5 ppm, reaching a 100% mortality rate at concentrations above 50 ppm. Structural differences between Boc-butenolide and butenolide affect the pharmacokinetics of the two compounds, leading to differences in potency and toxicity towards the larvae.

2.3. Release Rate of Boc-Butenolide from the Coatings

Figure 7 shows the release rate of different concentrations of Boc-butenolide and butenolide for at least 90 d. Generally, the amount of compounds released from the coatings at a particular time is positively correlated with the initial concentration of the compounds in the coatings. The release rate could be controlled by changing the concentration of antifoulant in the coatings. The initial release rate of Boc-butenolide (150 µg/cm^2/day) was much higher than that of butenolide (45 µg/cm^2/day) for 10 wt% samples. A possible explanation is the hydrophilicity difference between Boc-butenolide and butenolide. A Boc-protecting-group was added to the side chain of butenolide. Thus, the Boc-butenolide was more hydrophilic with the added highly electronegative N and O atoms of the Boc group and easier to dissolve in seawater, thereby resulting in a high initial release rate. A huge decrease in the release of antifoulant from the coatings for both Boc-butenolide and butenolide was found after 1 month. Notably, the release of Boc-butenolide from the coatings for all four concentrations was much lower than that of butenolide after 1 month. This finding might be due to the fact that a steady release in the later stage cannot be supported after a huge initial release of Boc-butenolide.

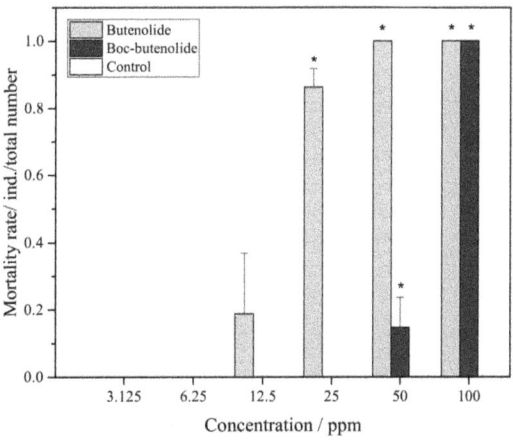

Figure 6. *H. elegans* larval mortality rate after Boc-butenolide and butenolide treatments. Asterisks indicate a significant difference from the control with $p < 0.05$.

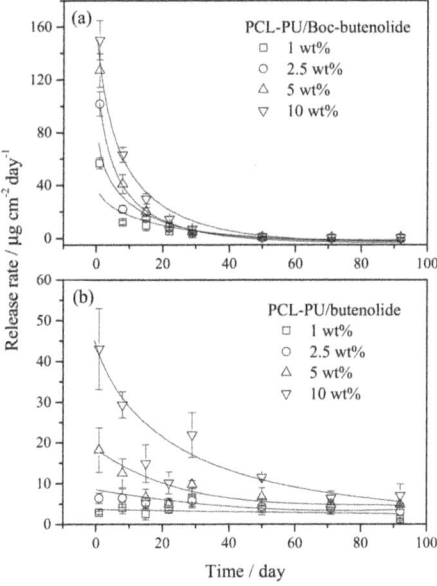

Figure 7. Release-rate measurement of (**a**) Boc-butenolide and (**b**) butenolide with PCL-PU matrix for 90 d.

PCL-PU polymer is biodegradable and environmentally friendly, and was applied as the polymer to develop the antifouling coating system in the present work. In the previous study, a PCL-PU/butenolide antifouling coating system was developed and test results showed that the polymer coating could be degraded in the sea [13]. In this experiment, PCL-PU/Boc-butenolide showed a large decrease in release rate when compared to that of PCL-PU/butenolide, which might be due to the compatibility of Boc-butenolide in PCL-PU and the relatively high solubility of Boc-butenolide in seawater. In future studies, more effort should be made in the improvement of the polymer structure so as to optimize the release performance of Boc-butenolide as an antifouling coating.

2.4. Field-Test Performance

A field test was conducted to evaluate the performance of the coatings in the marine environment. Figures 8 and 9 show the images and the relative coverage of the panels coated with different concentrations of Boc-butenolide or butenolide with PCL-PU as a polymer matrix. After 1 month of exposure, all of the coatings with antifoulants remained almost fouling-free, with less than 10% coverage. Approximately 80% biofilm coverage was observed on the control panels. All of the panels treated with the coatings showed good antifouling performances, indicating the effectiveness of Boc-butenolide and butenolide as antifoulants. This finding is consistent with the larval settlement results, suggesting that the compounds can prevent larval attachment.

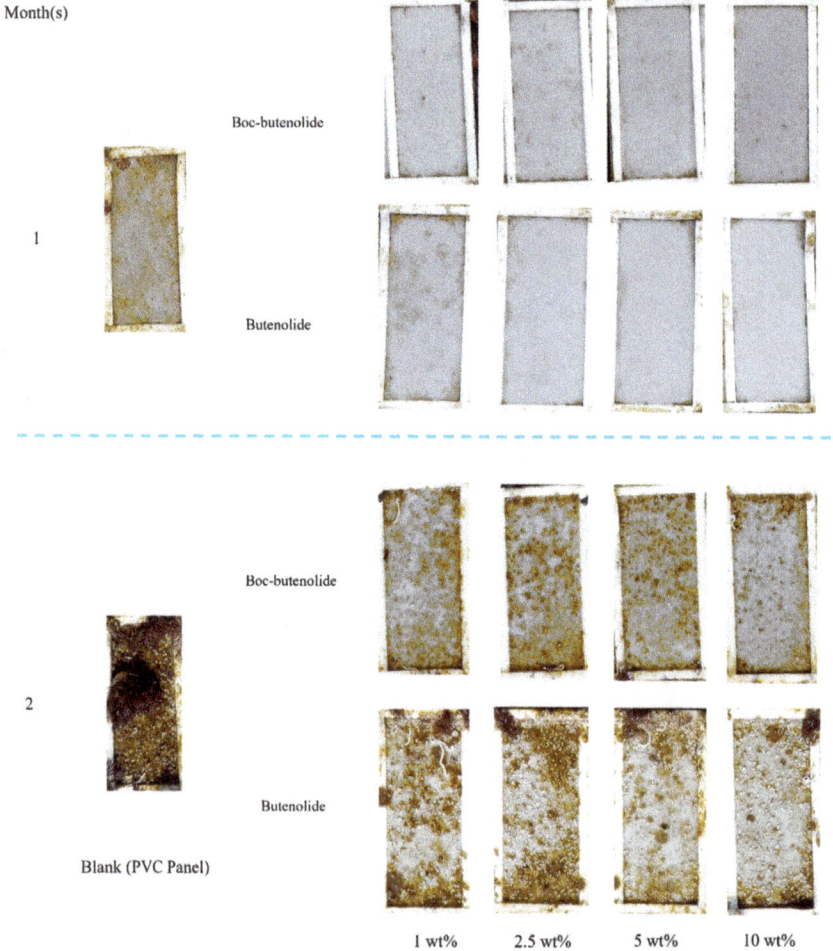

Figure 8. Field test of various concentrations of Boc-butenolide and butenolide with PCL-PU matrix for 2 months. From left to the right, the control, 1, 2.5, 5 and 10 wt% of Boc-butenolide (**top**) or butenolide (**bottom**) are presented. The test was continued for 2 months and retrieved at monthly intervals.

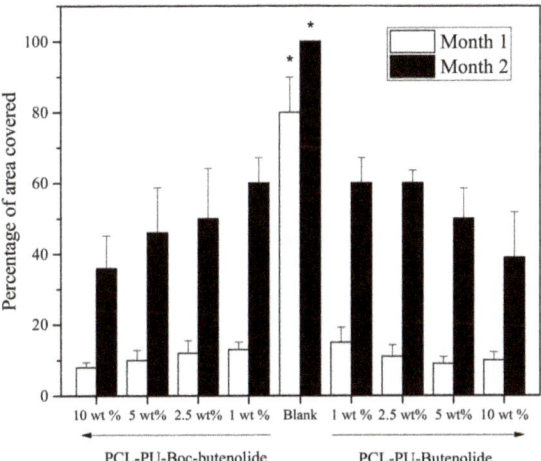

Figure 9. Percentage of area covered with biofoulers for different coatings during a period of 2 months. From left to right, PCL-PU with 10, 5, 2.5 and 1 wt% Boc-butenolide, control and PCL-PU with 1, 2.5, 5 and 10 wt% butenolide are presented. Asterisks indicate a significant difference between the samples within 1 month ($p < 0.05$).

In the second month's results, the coatings with higher concentrations of Boc-butenolide or butenolide showed better antifouling abilities (Figure 9). Performance levels of both Boc-butenolide and butenolide were similar. These results were consistent with the release rate and larval attachment results mentioned above. Although Boc-butenolide was less potent in preventing larval settlement at similar nominal concentrations in the laboratory studies, its huge amount of initial release helped to compensate for its lack of potency, resulting in an antifouling performance similar to that of butenolide in the field test.

The differences in effectiveness and toxicity between Boc-butenolide and butenolide are possibly due to their structural difference. Considering that a Boc group was added to the carbon side chain of butenolide in Boc-butenolide, its structure was large and bulky. Molecular weight and hydrophilicity can affect the pharmacokinetics of the compounds, especially regarding their absorption by organisms [14]. Generally, a large molecule containing electronegative atoms, such as N or O, is more hydrophilic and is difficult to be absorbed or become bioavailable to the organisms. Therefore, Boc-butenolide shows a lower effectiveness when compared with butenolide. The difference in effectiveness was obvious at 25 ppm. At the same time, as Boc-butenolide has a lower absorption or bioavailability, it also shows no or relatively low toxic effects to the treated larvae. The structural modification of butenolide changes the physical and chemical properties of the original compound. For instance, Boc-butenolide is odourless and with a lower toxicity towards the larvae compared with butenolide. Boc-butenolide's chemical stability is also increased, as the Boc group is stable towards most nucleophiles and bases. These changes in physical and chemical properties can be beneficial when designing effective antifouling coatings and also when considering the environmental impact for actual use.

From the release-rate results, an exponential decrease in Boc-butenolide release into the seawater throughout the test period was observed. This result may be due to the high hydrophilicity of Boc-butenolide, which allows it to dissolve more easily in the seawater and achieve a high release rate. The release rate can be improved through the structural modifications of Boc-butenolide. Changes in physical and chemical properties, such as the melting point and hydrophilicity, can be achieved by structural modification [12]. For instance, the water solubility of Boc-butenolide can be reduced by a slight structural modification. Another method for optimising the controlled release of Boc-butenolide in seawater is by developing a suitable polymer as a binder. For example, the antifouling compound could chemically bind to the polymer chain, e.g., in tributyltin-SPC antifouling coatings [15,16]. The release of biocide would then be controlled by the hydrolysis of the polymer, thereby controlling the release rate of the biocide.

3. Materials and Methods

3.1. Chemicals and Seawater

All chemical reagents used in this study, unless otherwise specified, were purchased from Sigma Aldrich (St. Louis, MO, USA) and VWR chemicals (Haasrode, Belgium). 5-Octylfuran-2(5H)-one (butenolide) and *tert*-butyl (5-(5-oxo-2,5-dihydrofuran-2-yl)pentyl)carbamate (Boc-butenolide) with a purity of >99% were purchased from ChemPartner (Shanghai, China) and used as received. Acetonitrile and methanol used were of HPLC grade.

Seawater was collected using a pump at the Coastal Marine Laboratory of Hong Kong University of Science and Technology. Filtered seawater (FSW) was obtained by filtering seawater through a 0.22 μm filter membrane from Millipore (Merck KGaA, Darmstadt, Germany). Artificial seawater (ASW) was prepared according to ASTM D114198 standards (2013) [17].

The stock concentrations of butenolide and Boc-butenolide were made by dissolving 100 mg of butenolide or Boc-butenolide in 1 mL of DMSO to make a stock of 100 mg/mL, stored at −20 °C. The butenolide and Boc-butenolide samples used in the larval settlement and mortality experiments were prepared by serial dilution of stock concentrations of butenolide and Boc-butenolide using ASW as the diluent, and the DMSO content in final samples were lower than 0.5‰ v/v.

3.2. Collection of Amphibalanus amphitrite Larvae Sample

Adult *A. amphitrite* colonies were collected from Tso Wo Hang Pier (22°23′32.1″ N 114°17′18.7″ E), Hong Kong, from April 2018 to June 2018. The adults were kept in a water tank with running seawater at the Coastal Marine Laboratory (the Hong Kong University of Science and Technology) for no more than a week before experimental use. Adults were induced to hatch under light sources for 1 h; the larvae were obtained using a method described previously by Harder et al. [18]. The nauplii larvae newly released from the adults were reared on diatom *Chaetoceros gracilis* Schütt. The seawater culture medium was replaced daily with fresh FSW and algae. The nauplii reached the competent stage, known as cyprid, after 4 d of incubation at approximately 28 °C.

3.3. Collection of Hydroides elegans Larvae Sample

Adult *H. elegans* colonies were collected from a fish farm at Yung Shue O, Hong Kong (22°24′ N, 114°21′ E) from March 2019 to April 2019. The adults were kept in a water tank with running seawater at the Coastal Marine Laboratory of Hong Kong University of Science and Technology for no more than 3 d before experimental use. The larvae were collected according to the methods described by Qian and Pechenik [19]. The tube of the adults was gently cracked with forceps to release the gametes. Oocytes were then mixed with the sperm and transferred into a new container with 500 mL FSW for fertilisation. Larvae were reared on microalga *Isochrysis galbana* (Tahitian strain) after hatching. The seawater culture medium was replaced daily with fresh FSW and algae, and the trochophore-stage larvae reached the competent stage after 5 d of incubation at approximately 25 °C.

3.4. Larvae Food and Cultivation

The diet for *A. amphitrite* and *H. elegans* cultivated in this study comprised *C. gracilis* and *Isochrysis galbana*, respectively. In the laboratory, the algae were cultured with Guillard's f/2 medium. The f/2 medium was prepared by adding designated amounts of $NaNO_3$, NaH_2PO_4 H_2O, trace metal and vitamin solutions into autoclaved FSW [20]. Na_2SiO_3 $9H_2O$ was added for the cultivation of *C. gracilis*. Algal stocks were then added into the culture medium in a 2 L Erlenmyer flask and subcultured bi-weekly. The cultures were bubbled and illuminated under 14 h/10 h light/dark cycle at 23 °C for incubation.

3.5. Settlement Bioassay of A. amphitrite

The test compounds were dissolved with a small amount of DMSO. The test compounds were used in six concentrations from 100 ppm to 3.125 ppm with 2-fold serial dilution. The same amount of DMSO was used as the negative control for all testing concentrations. Approximately 20 ± 2 individual *A. amphitrite* cyprids were placed into each well of the 24-well polystyrene culture plate containing 2 mL of FSW and were subjected to different treatments. For all treatments and controls, three replicates were performed. The plates were then incubated at 25 °C in darkness. After 48 h, the number of settled and swimming larvae were counted using a Leica MZ6 microscope, and possible toxic effects were noted.

3.6. Settlement Bioassay of H. elegans

The test compounds were dissolved with a small amount of DMSO. The test compounds were used at six different concentrations with a 2-fold serial dilution from 100 ppm to 3.125 ppm. The same amount of DMSO was used as the negative control for all testing concentrations. Approximately 10 ± 2 individual *H. elegans* larvae were placed into each well of a 24-well polystyrene culture plate that contained 2 mL of FSW with different concentrations of the test solution. Approximately 10^{-4} molarity of 3-isobutyl-l-methylxanthine was added into each well as an inducer for the settlement of *H. elegans* larvae [7]. The plates were then incubated at 25 °C in darkness. After 24 h, the number of settled and swimming larvae were counted using a Leica MZ6 microscope, and possible toxic effects were noted.

3.7. Determination of Working Concentration and Stability Using High-Performance Liquid Chromatography (HPLC)

The measurement and analysis of butenolide and Boc-butenolide were performed according to previous reports [13,21,22]. The preparation of nominal concentrations for butenolide and Boc-butenolide was described in the section of "Chemicals and seawater". The calibration standards were prepared by serial dilutions of stock concentrations of butenolide and Boc-butenolide using methanol as the diluent, and the DMSO content in all calibration standard samples was lower than 0.5‰ v/v. The stock concentrations of butenolide and Boc-butenolide were made by dissolving 500 mg of butenolide or Boc-butenolide in 1 mL of DMSO to make a stock of 500 mg/mL and stored at −20 °C. The working concentrations of butenolide and Boc-butenolide samples used in settlement bioassay were measured by reverse-phase HPLC using a Waters 2695 separation module coupled to a Waters 2669 photo-diode array (PDA) detector according to the peak area at 210 nm (Waters Corporation, Taunton, MA, USA). Identification of butenolide and Boc-butenolide was determined based on their retention times (butenolide, 11 ± 0.1 min; Boc-butenolide, 6.8 ± 0.1 min). The samples were tested with a 20 min gradient of 50–99% aqueous acetonitrile (ACN) containing 0.05% v/v trifluoroacetic acid (TFA) at a flow of 1 mL/min. The working concentrations of butenolide and Boc-butenolide were calculated according to their standard curves using peak areas plotted against known quantities of standards. The recoveries for butenolide and Boc-butenolide were 90.9% and 99.5%, respectively.

The stability of Boc-butenolide was measured by the concentration changes of Boc-butenolide in ASW throughout 3 months. The starting nominal concentration of Boc-butenolide was 200 ppm. At every time point, 5 mL of the solution was drawn and mixed with 10 mL dichloromethane (DCM). The DCM fraction with the analyte was dried under nitrogen gas, redissolved reconcentrated in 1 mL of methanol and subjected to above HPLC analysis.

3.8. Preparation of Polymer/Antifoulant Coatings

The polymer/antifoulant coatings were prepared using the solution casting method described by Ding et al. [23]. The coating was prepared by dissolving poly(ε-caprolactone)-polyurethane (PCL-PU) [13] and butenolide or Boc-butenolide with different proportions (i.e., 95 wt% polymer and 5 wt% antifoulant for 5% antifoulant coating) in xylene, the mixture was then stirred vigorously until all solids dissolved, thereby forming a uniform solution. The coating solution was applied onto the surface of the panels, which were either epoxy panel (25 mm × 75 mm) for release rate determination or PVC panels (53 mm × 125 mm) for the field test. The panels were then placed under room temperature for 7 days until all solvents evaporated, and a continuous coating was formed.

3.9. Determination of Antifoulant Release Rate from the Coatings

The release rate of butenolide was determined by HPLC for quantification. The polymer/antifoulant coatings were prepared on an epoxy panel (25 mm × 75 mm) according to the above procedure. The coated panels were then placed into ASW. At certain time points (days 1, 8, 15, 22, 29, 50, 71 and 92 after immersion onto ASW), the panels were transferred into separate containers, which filled with 100 mL of fresh ASW. After 24 h immersion, the analyte in ASW was extracted with equal portion of dichloromethane (DCM). The DCM fraction with the analyte was dried under nitrogen gas, reconcentrated in 200 µL of methanol and subjected to HPLC analysis (Waters 2695, Taunton, MA, USA) using a reversed-phase system with a C18 column (Phenomenex Luna C18(2), 250 × 4.6 mm, 5 microns, Torrance, CA, USA) and a photodiode array detector (Waters 2998, Taunton, MA, USA) operated at 210 nm [13,21,22].

3.10. Field Test

The field tests were conducted in a fish farm in Yung Shue O, Hong Kong (114°21′ E, 22°24′ N) from January 2018 to March 2018. PVC panels (53 mm × 125 mm) covered with coatings were immersed in seawater at a depth of 1 m from the surface. The panels were retrieved once monthly, the dirt on the panels was removed by washing the panel gently with seawater before being photographed. The panels were placed back into the sea for monitoring. The antifouling potential of different panels were compared to determine the efficiency of the coatings. The estimation of the panel fouling coverage was achieved by ImageJ (National Institutes of Health, Bethesda, MD, USA) [24]. The percentage of area covered by foulers was calculated from the ratio of total fouling area to the panel area, in which the area was highlighted via the threshold function of ImageJ. IBM SPSS Statistics 22 was used for all statistical analyses. One-way ANOVA was used after initial analyses of heterogeneity and variance of the dataset with Levene's test followed by Tukey's post hoc test. Significance was defined as a p-value lower than 0.05.

4. Conclusions

The structure of butenolide was modified to Boc-butenolide to solve the problems of low melting point and smelliness of butenolide. *A. amphitrite* and *H. elagans* larval settlement bioassay results indicated that Boc-butenolide has similar antifouling ability against macrofoulers but with lower toxicity at high concentration. Boc-butenolide was released from the coatings and demonstrated antifouling ability for at least 2 months (as long as Boc-butenolide was released from coating). The release rate decreased with the increase in concentration of Boc-butenolide in the coatings. Our experiment demonstrated that Boc-butenolide exhibited good antifouling ability and could be a substitute compound for antifouling paints, and future efforts should focus on developing Boc-butenolide as a non-toxic antifouling compound with improved controlled release in the marine environment.

Author Contributions: Conceptualization and methodology, P.-Y.Q., H.Y.C., J.C. and C.M.; investigation, H.Y.C. and X.L.; formal analysis, H.Y.C. and J.C.; resources, P.-Y.Q. and C.M.; writing—original draft preparation, H.Y.C., J.C., X.L. and P.-Y.Q.; writing—review and editing, H.Y.C., J.C., X.L., C.M.

and P.-Y.Q.; supervision and funding acquisition, P.-Y.Q. All authors have read and agreed to the published version of the manuscript.

Funding: This research work was financially supported by the Hong Kong Branch of Southern Marine Science and Engineering Guangdong Laboratory (Guangzhou) (SMSEGL20SC01).

Institutional Review Board Statement: Not applicable.

Informed Consent Statement: Not applicable.

Data Availability Statement: The data presented in this study are available in the main text.

Acknowledgments: Special thanks to Lisa SOO at the Department of Ocean Science at The Hong Kong University of Science and Technology for her technical support in this project.

Conflicts of Interest: The authors declare the following competing interest: This work has been submitted for the U.S. provisional patent application (No. P1964US00).

References

1. Gipperth, L. The legal design of the international and European Union ban on tributyltin antifouling paint: Direct and indirect effects. *J. Environ. Manag.* **2009**, *90*, 86–95. [CrossRef] [PubMed]
2. Qian, P.Y.; Xu, Y.; Fusetani, N. Natural products as antifouling compounds: Recent progress and future perspectives. *Biofouling* **2010**, *26*, 223–234. [CrossRef] [PubMed]
3. Fusetani, N. Antifouling marine natural products. *Nat. Prod. Rep.* **2011**, *28*, 400–410. [CrossRef] [PubMed]
4. Qian, P.Y.; Li, Z.; Xu, Y.; Li, Y.; Fusetani, N. Mini-review: Marine natural products and their synthetic analogs as antifouling compounds: 2009–2014. *Biofouling* **2015**, *31*, 101–122. [CrossRef] [PubMed]
5. Liu, L.L.; Wu, C.H.; Qian, P.Y. Marine natural products as antifouling molecules—A mini-review (2014–2020). *Biofouling* **2020**, *36*, 1210–1226. [PubMed]
6. Dobretsov, S.; Dahms, H.U.; Qian, P.Y. Inhibition of biofouling by marine microorganisms and their metabolites. *Biofouling* **2006**, *22*, 43–54. [CrossRef] [PubMed]
7. Xu, Y.; He, H.; Schulz, S.; Liu, X.; Fusetani, N. Potent antifouling compounds produced by marine *Streptomyces*. *Bioresour. Technol.* **2010**, *101*, 1331–1336. [CrossRef] [PubMed]
8. Dahms, H.U.; Ying, X.; Pfeiffer, C. Antifouling potential of cyanobacteria: A mini-review. *Biofouling* **2006**, *22*, 317–327. [CrossRef] [PubMed]
9. Qian, P.Y.; Lau, S.C.; Dahms, H.U.; Dobretsov, S.; Harder, T. Marine biofilms as mediators of colonization by marine macroorganisms: Implications for antifouling and aquaculture. *Mar. Biotechnol.* **2007**, *9*, 399–410. [CrossRef] [PubMed]
10. Almeida, J.R.; Vasconcelos, V. Natural antifouling compounds: Effectiveness in preventing invertebrate settlement and adhesion. *Biotechnol. Adv.* **2015**, *33*, 343–357. [CrossRef] [PubMed]
11. Li, Y.; Zhang, F.; Xu, Y.; Matsumura, K.; Han, Z. Structural optimization and evaluation of butenolides as potent antifouling agents: Modification of the side chain affects the biological activities of compounds. *Biofouling* **2012**, *28*, 857–864. [CrossRef] [PubMed]
12. Guha, R. On exploring structure-activity relationships. *Methods Mol. Biol.* **2013**, *993*, 81–94. [PubMed]
13. Ma, C.; Zhang, W.; Zhang, G.; Qian, P.Y. Environmentally friendly antifouling coatings based on biodegradable polymer and natural antifoulant. *ACS Sustain. Chem. Eng.* **2017**, *5*, 6304–6309.
14. Turfus, S.C.; Delgoda, R.; Picking, D.; Gurley, B.J. Pharmacokinetics. In *Pharmacognosy*, 1st ed.; Simone, B., Rupika, D., Eds.; Academic Press: Cambridge, MA, USA, 2017; pp. 495–512.
15. Kiil, S.; Weinell, C.E.; Yebra, D.M.; Dam-Johansen, K. Marine biofouling protection: Design of controlled release antifouling paints. In *Computer Aided Chemical Engineering*; Ka, M.N., Rafiqul, G., Kim, D.-J., Eds.; Elsevier: Amsterdam, The Netherlands, 2007; pp. 181–238.
16. Bressy, C.; Margaillan, A.; Faÿ, F.; Linossier, I.; Réhel, K. 18—Tin-free self-polishing marine antifouling coatings. In *Advances in Marine Antifouling Coatings and Technologies*; Claire, H., Diego, Y., Eds.; Woodhead Publishing: Cambridge, UK, 2009; pp. 445–491.
17. ASTM. *Standard Practice for the Preparation of Substitute Ocean Water*; ASTM D1141-98; ASTM International: West Conshohocken, PA, USA, 2013.
18. Harder, T.N.; Thiyagarajan, V.; Qian, P.Y. Effect of cyprid age on the settlement of *Balanus amphitrite* darwin in response to Natural Biofilms. *Biofouling* **2001**, *17*, 211–219. [CrossRef]
19. Qian, P.Y.; Pechenik, J.A. Effects of larval starvation and delayed metamorphosis on juvenile survival and growth of the tube-dwelling polychaete *Hydroides elegans* (Haswell). *J. Exp Mar. Biol. Ecol.* **1998**, *227*, 169–185. [CrossRef]
20. Guillard, R.R.L.; Ryther, J.H. Studies of marine planktonic diatoms. I. Cyclotella nana Hustedt, and Detonula confervacea (cleve) Gran. *Can. J. Microbiol.* **1962**, *8*, 229–239. [CrossRef] [PubMed]
21. ASTM. *Standard Test Method for Determination of Organic Biocide Release Rate from Antifouling Coatings in Substitute Ocean Water*; ASTM D6903-07; ASTM International: West Conshohocken, PA, USA, 2013.

22. Chen, L.; Xu, Y.; Wang, W.; Qian, P.Y. Degradation kinetics of a potent antifouling agent, butenolide, under various environmental conditions. *Chemosphere* **2015**, *119*, 1075–1083. [CrossRef]
23. Ding, W.; Ma, C.; Zhang, W.; Chiang, H.; Tam, C. Anti-biofilm effect of a butenolide/polymer coating and metatranscriptomic analyses. *Biofouling* **2018**, *34*, 111–122. [CrossRef] [PubMed]
24. Schneider, C.A.; Rasband, W.S.; Eliceiri, K.W. NIH Image to ImageJ: 25 years of image analysis. *Nat. Methods* **2012**, *9*, 671–675. [CrossRef] [PubMed]

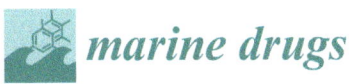

Article

Discovery of Antibiofilm Activity of Elasnin against Marine Biofilms and Its Application in the Marine Antifouling Coatings

Lexin Long [1,2], Ruojun Wang [2], Ho Yin Chiang [2], Wei Ding [3], Yong-Xin Li [4,*], Feng Chen [5,*] and Pei-Yuan Qian [2,*]

1. SZU-HKUST Joint PhD Program in Marine Environmental Science, Shenzhen University, Shenzhen 518000, China; llongaa@connect.ust.hk
2. Department of Ocean Science and Hong Kong Branch of Southern Marine Science and Engineering Guangdong Laboratory, Guangzhou, The Hong Kong University of Science and Technology, Clear Water Bay, Kowloon, Hong Kong 999077, China; rwangaw@connect.ust.hk (R.W.); hychiang@connect.ust.hk (H.Y.C.)
3. Colleague of Marine Life Science, Ocean University of China, 5 Yushan Road, Qingdao 266100, China; dingwei@ouc.edu.cn
4. Department of Chemistry, The University of Hong Kong, Pokfulam, Hong Kong 999077, China
5. Institute for Advanced Study, Shenzhen University, Shenzhen 518060, China
* Correspondence: yxpli@hku.hk (Y.-X.L.); sfchen@szu.edu.cn (F.C.); boqianpy@ust.hk (P.-Y.Q.)

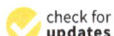

Citation: Long, L.; Wang, R.; Chiang, H.Y.; Ding, W.; Li, Y.-X.; Chen, F.; Qian, P.-Y. Discovery of Antibiofilm Activity of Elasnin against Marine Biofilms and Its Application in the Marine Antifouling Coatings. *Mar. Drugs* 2021, 19, 19. https://doi.org/10.3390/md19010019

Received: 27 November 2020
Accepted: 30 December 2020
Published: 5 January 2021

Publisher's Note: MDPI stays neutral with regard to jurisdictional claims in published maps and institutional affiliations.

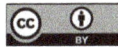

Copyright: © 2021 by the authors. Licensee MDPI, Basel, Switzerland. This article is an open access article distributed under the terms and conditions of the Creative Commons Attribution (CC BY) license (https://creativecommons.org/licenses/by/4.0/).

Abstract: Biofilms are surface-attached multicellular communities that play critical roles in inducing biofouling and biocorrosion in the marine environment. Given the serious economic losses and problems caused by biofouling and biocorrosion, effective biofilm control strategies are highly sought after. In a screening program of antibiofilm compounds against marine biofilms, we discovered the potent biofilm inhibitory activity of elasnin. Elasnin effectively inhibited the biofilm formation of seven strains of bacteria isolated from marine biofilms. With high productivity, elasnin-based coatings were prepared in an easy and cost-effective way, which exhibited great performance in inhibiting the formation of multi-species biofilms and the attachment of large biofouling organisms in the marine environment. The 16S amplicon analysis and anti-larvae assay revealed that elasnin could prevent biofouling by the indirect impact of changed microbial composition of biofilms and direct inhibitory effect on larval settlement with low toxic effects. These findings indicated the potential application of elasnin in biofilm and biofouling control in the marine environment.

Keywords: elasnin; biofilms; marine; biofouling; natural products

1. Introduction

A biofilm is a microbial community attached to a surface [1]. It consists of microbial cells massed in the matrix of extracellular polymeric substances, which contain a large variety of biopolymers such as proteins, nucleic acids, lipids, and other substances [2]. Biofilms can be made up of a single microbial species or multiple species that colonize biotic or abiotic surfaces [3,4]. The elaborate biofilm architecture protects the microbes in biofilms and provides spatial proximity and internal homeostasis needed for growth and differentiation [3–5]. This composition makes microbial cells more resistant than their planktonic counterparts to diverse external insults such as antimicrobial treatment, poisons, protozoans, and host immunity [6,7]. For example, biofilms can render organisms 10- to 1000-fold less susceptible to antimicrobial agents; furthermore, organisms in multi-species biofilms are less susceptible to antimicrobial treatment than those in mono-species biofilms because of their complex interactions [6,8,9].

In the marine environment, biotic and abiotic surfaces are rapidly colonized by microorganisms and subsequent biofilm formation composed of bacteria, diatoms, fungi, unicellular algae, and protozoa [5,10], which creates a big problem for humans. Marine biofilms are critical in inducing biofouling and biocorrosion in the marine environment.

Biofilms are important to habitat selection and settlement of many sessile marine organisms; for example, invertebrate larvae can distinguish biofilms composed of different microbial community structures to settle on or not [11–13]. The metabolites produced by microorganisms such as hydrogen sulfide, various acids, and ammonia destroy various materials. Every year, biofouling and biocorrosion contribute to enormous economic losses worldwide in industries, including heat exchange, oil and gas processing, storage and transportation, and drinking and wastewater industries [14–16]. Moreover, the persistence and transmission of harmful or pathogenic microorganisms and their genetic determinants within the marine biofilms pose a great threat to human beings [5].

Given the continuous increase in economic loss and the potential threats caused by the formation of marine biofilms, effective and economic control methods are necessary. At present, antibiofilm/antifouling coatings are the widely used and are an easy control method in the marine environment. However, the chemical inhibitors used in traditional coatings, such as amines, amides, organic tin, and cuprous oxide, are toxic and harmful, have no favorable environmental profile, and can be bioaccumulated. Increasing attention is focused on the use of natural products to develop effective and less hazardous coatings. Natural compounds with antibiofilm activities generated from the metabolic mechanism of microorganisms can be an ideal substitute for the traditional chemical biocides, presenting environmentally friendly properties such as low toxicity and biodegradability. However, insufficient productivity and difficulty in synthesis limit the development of naturally synthesized compounds [14,16,17].

Among the marine biofilms, as the early colonizers, bacteria are an important factor in determining the structure and function of a mature biofilm [5,14,18]. Therefore, bacteria from marine biofilms can be great targets for the discovery of antibiofilm compounds. In the present study, we used bacteria isolated from marine biofilms to screen for antibiofilm compounds, which led to the discovery of the potent antibiofilm activity of elasnin. With high productivity, elasnin-based coatings were consequently prepared, and their activities against natural multispecies marine biofilms were assessed in the field test.

2. Results

2.1. Isolation and Identification of Biofilm Inhibition Compounds

During our screening project, secondary metabolites produced by *Streptomyces mobaraensis* DSM 40847 (Figure 1b) exhibited strong biofilm inhibition activity against marine bacteria *Staphylococcus aureus* B04. Fractionation coupled with biofilm inhibition assay led to the identification of the main bioactive compound fraction 16 (Figure S1), which was produced at a high yield (approximately 332 mg/L), thereby achieving the maximum productivity after 2 days of incubation. Fraction 16 was subsequently purified using high-performance liquid chromatography (HPLC) and structurally characterized as a known compound elasnin using ultra-performance liquid chromatography-tandem mass spectrometry (UPLC–MS/MS) and nuclear magnetic resonance (NMR) spectroscopy (Figure 1, Supplementary Materials Figures S2 and S6 and Table S2).

Fraction 16: Appearance: colorless, viscous oil; UV (λmax): 291 nm; ^{1}H NMR (500 MHz, DMSO-d_6):δ0.80 (t, 3H), δ0.83 (t, 3H), δ0.86 (t, 3H), δ0.90 (t, 3H), 1.04~1.45 (overlapped, 18H), 1.61 (m, H, H$_a$-13), 1.86 (m, H, H$_b$-13), 2.32~2.47 (m, 6H), 3.87 (dd, 1H, J = 8.8, 5.7 Hz, H-6), 10.49 (s, 1H, 3-OH); ^{13}C NMR (150 MHz, DMSO-d_6): δ13.8, 13.8, 13.8, 13.8, 22.0, 22.1, 22.1, 22.1, 22.8, 22.8, 23.9, 27.6 (C-13), 28.9, 30.0, 30.5, 31.5, 39.8 (C-8), 52.8 (C-6), 103.1 (C-2), 114.2 (C-4), 154.5 (C-5), 163.6 (C-3), 163.8 (C-1), 206.8 (C-7); LC-ESI-MS: (m/z) [M + H]$^+$ 393.3.

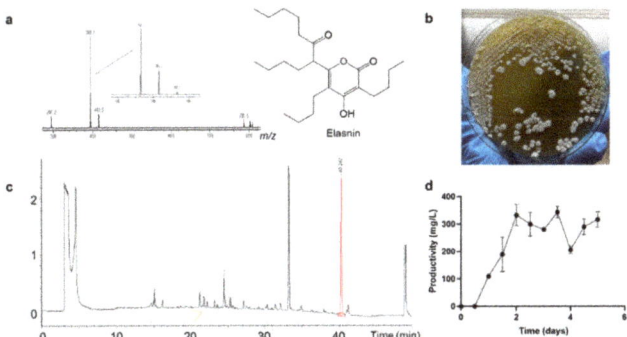

Figure 1. Elasnin was produced by *Streptomyces mobaraensis* DSM 40847 with high yield. (**a**) Mass spectra (ESI) and structure of elasnin; (**b**) growth of *S. mobaraensis* DSM 40847 on the GYM (Table S1) agar plate; (**c**) high-performance liquid chromatography (HPLC) analysis of the crude extracts of *S. mobaraensis* DSM 40847; (**d**) time course of the production of elasnin in AM4 medium at 30 °C.

2.2. Elasnin Could Inhibit the Biofilm Formation of Multiple Strains of Bacteria Isolated from Marine Biofilms

Ten strains isolated from marine biofilms—*Vibrio alginolyticus* B1, *Erythrobacter* sp. HKB8, *Ruegeria* B32, *S. aureus* B04, *S. hominis* N32, *S. arlettae* OM, *Microbacterium esteraromaticum* N22, *Idiomarina sediminum* N28, *Pseudoalteromonas* L001, and *Escherichia coli* N57—were used as targets in the minimum biofilm inhibitory concentration (MBIC) assay and minimal inhibitory concentration (MIC) assay. The MBIC is the lowest concentration of a compound that resulted in a certain reduction in the attached cells while the MIC is the lowest concentration needed for inhibiting the visible growth of planktonic cells. Among the ten strains, seven successfully formed biofilms during the test, and three (*V. alginolyticus* B1, *Erythrobacter* sp. HKB8, and *Ruegeria* B32) cannot form biofilms under the testing situation. For the seven biofilm-forming strains, the biofilms of four Gram-positive strains were sensitive to elasnin treatment with $MBIC_{90}$ of 2.5 to 5 µg/mL and $MBIC_{50}$ of 1.25 to 5 µg/mL, whereas the $MBIC_{90}$ and $MBIC_{50}$ of elasnin against Gram-negative strains ranged from 5 to 10 µg/mL and 1.25 to 10 µg/mL, respectively (Figure 2a). The MICs of nine strains were determined except for *Microbacterium esteraromaticum* N22 due to its inability to grow under the testing conditions. Elasnin inhibited the planktonic cells of *S. aureus* B04 and *Idiomarina sediminum* N28 from growing with MICs of 5 to 10 µg/mL while for other strains the MICs of elasnin were above 10 µg/mL (Figure 2b). Overall, comparing to antimicrobial activity, elasnin shows more significant efficiency in inhibiting biofilm formation.

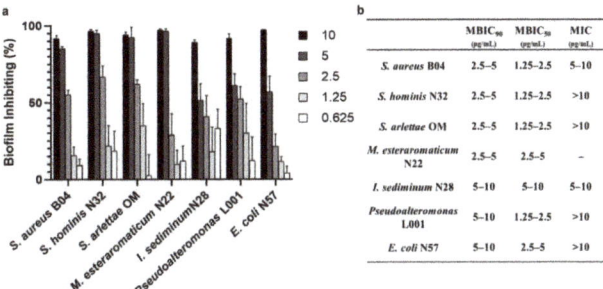

Figure 2. Antibiofilm activities of elasnin against bacteria isolated from marine biofilms. (**a**) Minimum concentration needed for inhibiting biofilm formation; (**b**) summary of minimum biofilm inhibitory concentration (MBICs) and minimal inhibitory concentration (MICs) of elasnin against test strains.

2.3. Preparation of Elasnin-Based Antibiofilm Coatings

Given the high antibiofilm efficiency and high productivity, elasnin-based antibiofilm coatings were prepared and immersed in a fish farm to evaluate their efficiency against natural marine biofilms. In the present study, we used a crude extract of *S. mobaraensis* DSM40847 that contained high concentrations of elasnin (=336.64 mg/L in n-hexane, Figure S7) instead of pure elasnin. The extracts were mixed with polyurethane (polymer) on the basis of poly ε-caprolactone and applied directly on the surface of glass slides. The concentrations of the coatings were calculated on the basis of the percentage of crude extracts in total coatings (polymer and crude extracts) by weight. As such, other compounds in low amounts in the fractionated extract might affect the results of our field testing. However, their effect should be negligible because we did not detect any significant effects of the minor compounds on the crude extracts (Figure S7) and the crude extracts has the same biofilm inhibition efficiency as elasnin shows (MBIC of 0.8–4 and 4–20 µg/mL to *S. aureus* B04 and *E. coli* N57, respectively).

2.4. Release Rate of Elasnin from Antibiofilm Coatings

The release rate of elasnin from the coatings was dependent on time and concentration during the 4 weeks observation (Figure 3c). In general, the release of elasnin was maintained at a low rate throughout the period; the higher the concentration, the faster the release of elasnin into the artificial seawater. The highest release rate of approximately 5 µg day^{-1} cm^{-2} occurred in the second week for the concentration of 10 wt%; for other concentrations, the maximum release rate was approximately 4 µg day^{-1} cm^{-2} in the first week. The release rate decreased over time and depended on the total amount of elasnin remaining in the coatings. After immersion for 4 weeks, the release rate dropped to approximately 1 µg day^{-1} cm^{-2} for the concentrations of 10 wt% and 5 wt% and 0.5 µg day^{-1} cm^{-2} for 1.5 wt% and 2.5 wt%.

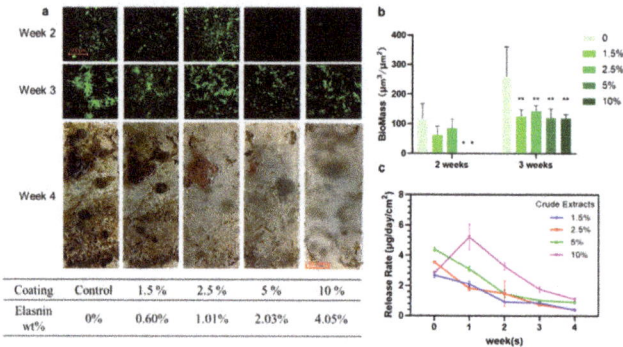

Figure 3. Antibiofilm (weeks 2 and 3) and antifouling (week 4) performance of elasnin-based antibiofilm coatings. (**a**) Confocal laser scanning microscopy (CLSM) images (weeks 2 and 3) of the coated surface (week 4); (**b**) Biomass of biofilms observed by CLSM. (**c**) Monitoring of the release rate of elasnin into the artificial seawater; Biomass is calculated using Comstat 2.1 on the basis of the CLSM images and values that are significantly different among elasnin-based antibiofilm coatings, and the control groups are indicated by asterisks: * for $p < 0.05$ and ** for $p < 0.01$.

2.5. Elasnin-Based Coatings Inhibited the Formation of Multi-Species Biofilms and the Attachment of Large Biofouling Organisms in the Marine Environment

The performance of the antibiofilm coatings was assayed every week from the second to the fourth week by direct and confocal laser scanning microscopy (CLSM) observation (Figure 3a). Based on the quantitative analysis of CLSM images, the average biofilm biomass on the slides without elasnin was 116.44 µm^3 µm^{-2} in the second week and 259.95 µm^3 µm^{-2} in the third week, whereas the average biomass of biofilms measured on

5 wt% and 10 wt% coating slides was less than 0.1 μm³ μm⁻² in the second week and less than 120 μm³ μm⁻² in the third week. For coatings with low concentrations (1.5 wt% and 2.5 wt%), no significant differences were observed with regard to average biomass (61.97 and 84.73 μm³ μm⁻², respectively) in the second week, but the biomass was significantly lower than that in the control (259.95 μm³ μm⁻²) in the third week, with an average biomass of approximately 125 and 145 μm³ μm⁻², respectively (Figure 3b). In the fourth week, slides coated with low concentrations of elasnin (1.5 wt%, 2.5 wt%, and control) were fouled by large marine organisms, whereas those coated with high concentrations of elasnin exhibited an anti-macrofouling activity and almost no larval settlement, except for a small area near the edges because of the edge effects commonly found on testing panels. Elasnin-based antibiofilm coatings inhibited the biofilm formation of multiple bacterial species in the first 2 weeks. However, after immersion for 4 weeks, the glass slides coated with low concentrations of elasnin were eventually covered with large biofouling organisms probably because of the low releasing rate of the elasnin after 3 weeks.

2.6. Elasnin Changed the Microbial Community Structure of Natural Marine Biofilms

Considering that the number of biofilms developed by the end of the second week was limited, and macrofoulers had overgrown by the end of the fourth week, only the 3 week-old biofilms developed on 10 wt% coatings and those on the control glass slides (coated with poly ε-caprolactone-based polyurethane only) were selected for 16S amplicon analysis to determine the changes in biofilm microbial community triggered by elasnin. A total of 3,000,000 16S rRNA gene sequences (500,000 per sample) were classified into 31 phyla (*Proteobacteria* were classified down to the class level). The microbial composition of the biofilms differed between the 10 wt% coatings and the control slides, as confirmed by alpha- and beta-diversity analysis. In the Bray–Curtis dissimilarity (beta-diversity) dendrogram (Figure 4a), the control and treatment groups were clustered separately on the basis of the differences in microbial abundance among the samples; the observed operational taxonomic units (OTUs) and Shannon diversity for the treated biofilm were significantly lower than those in the control group (Figure 4b), indicating that species richness and diversity in the treated biofilms were reduced.

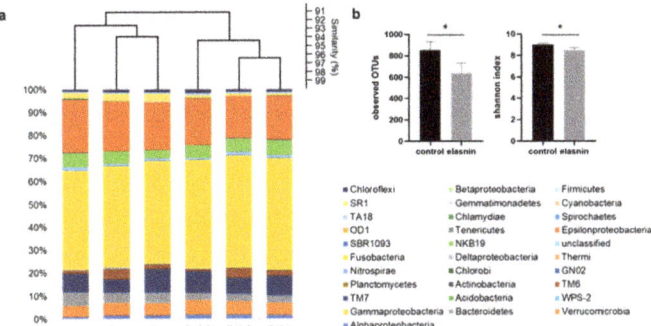

Figure 4. Composition analysis of biofilms grown on the control slides (without crude extracts) and treatment slides (with 10% CR coatings). (**a**) Similarity comparison of microbial compositions among biofilms on control slides (C-1,2,3) and 10 wt% elasnin-based coatings (E10-1,2,3) based on the beta-diversity (Bray–Curtis) at the phylum level. (**b**) Alpha-diversity of biofilms at the phylum level. The difference between the two types of biofilms is calculated using Student's t-test and is indicated by an asterisk: * for $p < 0.05$.

2.7. Elasnin Inhibited the Larval Settlement of Balanus Amphitrite with a Low Toxic Effect

The antilarval settlement activity of elasnin was measured using *B. amphitrite*, and its possible toxic effects were preliminarily assessed by the mortality rate. When the larvae were exposed to elasnin for 24 h, the larval settlement was significantly inhibited at concentrations above 12.5 µg/mL. No increase in mortality rate was observed at a concentration range from 6.25 to 50 µg/mL compared with the control groups (Figure 5a). After 48 h exposure to elasnin, the settlement inhibition was slightly reduced for the concentration of 25 µg/mL, whereas for the concentration of 50 µg/mL, the inhibitory effect was significant. An increased mortality rate of around 65% and reduced vitality of larva were observed at concentrations of 50 µg/mL after 48 h exposure, but no significant changes were exhibited in the mortality rate for other concentrations of the group compared with the control (Figure 5b).

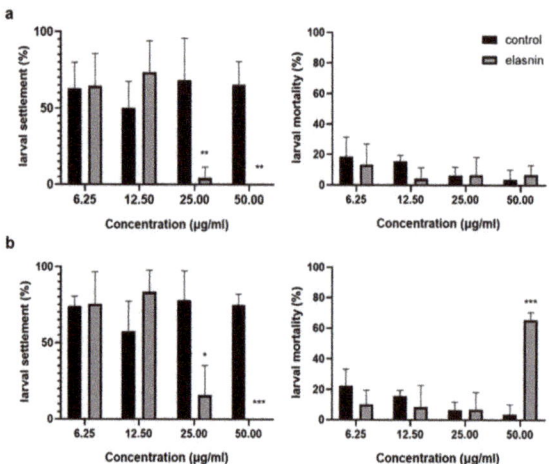

Figure 5. Effect of elasnin on the percentage of larval settlement and mortality rate of *B. amphitrite* after treatment for (**a**) 24 h and (**b**) 48 h. The differences between the control and treatment groups are calculated using Student's t-test and are indicated by asterisks: * for $p < 0.05$, ** for $p < 0.01$, and *** for $p < 0.001$.

3. Discussion

Here, we used bacteria isolated from marine biofilms to screen for the antibiofilm compounds that targeted the marine biofilms, which led to the discovery of the antibiofilm activity of elasnin. Elasnin-based coatings were then prepared with simple and cost-effective methods, and its efficiency against multi-species biofilms was tested in the natural marine environment.

The predictive validity of the screening assay is an important determinant of the success of drug discovery [19,20]. Marine biofilms are complex mixed-species microbial communities with specific intraspecies and interspecies communication and interaction [21,22]. Therefore, the simulation of the marine biofilm formation is difficult under laboratory conditions. In accelerating and simplifying the screening for antibiofilm compounds against marine biofilms with high predictive validity, bacteria isolated from marine biofilms were selected as the target for the bioassay. Consequently, the potential inhibitory activity of elasnin against marine biofilms was discovered during screening. Seven out of ten strains of bacteria isolated from marine biofilms had successfully formed biofilms under the testing situation, and elasnin showed great inhibiting efficiency against all biofilm-forming strains. The inhibiting efficiency of elasnin-based coatings against natural marine biofilms was then validated in the field test, which indicated a great predictive validity of our screening assays.

Elasnin was first discovered in 1978 as a new elastase inhibitor with low toxicity in mice and high selectivity for human granulocyte elastase [23], and its antimicrobial and antibiofilm activities have never been discovered. Based on the test results in the present study, elasnin not only inhibited the biofilm formation of both mono- and multispecies biofilms but also inhibited the settlement of large biofouling organisms. The 16S amplicon analysis revealed that the species richness and diversity of biofilms on the elasnin-based coatings were reduced, which might indirectly inhibit the settlement of biofouling organisms because the changed microbial compositions of the biofilms might not be suitable for them to settle on. In addition, the antilarval-settlement assay showed that elasnin could inhibit larval settlement, which had low toxicity. Considering the effective concentration of elasnin and the water mobility in the marine environment, the toxic effect of elasnin should be negligible, although a high mortality rate was recorded under the high concentration after 48 h exposure. However, the present study only superficially assessed the potential toxic effect of elasnin by the mortality rate of the larva, and its environmental impact should be further explored.

In addition, the wide-type strain *S. mobaraensis* DSM 40847 produced elasnin in substantial quantity (0.33 g/L), which was considered as a new industrial-producing strain of antibiofilm agents. Low product yield has always been a limitation for the development and commercial applications of newly discovered biologically active compounds. The fermentation of this bacterium would address the supply problem that often limited natural products from biotechnical development, leading to the late-stage development of elasnin. Subsequently, elasnin-based coatings were easily prepared with low expenditures. During a 4 week observation, the coatings (10 wt%) inhibited the biofilm formation in the first 2 weeks and the larval settlement in the last 2 weeks. Coatings began to lose their effectiveness after the third week in the field probably because of the reduced release rate of elasnin. Since 2008, when tributyltin (TBT) was restricted by the implementation of the International Maritime Organization Treaty on biocides, the development of efficient and environmentally friendly surface coatings became a hot topic. Collectively, originating from nature, elasnin showed great antibiofilm and antifouling activities with low toxic effects; combined with the low cost of supply, elasnin could provide a new selection for the development of antibiofilm and antifouling materials.

In the present study, we identified a potent antibiofilm compound, namely, elasnin, from the strain *S. mobaraensis* DSM 40847 in the course of our screening program using bacteria isolated from marine biofilms. With high productivity, elasnin-based antibiofilm coatings were easily prepared, which presented a favorable performance in inhibiting the biofilm formation and attachment of macro-foulers in the marine environment. The 16S amplicon and antilarval settlement assays revealed that the antifouling performance of elasnin-based coatings might be caused by the indirect effect of elasnin on biofilm's microbial compositions and its direct inhibitory effect on the larval settlement. With low toxicity, high efficiency, and high productivity, elasnin showed great potential in the applications of biofilm and biofouling control in the marine environment.

4. Materials and Methods

4.1. Strains, Culture Media, and Chemicals

Streptomyces mobaraensis DSM 40847 was purchased from the German Collection of Microorganisms and Cell Cultures (DSMZ, Braunschweig, Germany). The marine bacteria *V. alginolyticus* B1, *Erythrobacter* sp. HKB8, *Ruegeria* B32, *S. aureus* B04, *S. hominis* N32, *S. arlettae* OM, *M. esteraromaticum* N22, *I. sediminum* N28, *Pseudoalteromonas* L001, and *E. coli* N57 were isolated from marine biofilms and obtained from the culture collection of our laboratory [24]. Soybean powder was purchased from Wugumf, Shenzhen, China. Soluble starch was purchased from Affymetrix, Santa Clara, CA, USA. Magnesium sulfate hydrate was purchased from Riedel-de-Haën, Seelze, Germany. Bacteriological peptone was obtained from Oxoid, Milan, Italy. Mueller-Hinton broth (MHB) was purchased from Fluka Chemie AG, Buchs, Switzerland. Phosphate-buffered saline (PBS) and 3-(4,5-dimethylthiazol-2-yl)-2,5-diphenyltetrazolium bromide (MTT) were purchased from Thermo Fisher Scientific Inc., San Jose, CA, USA. Lysogeny broth (LB), glucose, and 1-butanol were purchased from VWR International Ltd., Leicestershire, UK. All other chemicals were supplied by Sigma-Aldrich Corporation, Saint Louis, MO, USA.

4.2. Bioactive Compound Isolation and Identification

Stock cultures of *S. mobaraensis* DSM 40847 were inoculated into 50 mL of AM4, AM5, and AM6 media (Table S1) containing glass beads (to break up globular colonies) and incubated at 30 °C on a rotary shaker (170 rpm). The culture broth was extracted with 1-butanol on days 3, 5, and 7. The crude extracts were dissolved in DMSO before storage and bioassay. Pure compounds were isolated by reversed-phase HPLC (Waters 2695, Milford, MA, USA) using a semi-prep C18 column (10 × 250 mm) that was eluted with a 55 min gradient of 5–95% aqueous acetonitrile containing 0.05% trifluoroacetic acid at a flow rate of 3 mL/min. The structure of elasnin was elucidated through NMR analysis of ^1H, ^1H-^1H-COSY, ^1H-^{13}C-HSQC, and ^1H-^{13}C-HMBC NMR spectra recorded on a Bruker AV500 NMR spectrometer (Bruker, Billerica, MA, USA) and ^{13}C-NMR spectra obtained with the Bruker DRX600 NMR Spectrometer (Bruker, Billerica, MA, USA) using dimethyl sulfoxide-d_6 (^1H-NMR DMSO-d_6: δH = 2.50 ppm; DMSO-d_6: δC = 39.50 ppm).

4.3. Productivity Monitoring and Extraction Efficiency Comparison

A stock culture of *S. mobaraensis* DSM 40847 was incubated in the AM4 medium. One milliliter of culture broth was collected every 12 h and extracted with 1 mL of 1-butanol, ethyl acetate, or n-hexane. The solvent for extraction was then removed by evaporation. The crude extract was dissolved in methanol and quantified through HPLC analysis with a Phenomenex Luna C18 column. The peak of elasnin was identified from the retention time, and its concentration was calculated on the basis of an established standard curve (Figure S9).

4.4. MBIC Assay and MIC Assay Against Marine Bacteria

MBICs were determined as previously described [25,26]. In brief, an overnight culture of test strains was diluted into approximately 10^7 CFU/mL with LB and 0.5% glucose and treated with various concentrations of elasnin (or only media for control) in 96-well cell culture plates. Then, the plates were incubated at 37 °C for 24 h and rinsed two times with 1 × PBS to remove non-adhering and planktonic cells. After rinsing, an MTT staining assay was conducted to measure viable cells in the biofilms because MTT could react with activated succinate dehydrogenase in the mitochondria of viable cells to form blue-violet formazan, which could be read at 570 nm after dissolving in DMSO. The $MBIC_{50}$ and $MBIC_{90}$ were defined as the lowest concentration needed for inhibiting 50% and 90% of biofilm formation individually. The biofilm inhibition efficiency was calculated using the following equation: Biofilm inhibition (%) = (OD_{570nm} of test compound) / (OD_{570nm} of control) × 100%. The experiments were performed in triplicate and repeated three times.

MICs were determined with test strains according to the Clinical and Laboratory Standards Institute guideline CLSI M100 (2018). Briefly, a 10^5 CFU/mL overnight culture of test strains was inoculated into MHB and treated with elasnin (or only media for control) at a series of concentrations. After incubation for 24 h, the minimum concentrations at which no bacterial growth was visible were recorded as the MICs. The experiments were performed in triplicate and repeated twice; vancomycin and kanamycin were used as a positive control in the experiments.

4.5. Elasnin-Based Antibiofilm Coating Preparation

A 4 L culture broth of *S. mobaraensis* DSM 40847 (incubated as previously described) was extracted using n-hexane to obtain a sufficient amount of high-elasnin-content crude extracts. The elasnin-based antibiofilm coatings were prepared following the same procedures as those described by Ma et al. (2017). For the 10 wt% coatings, polymer (0.90 g, 90 wt%) and crude extracts (0.10 g, 10 wt%) were dissolved by vigorously stirring xylene and tetrahydrofuran (v:v = 1:2) at 25 °C. After mixing, a glass slide was coated with the solution and left to dry at room temperature for a week to remove the solvent. The same procedure was used in preparing coatings with different concentrations of crude extracts.

4.6. Field Test and Release Rate Determination

Coated glass slides were submerged in seawater at a fish farm in Yung Shue O, Hong Kong (114°21′ E, 22°24′ N) for 2 to 4 weeks. Afterward, the glass slides were retrieved and transported back to the laboratory in a cooler with in situ seawater and were washed two times using an autoclave and 0.22 µm filtered seawater (FSW) to remove loosely attached particles and cells. The slides were then stained using the FilmTracer™ LIVE/DEAD Biofilm Viability kit and investigated under CLSM (Zeiss LSM710, Carl Zeiss, Oberkochen, Germany). Moreover, the release rate of elasnin was determined by measuring its concentration using HPLC under static conditions. The coated panels were immersed in 100 mL of sterilized artificial seawater held in a measuring container. Ten milliliters of seawater was collected after immersion for 24 h, and elasnin was extracted with the same volume of dichloromethane, which was then removed under nitrogen gas. After drying, the extract was resuspended in 100 mL of methanol and underwent HPLC analysis. The release rate was measured every week for 4 straight weeks, and each concentration was tested in duplicate.

4.7. DNA Extraction, 16S rRNA Gene Sequencing, and Analyses

Biofilm samples on the coated slide surface were collected with autoclaved cotton and stored in DNA storage buffer (10 mM Tris-HCl; 0.5 mM EDTA, pH 8.0) at −80 °C. Before the extraction, samples were vortexed several times to release the microbial cells into the DNA storage buffer. All the samples were then subjected to centrifugation at 10,000 rpm for 1 min, and the supernatant was discarded. After continuous treatment with 10 mg/mL of lysozyme and 20 mg/mL of proteinase K, DNA was extracted from the treated microbial cells with a microbial genomic DNA extraction kit (Tiangen Biotech, Beijing, China) following the manufacturer's protocol.

The quality of DNA samples was controlled using NanoDrop (which tested DNA purity, OD260/OD280) and agarose gel electrophoresis (which tested DNA degradation and potential contamination). The hypervariable V3-V4 region (forward primer: 5′-CCTAYGGGRBGCASCAG-3′; reverse primer: 5′-GGACTACNNGGGTATCTAAT-3′) of prokaryotic 16S rRNA genes was used to amplify DNA from biofilms by polymerase chain reaction (PCR). The PCR products were purified before library construction and sequenced at Novogene (Beijing, China) on the NovaSeq 6000 System. The read length was 250 bp, and each pair of reads had a 50 bp overlapping region. The paired-end reads were subjected to quality control using the NGS QC Toolkit (version 2.0, The National Institute of Plant Genome Research, New Delhi, India) [27]. The 16S rRNA gene amplicon data were analyzed using the software package QIIME2 and then merged using Q2_manifest_maker.py in QIIME2 [28]. The low-quality reads and chimeras were removed using dada2 commands in QIIME2. A total of 500,000 filtered reads for each sample were selected to normalize the uneven sequencing depth. OTUs were classified de novo from the pooled reads at 97% sequence similarity using a classifier trained by the Naive Bayes method. Representative sequences were then recovered using the feature-classifier classify-sklearn script in QIIME2. The alpha-diversity analyses (observed OTUs and Shannon diversity) were performed using the script "qiime diversity alpha" in QIIME2. Beta-diversity based on the Bray–Curtis distances was conducted by the cluster analysis in the software PAST (version 3.0) [29]. Furthermore, the taxonomic structure was drawn in Excel wo (Office 365 MSO 64-bit) on the basis of the relative abundance.

4.8. Antilarval-Settlement Assay

The direct antilarval-settlement assay was conducted using cyprids of the barnacle *B. amphitrite* Darwin as described previously [30–33]. In brief, adult *B. amphitrite* (Darwin) were collected from the intertidal zone in Pak Sha Wan, Hong Kong (22°19′ N, 114°16′ E) and raised to competence for experiments. Elasnin was dissolved in DMSO and diluted into four concentrations from 50 to 6.25 µg/mL with a twofold serial dilution. DMSO was used as a negative control. About 10 ± 2 *B. amphitrite* cyprids were inoculated into each well of a 24-well polystyrene culture plate that contained 2 mL of 0.22 µm FSW with different treatments. For all treatments and controls, three replicates were performed. The plates were then incubated at 25 °C in darkness. After 24 and 48 h, the number of settled and swimming larvae was counted using a Leica MZ6 microscope (Leica Microsystems, Wetzlar, Germany), and possible toxic effects were also noted.

4.9. Statistical Analyses

Statistical analyses for all data were performed using the GraphPad Prism 8.0.2 software (San Diego, CA, USA). The composition of the biofilm on the coatings was compared with that in the control groups using Student's t-test.

5. Patents

The authors declare the following competing interests: This work has been submitted for the U.S. Patent Application (No. 16999437) and Chinese Patent application (No. 202010850564.X).

Supplementary Materials: The following are available online at https://www.mdpi.com/1660-3397/19/1/19/s1, Table S1: Media used in this study, Figure S1: Bioactivities of crude extract of the secondary metabolites produced by *S. mobaraensis* DSM 40847 (incubated with AM4 media and extracted with 1-butanol) and 20 fractions of it. Fraction 17 and 15 are the analogs of franction 16 (elasnin), Figure S2: ^{13}C-NMR analysis of bioactive fraction 16 (Elasnin), Figure S3: ^{1}H-NMR analysis of bioactive fraction 16 (Elasnin), Figure S4: ^{1}H-^{1}H COSY of bioactive fraction 16 (Elasnin), Figure S5: ^{1}H-^{13}C HSQC of bioactive fraction 16 (Elasnin), Figure S6: ^{1}H-^{13}C HMBC of bioactive fraction 16 (Elasnin), Table S2 ^{13}C-NMR (150 MHz, DMSO-d_6), ^{1}H-NMR (500 MHz, DMSO-d_6) and HMBC correlations of compound Fraction 16 (DMSO-d_6) and comparisons between Elasnin (Omura, Nakagawa et al. 1979), Figure S7: HPLC profile of high-elasnin-content crude extracts and productivity of crude extracts/elasnin by using different extraction solvent, Figure S8: Microbial compositions of biofilms on control slides (C-1,2,3) and 10 wt% elasnin-based (E10-1,2,3) coatings at the genus level, Figure S9: Stand curve of elasnin acquired by HPLC.

Author Contributions: L.L. contributed to the experiment design, performed all the experiments, interpreted the data, and prepared the manuscript. R.W. performed the experiments of DNA extraction, 16S amplicon analysis, wrote related methods in the manuscript, and commented on the manuscript. H.Y.C. performed the antilarval-settlement assay, assisted in the coating preparation and field test, and commented on the manuscript. R.W. and W.D. isolated the bacteria from marine biofilms. Y.-X.L. designed and supervised this study, discussed the results and implications at all stages, and edited the manuscript. F.C. and P.-Y.Q. supervised this study, gave technical support and conceptual advice, and edited the manuscript. All authors have read and agreed to the published version of the manuscript.

Funding: This work was financially supported by the National Key R&D Program of China (2018YFA0903200), China Ocean Mineral Resources Research and Development Association (COMRRDA17SC01), the Hong Kong Branch of Southern Marine Science and Engineering Guangdong Laboratory (Guangzhou) (SMSEGL20SC01 and GML2019ZD0409) and a CRF grant from HKSAR government (C6026-19G-A).

Institutional Review Board Statement: Not applicable.

Informed Consent Statement: Not applicable.

Data Availability Statement: The data presented in this study are available in the main text and the supplementary materials of this article.

Acknowledgments: Special thanks to Weipeng Zhang of the College of Marine Life Science at Ocean University for helping to isolate the bacteria from marine biofilms and Rui Feng of the Division of Life Science at the Hong Kong University of Science and Technology for assisting in doing NMR analysis.

Conflicts of Interest: The authors declare no conflict of interest.

References

1. O'Toole, G.; Kaplan, H.B.; Kolter, R. Biofilm formation as microbial development. *Annu. Rev. Microbiol.* **2000**, *54*, 49–79. [CrossRef]
2. Flemming, H.C.; Wingender, J. The biofilm matrix. *Nat. Rev. Microbiol.* **2010**, *8*, 623–633. [CrossRef] [PubMed]
3. Davey, M.E.; O'Toole, G.A. Microbial biofilms: From ecology to molecular genetics. *Microbiol. Mol. Biol. Rev.* **2000**, *64*, 847–867. [CrossRef] [PubMed]
4. Hall-Stoodley, L.; Costerton, J.W.; Stoodley, P. Bacterial biofilms: From the natural environment to infectious diseases. *Nat. Rev. Microbiol.* **2004**, *2*, 95–108. [CrossRef] [PubMed]
5. Dang, H.; Lovell, C.R. Microbial surface colonization and biofilm development in marine environments. *Microbiol. Mol. Biol. Rev.* **2016**, *80*, 91–138. [CrossRef] [PubMed]
6. Antunes, L.C.M.; Ferreira, R.B.R. Biofilms and bacterial virulence. *Rev. Med. Microbiol.* **2011**, *22*, 12–16. [CrossRef]
7. Lopez, D.; Vlamakis, H.; Kolter, R. Biofilms. *Cold Spring Harb. Perspect. Biol.* **2010**, *2*, a000398. [CrossRef]
8. Davies, D. Understanding biofilm resistance to antibacterial agents. *Nat. Rev. Drug Discov.* **2003**, *2*, 114–122. [CrossRef]
9. Hengzhuang, W.; Wu, H.; Ciofu, O.; Song, Z.; Hoiby, N. Pharmacokinetics/pharmacodynamics of colistin and imipenem on mucoid and nonmucoid *Pseudomonas aeruginosa* biofilms. *Antimicrob. Agents Chemother.* **2011**, *55*, 4469–4474. [CrossRef]
10. Qian, P.Y.; Lau, S.C.; Dahms, H.U.; Dobretsov, S.; Harder, T. Marine biofilms as mediators of colonization by marine macroorganisms: Implications for antifouling and aquaculture. *Mar. Biotechnol.* **2007**, *9*, 399–410. [CrossRef]
11. Lau, S.C.K.; Thiyagarajan, V.; Cheung, S.C.K.; Qian, P.Y. Roles of bacterial community composition in biofilms as a mediator for larval settlement of three marine invertebrates. *Aquat. Microbial. Ecol.* **2005**, *38*, 41–51. [CrossRef]
12. Hung, O.S.; Thiyagarajan, V.; Wu, R.S.S.; Qian, P.Y. Effect of ultraviolet radiation on biofilms and subsequent larval settlement of *Hydroides elegans*. *Mar. Ecol. Prog. Ser.* **2005**, *304*, 155–166. [CrossRef]
13. Dobretsov, S.; Qian, P.-Y. Facilitation and inhibition of larval attachment of the bryozoan *Bugula neritina* in association with mono-species and multi-species biofilms. *J. Exp. Mar. Biol. Ecol.* **2006**, *333*, 263–274. [CrossRef]
14. De Carvalho, C.C.C.R. Marine biofilms: A successful microbial strategy with economic implications. *Front. Mar. Sci.* **2018**, *5*. [CrossRef]
15. Lehaitre, M.; Delauney, L.; Compère, C. Biofouling and underwater measurements. In *Real-Time Observation Systems for Ecosystem Dynamics and Harmful Algal Blooms: Theory, Instrumentation and Modelling*; Unesco Publishing: Paris, France, 2008; pp. 463–493.
16. Plaza, G.; Achal, V. Biosurfactants: Eco-friendly and innovative biocides against biocorrosion. *Int. J. Mol. Sci.* **2020**, *21*, 2152. [CrossRef] [PubMed]
17. Gu, Y.; Yu, L.; Mou, J.; Wu, D.; Xu, M.; Zhou, P.; Ren, Y. Research strategies to develop environmentally friendly marine antifouling coatings. *Mar. Drugs* **2020**, *18*, 371. [CrossRef]
18. Dang, H.; Li, T.; Chen, M.; Huang, G. Cross-ocean distribution of Rhodobacterales bacteria as primary surface colonizers in temperate coastal marine waters. *Appl. Environ. Microbiol.* **2008**, *74*, 52–60. [CrossRef]
19. Moffat, J.G.; Vincent, F.; Lee, J.A.; Eder, J.; Prunotto, M. Opportunities and challenges in phenotypic drug discovery: An industry perspective. *Nat. Rev. Drug Discov.* **2017**, *16*, 531–543. [CrossRef]
20. Scannell, J.W.; Bosley, J. When quality beats quantity: Decision theory, drug discovery, and the reproducibility crisis. *PLoS ONE* **2016**, *11*, e0147215. [CrossRef]
21. Pollet, T.; Berdjeb, L.; Garnier, C.; Durrieu, G.; Le Poupon, C.; Misson, B.; Jean-Francois, B. Prokaryotic community successions and interactions in marine biofilms: The key role of Flavobacteriia. *FEMS Microbiol. Ecol.* **2018**, *94*. [CrossRef]
22. Salta, M.; Wharton, J.A.; Blache, Y.; Stokes, K.R.; Briand, J.F. Marine biofilms on artificial surfaces: Structure and dynamics. *Environ. Microbiol.* **2013**, *15*, 2879–2893. [CrossRef] [PubMed]
23. Ohno, H.; Saheki, T.; Awaya, J.; Nakagawa, A.; Omura, S. Isolation and characterization of elasnin, a new human granulocyte elastase inhibitor produced by a strain of Streptomyces. *J. Antibiot.* **1978**, *31*, 1116–1123. [CrossRef] [PubMed]
24. Wang, R.; Ding, W.; Long, L.; Lan, Y.; Saha, S.; Wong, Y.H.; Sun, J.; Li, Y.; Zhang, W.; Qian, P.-Y. Exploring the influence of signal molecules on marine biofilm development. *Front. Microbiol.* **2020**, *11*, 2927. [CrossRef]
25. Yin, Q.; Liang, J.; Zhang, W.; Zhang, L.; Hu, Z.L.; Zhang, Y.; Xu, Y. Butenolide, a marine-derived broad-spectrum antibiofilm agent against both gram-positive and gram-negative pathogenic bacteria. *Mar. Biotechnol.* **2019**, *21*, 88–98. [CrossRef] [PubMed]
26. Nair, S.; Desai, S.; Poonacha, N.; Vipra, A.; Sharma, U. Antibiofilm activity and synergistic inhibition of *Staphylococcus aureus* biofilms by bactericidal protein P128 in combination with antibiotics. *Antimicrob. Agents Chemother.* **2016**, *60*, 7280–7289. [CrossRef]
27. Patel, R.K.; Jain, M. NGS QC Toolkit: A toolkit for quality control of next generation sequencing data. *PLoS ONE* **2012**, *7*, e30619. [CrossRef]
28. Bolyen, E.; Rideout, J.R.; Dillon, M.R.; Bokulich, N.A.; Abnet, C.C.; Al-Ghalith, G.A.; Alexander, H.; Alm, E.J.; Arumugam, M.; Asnicar, F.; et al. Reproducible, interactive, scalable and extensible microbiome data science using QIIME 2. *Nat. Biotechnol.* **2019**, *37*, 852–857. [CrossRef]
29. Hammer, Ø.; Harper, D.A.; Ryan, P.D. PAST: Paleontological statistics software package for education and data analysis. *Palaeontol. Electron.* **2001**, *4*, 9.
30. Qian, P.Y.; Pechenik, J.A. Effects of larval starvation and delayed metamorphosis on juvenile survival and growth of the tube-dwelling polychaete *Hydroides elegans* (Haswell). *J. Exp. Mar. Biol. Ecol.* **1998**, *227*, 169–185. [CrossRef]

31. Harder, T.N.; Thiyagarajan, V.; Qian, P.Y. Effect of cyprid age on the settlement of *Balanus amphitrite* darwin in response to natural biofilms. *Biofouling* **2001**, *17*, 211–219. [CrossRef]
32. Thiyagarajan, V.; Harder, T.; Qiu, J.-W.; Qian, P.-Y. Energy content at metamorphosis and growth rate of the early juvenile barnacle *Balanus amphitrite*. *Mar. Biol.* **2003**, *143*, 543–554. [CrossRef]
33. Gao, C.H.; Tian, X.P.; Qi, S.H.; Luo, X.M.; Wang, P.; Zhang, S. Antibacterial and antilarval compounds from marine gorgonian-associated bacterium *Bacillus amyloliquefaciens* SCSIO 00856. *J. Antibiot.* **2010**, *63*, 191–193. [CrossRef] [PubMed]

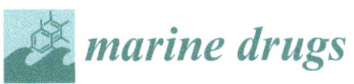

Article

Flavonoid Glycosides with a Triazole Moiety for Marine Antifouling Applications: Synthesis and Biological Activity Evaluation

Daniela Pereira [1,2,†], Catarina Gonçalves [2,†], Beatriz T. Martins [1], Andreia Palmeira [1,2], Vitor Vasconcelos [2,3], Madalena Pinto [1,2], Joana R. Almeida [2,*], Marta Correia-da-Silva [1,2,*] and Honorina Cidade [1,2]

1. Laboratório de Química Orgânica e Farmacêutica, Departamento de Ciências Químicas, Faculdade de Farmácia, Universidade do Porto, R. Jorge de Viterbo Ferreira 228, 4050-313 Porto, Portugal; dmpereira@ff.up.pt (D.P.); beatriz.martins@itqb.unl.pt (B.T.M.); apalmeira@ff.up.pt (A.P.); madalena@ff.up.pt (M.P.); hcidade@ff.up.pt (H.C.)
2. CIIMAR—Centro Interdisciplinar de Investigação Marinha e Ambiental, Avenida General Norton de Matos, S/N, 4450-208 Matosinhos, Portugal; catarina.goncalves@ciimar.up.pt (C.G.); vmvascon@fc.up.pt (V.V.)
3. Departamento de Biologia, Faculdade de Ciências, Universidade do Porto, Rua do Campo Alegre S/N, 4169-007 Porto, Portugal
* Correspondence: jalmeida@ciimar.up.pt (J.R.A.); m_correiadasilva@ff.up.pt (M.C.-d.-S.)
† These authors contributed equally to this work.

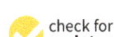

Abstract: Over the last decades, antifouling coatings containing biocidal compounds as active ingredients were used to prevent biofouling, and eco-friendly alternatives are needed. Previous research from our group showed that polymethoxylated chalcones and glycosylated flavones obtained by synthesis displayed antifouling activity with low toxicity. In this work, ten new polymethoxylated flavones and chalcones were synthesized for the first time, including eight with a triazole moiety. Eight known flavones and chalcones were also synthesized and tested in order to construct a quantitative structure-activity relationship (QSAR) model for these compounds. Three different antifouling profiles were found: three compounds (**1b**, **11a** and **11b**) exhibited anti-settlement activity against a macrofouling species (*Mytilus galloprovincialis*), two compounds (**6a** and **6b**) exhibited inhibitory activity against the biofilm-forming marine bacteria *Roseobacter litoralis* and one compound (**7b**) exhibited activity against both mussel larvae and microalgae *Navicula* sp. Hydrogen bonding acceptor ability of the molecule was the most significant descriptor contributing positively to the mussel larvae anti-settlement activity and, in fact, the triazolyl glycosylated chalcone 7b was the most potent compound against this species. The most promising compounds were not toxic to *Artemia salina*, highlighting the importance of pursuing the development of new synthetic antifouling agents as an ecofriendly and sustainable alternative for the marine industry.

Keywords: flavonoids; synthesis; click chemistry; biofouling; antifouling; eco-friendly alternatives

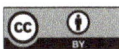

1. Introduction

Marine biofouling, resulting from the accumulation of marine micro and macroorganisms on submerged surfaces, has been a huge problem for maritime industries, causing several technical and economic problems, including corrosion of materials and the increase in fuel consumption. Moreover, marine biofouling is associated with environmental and health problems, due to an increase in gas emissions and the spread of invasive species [1,2].

Biocidal paints containing organotin compounds, namely tributyltin (TBT), were widely used for decades in the maritime industry to prevent biofouling. However, due to their negative effect on the environment and on live organisms, these substances were completely banned in 2008 by the international maritime organization [3]. Since then, some booster biocides, such as Irgarol 1051 or Sea-nine 211, in combination with copper, have been used; nevertheless, even these compounds have demonstrated toxicity on living organisms.

Therefore, it is imperative to find new antifouling (AF) compounds with environmentally safe characteristics [4–6]. Several non-toxic marine natural products with AF activity have been reported; among them, some flavonoids presented potential AF activity and low toxicity, suggesting their potential as new lead compounds for the development of new AF agents [7].

Previous works from our group reported some glycosylated flavones [8] and chalcones [9] with potential AF activity. Interestingly, when comparing the anti-settlement activity against *Mytilus galloprovincialis* of previously described chalcones, it seemed that the presence of a polymethoxylated B-ring could be important for this activity [9]. Moreover, the introduction of a triazole moiety is associated with an increase in AF activity [10]. In fact, over the last decade, there has been a great interest in the synthesis of 1,2,3-triazoles due to the fact of these moieties behaved as more than passive linkers. They carried favorable physicochemical properties, showing importance to biological activity [11,12]. This approach has been used to generate a vast array of compounds with biological potential [13–16], namely with AF activity [10,17,18]. Moreover, some antimicrobial agents are based on nitrogen heterocycles, including the triazole-based biocides fluconazole and itraconazole, which suggest their potential to act as AF agents [10].

Based on this, the present work aims to synthesize new potential AF polymethoxylated chalcone and flavone derivatives with glycosyl groups incorporating a 1,2,3-triazole moiety using a click chemistry approach. The potential of synthesized compounds as benign AF agents was assessed against the adhesive larvae of the macrofouling mussel *Mytilus galloprovincialis* and the biofilm-forming marine bacteria *Cobetia marina*, *Vibrio harveyi*, *Pseudoalteromonas atlantica*, *Halomonas aquamarina* and *Roseobacter litoralis*. The most promising compounds were submitted to complementary assays to evaluate their viability as AF agents, including the evaluation of possible mechanisms of action related with adhesion and neurotransmission pathways. These compounds were also tested for anti-microalgal activity towards *Navicula* sp. and general ecotoxicity using nauplii of the marine shrimp *Artemia salina*.

2. Results and Discussion
2.1. Synthesis and Structure Elucidation

A series of four glycosylated flavones and four glycosylated chalcones bearing a 1,2,3-triazole moiety was synthesized. To prepare glycosylated flavones (Scheme 1), flavones **1a** and **1b**, used as building blocks, were synthesized by the Mentzer synthesis, through direct thermal cyclocondensation of phloroglucinol and β-ketoesters, with good yields, as described by Seijas et al. [19]. However, instead of a microwave (MW) irradiation, the synthesis of flavones **1a** and **1b** was performed in a muffle furnace. After, the propargylation of flavones **1a** and **1b** was achieved with propargyl bromide, giving rise to flavones **2a** and **2b** with 66% and 55% yield, respectively. Copper(I)-catalysed azide alkyne cycloaddition (CuAAC), commonly referred as click chemistry, was developed by the Sharpless and Meldal groups in 2002, and is the most useful reaction for the regioselective synthesis of 1,4-disubstituted-1,2,3-triazole ring [20,21]. This involves a reaction of a terminal alkyne and an aliphatic azide using copper (I) as a catalyst in low-time and mild conditions, with high yields and few by-products [20–22]. Therefore, the incorporation of the triazole linked glycosidic moiety in flavones **2a** and **2b** was accomplished by CuAAC under MW irradiation, giving rise to flavones **3a**, **3b**, **4a** and **4b** with 49–82% yield (Scheme 1).

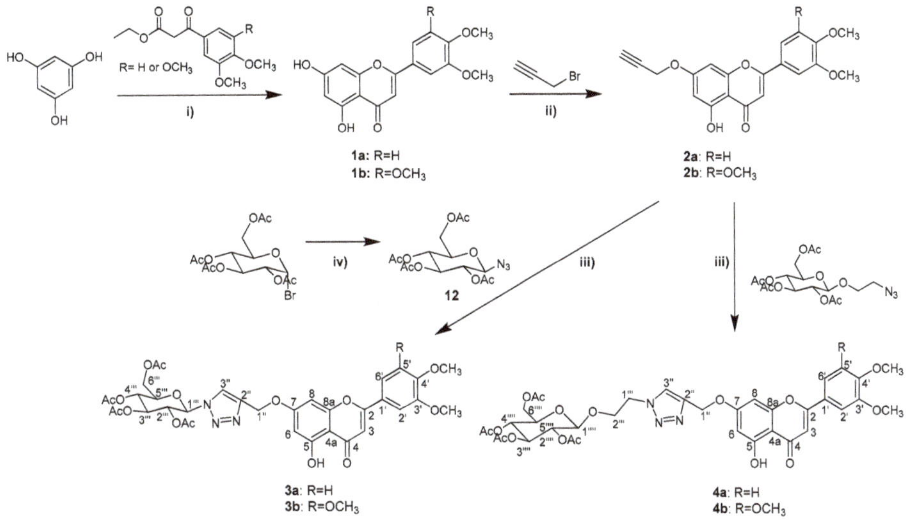

Scheme 1. Synthesis of flavones **1a–1b**, **2a–2b**, **3a–3b** and **4a–4b**. (i) 240 °C, 60–80 min, 74–77%; (ii) Cs_2CO_3, tetrabutylammonium bromide (TBAB), acetone, 60 °C, 6 h, 55–66%; (iii) Sodium ascorbate, $CuSO_4.5H_2O$, tetrahydrofuran (THF):water, microwave (MW), 30 min, 49–82%; (iv) NaN_3, acetone:water, r.t., 3 h, 72%.

The first step in the synthetic process to obtain glycosylated chalcones (Scheme 2) was the propargylation of 2,4-dihydroxyacetophenone with propargyl bromide. As for the synthesis of flavones **2a–2b**, firstly this reaction was accomplished with propargyl bromide, in the presence of anhydrous Cs_2CO_3 and tetrabutylammonium bromide (TBAB). Nevertheless, in addition to the desired 4-O-monosubstituted acetophenone (**5**), the 2,4-disubstituted acetophenone was obtained. Therefore, this reaction was performed in the presence of anhydrous K_2CO_3, as described by Zhao et al. [23], with slight modifications, and the 4-O-monosubstituted acetophenone (**5**) was successfully obtained as expected, with a 76% yield. Afterwards, the base-catalysed aldol reaction of this propargylated acetophenone with benzaldehydes afforded chalcones **6a** and **6b** with moderate yields, which were subsequently submitted to MW assisted CuAAC with azide sugar derivatives, affording triazole linked glycosylated chalcones **7a**, **7b**, **8a** and **8b** with 45–65% yield.

In order to perform structure–activity relationship studies, structure related non-glycosylated chalcones were also synthesized (Scheme 3). Firstly 2,4-dihydroxyacetophenone was protected with methoxymethyl chloride affording **9** with 84% yield. Chalcones **10a** and **10b** were prepared by base-catalyzed aldol reaction of **9** and 3,4-dimethoxy- and 3,4,5-trimethoxybenzaldehyde with 33% and 47% yield, respectively, as described before [24,25], with slight modifications. Chalcones **11a** and **11b** were obtained with moderate yields by deprotection of methoxymethyl group at C-4' of intermediate chalcones **10a** and **10b**, as described by Loureiro et al. [26].

The 2,3,4,6-tetra-O-acetyl-β-D-glucopyranosyl azide (**12**), used as a building block for the synthesis of glycosylated derivatives **3a**, **3b**, **7a** and **7b**, was synthesized from 2,3,4,6-tetra-O-acetyl-α-D-glucopyranosyl bromide and sodium azide, as described by Adesoye et al. [27], with 72% yield.

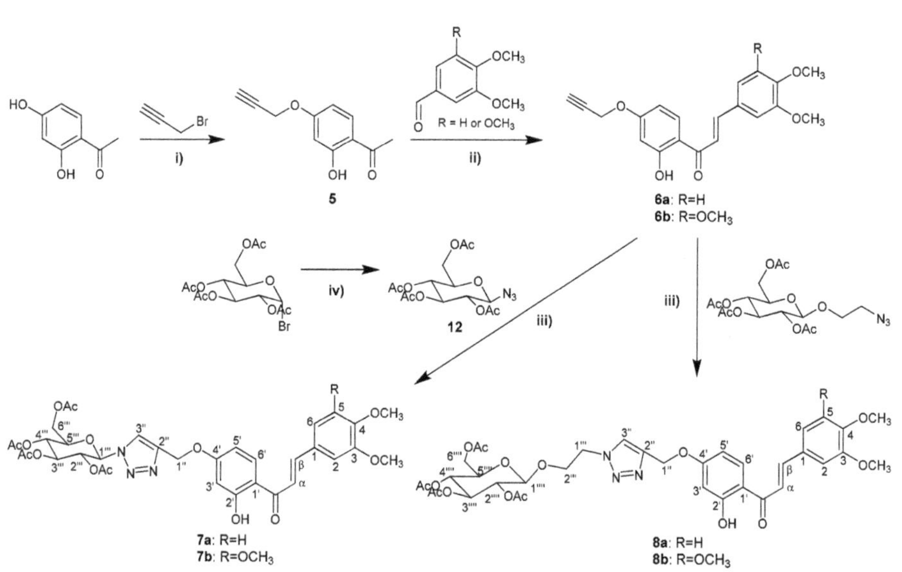

Scheme 2. Synthesis of chalcones **6a–6b**, **7a–7b** and **8a–8b**. (i) K$_2$CO$_3$, acetone, 60 °C, 1 h, 76%; (ii) 40% NaOH, methanol, microwave (MW), 3 h, 41–43%; (iii) Sodium ascorbate, CuSO$_4$.5H$_2$O, tetrahydrofuran (THF):water, microwave (MW), 1 h, 45–65%; (iv) NaN$_3$, acetone:water, r.t., 3 h, 72%.

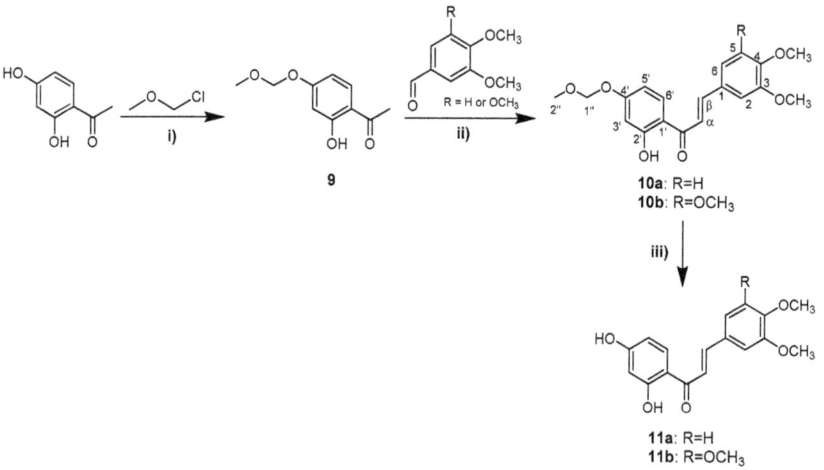

Scheme 3. Synthesis of chalcones **10a–10b** and **11a–11b**. (i) K$_2$CO$_3$, acetone, 60 °C, 1 h, 84%; (ii) 40% NaOH, methanol, microwave (MW), 4 h, 33–47%; (iii) p-Toluenesulfonic acid (PTSA), methanol, 50 °C, 5 h, 24–31%.

The newly synthesized compounds, **2a**, **2b**, **3a**, **3b**, **4a**, **4b**, **7a**, **7b**, **8a** and **8b** were characterized by high resolution mass spectrometry (HRMS) and nuclear magnetic resonance (NMR). The coupling constants of the vinylic system ($J_{H\alpha\text{-}H\beta}$ = 15.5–15.3 Hz) confirm the (E)-configuration for all synthesized chalcones. The NMR spectra of the newly synthesized compounds **3a**, **3b**, **4a**, **4b**, **7a**, **7b**, **8a** and **8b** showed characteristic signals for the flavone scaffold and chalcone precursors. Additionally, signals of a triazole ring (δH-3″ 8.61–7.73 s, δC2″ 144.1–141.6 and δC3″ 125.2–121.5) and a glycosyl moiety were observed. The position of the triazole ring on these compounds was evidenced by the correlation found in the heteronuclear multiple bond correlation (HMBC) spectra between the proton signals of H-1″ and the carbon signals of C-2″ and C-3″.

2.2. Mussel (Mytilus galloprovincialis) Larvae Anti-Settlement Activity

Mussels are one of the main macrofouling organisms present on ships and submerged maritime structures worldwide; thus, they are a target species used in settlement inhibition bioassays [28,29]. Due to the presence of a muscular sensory foot, mussel plantigrade larvae are highly specialized in adhesion to the submerged surfaces and the fixation is made through the production of byssal threads [30], which constitutes the endpoint of this bioassay. Therefore, for the evaluation of the AF activity of the compounds towards macrofouling species, the ability of the synthetized flavonoids to inhibit the settlement of *Mytilus galloprovincialis* larvae at 50 µM was assessed. In this screening bioassay, in addition to glycosylated flavones **3a**, **3b**, **4a** and **4b** and chalcones **7a**, **7b**, **8a** and **8b**, non-glycosylated flavones **1a–b** and **2a–b** and chalcones **6a–b**, **10a–b** and **11a–b** were tested in order to perform SAR studies. Results showed that among 18 tested flavonoids (10 chalcones and 8 flavones), seven chalcones (**6a**, **6b**, **7b**, **8a**, **8b**, **11a** and **11b**) and only three flavones (**1b**, **4a** and **4b**) presented a percentage of settlement ≤ 40%, suggesting that chalcone scaffold seems to be more promising for anti-settlement activity. These 10 compounds were further selected for dose–response studies in order to determine LC_{50}/EC_{50} values.

Among these, three chalcones (**7b**, **11a**, **11b**) and one flavone (**1b**) revealed effective anti-settlement activity ($EC_{50} < 25$ µg/mL), with triazolyl glycosylated chalcone **7b** being the most potent ($EC_{50} = 3.28$ µM; 2.43 µg·mL^{-1}), showing the highest therapeutic ratio (> 60.98) (Table 1).

Table 1. Antifouling (AF) effectiveness and toxicity parameters of flavones **1b**, **4a** and **4b** and chalcones **6a**, **6b**, **7b**, **8a**, **8b**, **11a** and **11b** towards mussel plantigrade larvae.

Compound	EC_{50} (µM)	EC_{50} (µg·mL^{-1})	LC_{50} (µM)	LC_{50}/EC_{50}
1b	8.34 (95% CI: 4.2–13.36)	2.87	> 200	> 23.98
4a	42.55 (95% CI: 34.90–52.80)	32.75	> 200	> 4.70
4b	48.22 (95% CI: 30.57–85.40)	38.56	> 200	> 4.15
6a	84.52 (95% CI: 45.07–267.02)	28.60	> 200	> 2.37
6b	85.56 (95% CI: 44.84–291.41)	31.52	> 200	> 2.34
7b	3.28 (95% CI: 1.97–4.74)	2.43	> 200	> 60.98
8a	35.83 (95% CI: 19.22–74.74)	27.07	> 200	> 5.58
8b	53.90 (95% CI: 29.98–126.88)	42.35	> 200	> 3.71
11a	18.10 (95% CI: 13.95–23.44)	5.44	> 200	> 11.05
11b	9.64 (95% CI: 3.85–17.22)	3.18	> 200	> 20.75

EC_{50}: minimum concentration that inhibited 50% of larval settlement; LC_{50}: median lethal dose; LC_{50}/EC_{50}: therapeutic ratio; CI: confidence interval. EC_{50} are recommend to be less than 25 µg/mL and therapeutic ratio higher than 15 for effective AF agents [31].

2.3. Quantitative Structure—Activity Relationship

Quantitative structure–activity relationship (QSAR) studies have been used for several years to point out small molecules' properties that are relevant for activity, and to forecast the activity of new compounds [32]. Therefore, a QSAR model was built to highlight the descriptors that are being relevant for anti-settlement activity against *M. galloprovincialis* plantigrades of the tested flavonoids. In this work, a 2D-QSAR model was elaborated using the Comprehensive Descriptors for Structural and Statistical Analysis (CODESSA 2.7.2) software package, which calculates approximately 500 descriptors. The heuristic method performs a pre-selection of descriptors by eliminating descriptors that are not available for each structure, that have a small variation in magnitude, that are correlated pairwise, and that have no statistical significance. The heuristic method is a very useful method for searching the best set of descriptors, without restrictions on the data set size [33].

The correlation coefficient (R^2), squared standard error (S^2), and Fisher's value (F) were used to evaluate the validity of regression equation [34]. As the rules of QSAR establish that there must be one descriptor for each five molecules used to build the model [34], three descriptors were used to build the QSAR equation. The multilinear regression analysis using Heuristic method for 15 compounds in the three-descriptor model is shown in Figure 1. The compounds are uniformly distributed around the regression line (Figure 1), which suggests that the obtained model has satisfactory predictive ability.

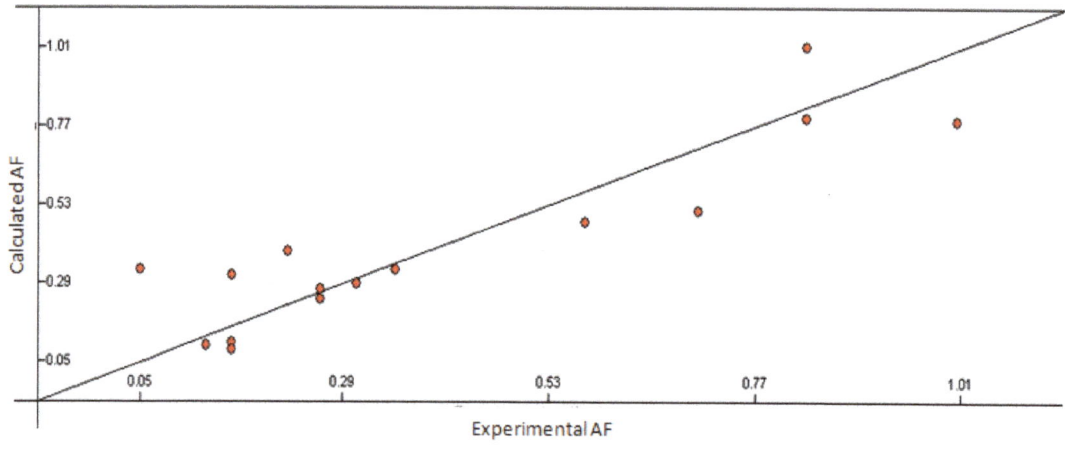

Nr	X	ΔX	t-test	Descriptor
0	0.3730	0.3417	1.0915	Intercept
1	0.1267	0.02264	5.5960	Hydrogen bonding acceptor ability of the molecule - HACA1
2	−0.9101	0.2645	−3.4416	Average Complementary Information content (order 2)
3	−0.2867	0.1532	−1.8721	Number of triple bonds

Figure 1. Quantitative structure-activity relationship (QSAR) model obtained with the heuristic method for 15 molecules with the CODESSA software (R^2 = 0.7945, F = 14.18, S^2 = 0.0243). X, ΔX and *t*-test are the regression coefficient of the linear model, standard errors of the regression coefficient, and the t significance coefficient of the determination, respectively. AF = antifouling activity.

The best QSAR equation had a R^2 of 0.7945, Fisher value of 14.18, and S^2 of 0.0243, which reveals that the proposed model has statistical validity [35]. The R^2 is higher than 0.6, which is an indicator of a good fit to the regression line [36], representing close to 80% of the total variance in AF activity shown by the test compounds. The QSAR model is significant at a 95% level, as shown by the Fisher F-test (F = 14.18), which is higher than the tabulated value (3.59), as desired for a statistically significant model [35]. The squared standard deviation S^2 is small and close to zero (s^2 = 0.0243), proving that the model is significant and has low variation about the regression line [37]. The reliability of the resulting QSAR model was explored using two different types of validation criteria: external validation by using a test set and internal validation by leave-one-out (LOO) cross-validation [38].

The model was able to predict the activity of an external test set with an average difference of 0.19 from the experimental value [39]. Moreover, the cross-validated R^2 (Q^2 = 0.5953) from the LOO internal validation process is higher than 0.5 and smaller than the overall R^2, as expected, and the difference between R^2 and Q^2 is lower than 0.3, which indicates that the model does not suffer from overfitting [40].

By interpreting the molecular descriptors in the regression model (Figure 1), it is possible to have some insight into structural characteristics that are likely to be responsible for AF activity of the studied compounds. There are three descriptors included in the regression model, which proved to be important features and provide statistically significant contributions to the QSAR equation.

As indicated by the higher t-test value, hydrogen bonding acceptor ability of the molecule (HACA1) is a charged partial surface area (CPSA) descriptor that appeared as the most significant descriptor for the obtained QSAR model, contributing positively to the AF activity [41]. HACA1 is determined by the equation:

$$HACA1 = \sum_A S_A \quad A \in X_{H-acceptor} \tag{1}$$

where S_A stands for solvent-accessible surface area of H-bonding acceptor atoms, selected by threshold charge. This descriptor proves the importance of the hydrogen bonding acceptor properties for the activity of the test compounds [42].

The topological descriptor average complementary information content of order 2 (CIC2) descriptor is predicted as being negatively implied in the AF activity of the test compounds [41]. The CIC2 descriptor represents the difference between the maximum possible complexity of a molecule and its real topological information. It belongs to the multi-graph information content indices and it describes neighborhood symmetry of second order [43]. The constitutional descriptor number of triple bonds is also responsible for a decrease in activity.

The molecular descriptors used in the QSAR model demonstrate that the mechanism underlying the AF activity of flavonoids is mainly related to their HACA1, and it may be prejudiced by topological CIC2 and by the presence of triple bonds. Interestingly, the triazolyl glycosylated chalcone **7b**, with the most promising anti-settlement activity, is one of the compounds with more hydrogen-bonding acceptors. In contrast, propargylated flavones **2a** and **2b** had a percentage of settlement higher than 40% at 50 µM, and therefore were not selected for dose–response studies and for the determination of the LC_{50}/EC_{50} values. Moreover, propargylated chalcones **6a** and **6b** showed the lowest activity. Overall, the examination of the molecular descriptors reported in this work can lead to a better understanding of the relation between the structure and AF activity of flavonoids.

2.4. Biofilm-Forming Marine Bacteria Growth Inhibitory Activity

Although the macrofouling species represent the most problematic component of fouling in terms of biomass and negative repercussions, the first micro-colonizers are also of extreme importance, since they represent the basis of the fouling community, and ultimately, they may modulate the colonization of further species by inducing or inhibiting species adhesion via biochemical cues [44]. Thus, synthesized flavonoids were further evaluated for their ability to inhibit the growth of five marine biofilm-forming bacteria, *Vibrio harveyi*, *Cobetia marina*, *Halomonas aquamarina*, *Pseudoalteromonas atlantica* and *Roseobacter litoralis*.

Results showed that only the bacterial growth of *Roseobacter litoralis* was meaningfully compromised by tested compounds, with significant inhibitory activity for propargylated chalcones **6a** and **6b** (Figure 2). These compounds were selected for concentration–response analysis (Figure 3).

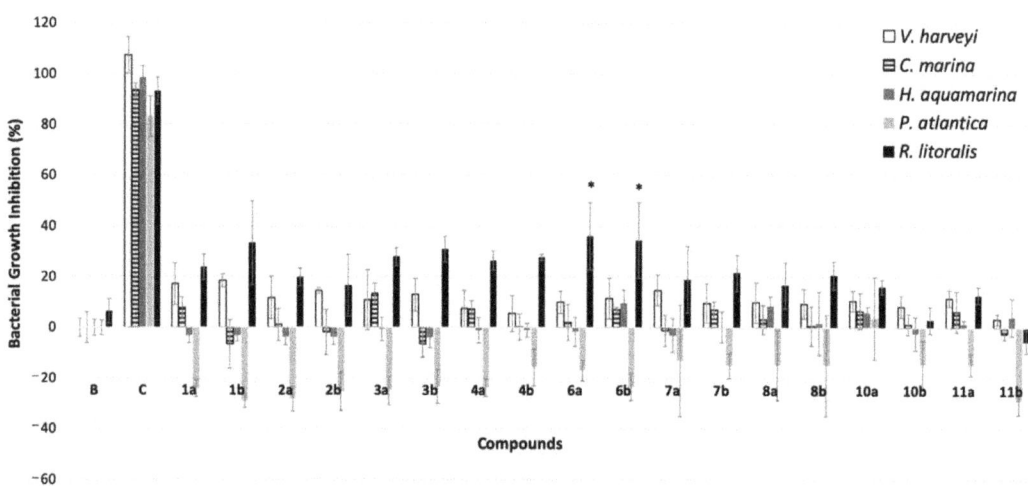

Figure 2. Bacterial growth inhibition screening of flavonoid derivatives (15 µM) towards five biofilm-forming marine bacteria: *Vibrio harveyi*, *Cobetia marina*, *Halomonas aquamarina*, *Pseudoalteromonas atlantica* and *Roseobacter litoralis*. B: Negative control with 1% dimethyl sulfoxide (DMSO); C: positive control with penicillin–streptomycin–neomycin-stabilized solution. * indicates significant differences at $p < 0.05$ (Dunnett test), against the negative control (B).

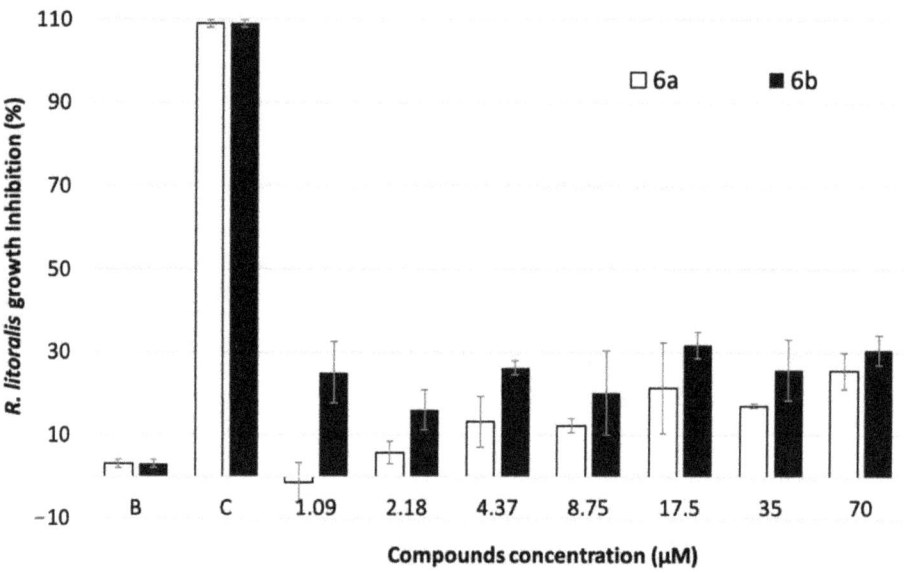

Figure 3. Concentration–response growth inhibition activity of compounds **6a** and **6b** towards *Roseobacter litoralis*. B: DMSO negative control; C: positive control with penicillin–streptomycin–neomycin-stabilized solution.

Compounds **6a** and **6b** presented low anti-bacterial activity towards *R. litoralis* with EC_{30} values of 135 and 83.5 µM, respectively.

2.5. Biofilm—Forming Marine Diatoms Growth Inhibitory Activity

The most promising compounds regarding anti-settlement activity (**1b**, **7b**, **11a**, **11b**) were further evaluated for their ability to inhibit the growth of the biofilm-forming microalgae *Navicula* sp. This marine diatom is a major biofouling species that very effectively colonizes submerged surfaces by secreting adhesive extracellular polymer substances (EPS), and thus is a good representative of fouling microalgae.

Only triazolyl glycosylated chalcone **7b** showed significant inhibitory activity with the concentration–response analyses revealing an EC_{50} value of 41.76 µM; 30.94 µg·mL^{-1}, suggesting the ability of this compound to act also as a promising AF agent against microfouling species.

2.6. In Vitro Acetylcholinesterase (AChE) and Tyrosinase (Tyr) Activities

The identification of the mechanism of action associated with AF activity remains a challenge for the scientific community. According to Qian et al. (2013) antifoulants appear to affect settlement through distinct pathways, which can be classified roughly into several categories such as inhibitors of ion channel function, inhibitors of quorum sensing, blockers of neurotransmission or inhibitors of adhesive production or release [45]. Moreover, some specific target molecules in fouling organisms have been determined, such as AChE, which seems to be involved in cholinergic neural signaling during the settlement [46]. It is known that the commercial booster biocide Sea-Nine 211 acts by this mechanism [47,48], as well as two natural compounds isolated from marine organisms, territrem A and pulmonarin [49,50]. For this reason, the ability of the most promising compounds to modulate the activity of AChE was evaluated (**1b**, **7b**, **11a** and **11b**). AChE activity was significantly induced for chalcones **7b** and **11b** (Figure 4). Induced AChE activity has been described as an exposure effect that is in some cases associated with apoptosis [51], and thus the specific target behind these compounds' bioactivity should be further explored in future work.

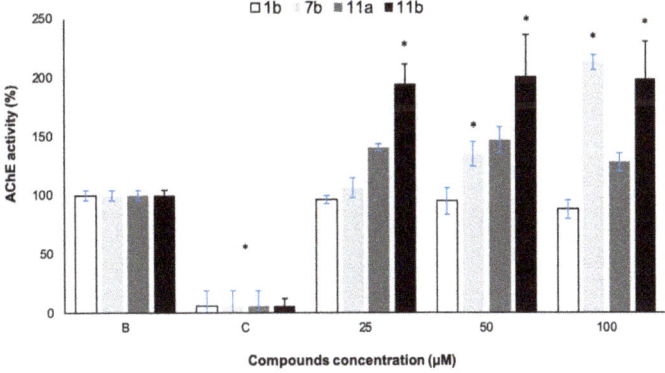

Figure 4. AChE activity of the most promising compounds **1b 7b**, **11a** and **11b**. B: Dimethyl sulfoxide (DMSO) (1% in water). C: Eserine (200 µM, water). * indicates significant differences at $p < 0.05$ (Dunnett test), against the negative control (B).

A well-known pathway in the production of biological adhesives of mussels is the 3,4-dihydroxyphenyl-L-alanine (L-DOPA) metabolism that functions in the production of DOPA-containing mussel byssal plaques by the action of Tyr that catalyses the conversion of DOPA precursor into DOPA residues [46,52]. Considering this, the most promising compounds in the inhibition of mussel adhesion were tested for their ability to inhibit Tyr (Figure 5). Results show that flavone **1b** is able to significantly decrease Tyr activity at all the concentrations tested, reaching 23.5% of inhibition at 100 µM. Therefore, the inhibition of this enzyme, with a crucial effect in the formation of mussel adhesive, could be one of the mechanisms involved in the inhibition of the mussel settlement. This also highlights a specific AF mode of action related with mussel adhesion and explains the absence of activity against bacteria and diatoms.

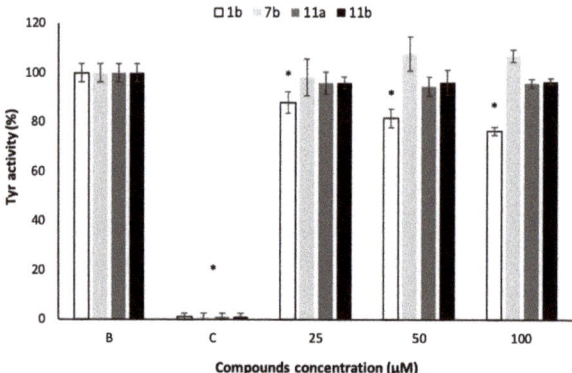

Figure 5. Tyr activity of the most promising compounds **1b**, **7b**, **11a** and **11b**. B: Dimethyl sulfoxide (DMSO) (1% in water). C: Kojic acid (1.4 mM, water). * indicates significant differences at $p < 0.05$ (Dunnett test), against the negative control (B).

2.7. Environmental Fate Parameters: Artemia Salina Ecotoxicity Bioassay

Ecotoxicity assays carried out on non-target organisms aim to understand how tested compounds can affect sensitive non-target organisms and influence the health status of the surrounding ecosystem [53]. *Artemia salina* is a species of small crustaceans that live in salty marine environments and are used as test organisms because of their easy culture, short generation time, cosmopolitan distribution and commercial availability of their eggs in latent form [54].

Ecotoxicity results showed that the most promising compounds **1b**, **7b**, **11a** and **11b** are non-toxic to *Artemia salina* (less than 10% mortality) at both concentrations tested (25 and 50 µM) (Figure 6), in contrast to the commercial AF agent ECONEA® which was previously shown by our group to cause 100% lethality at the same concentrations and conditions [9]. These results suggest that any of the tested compounds could be a good alternative, being more environmentally compatible antifoulants.

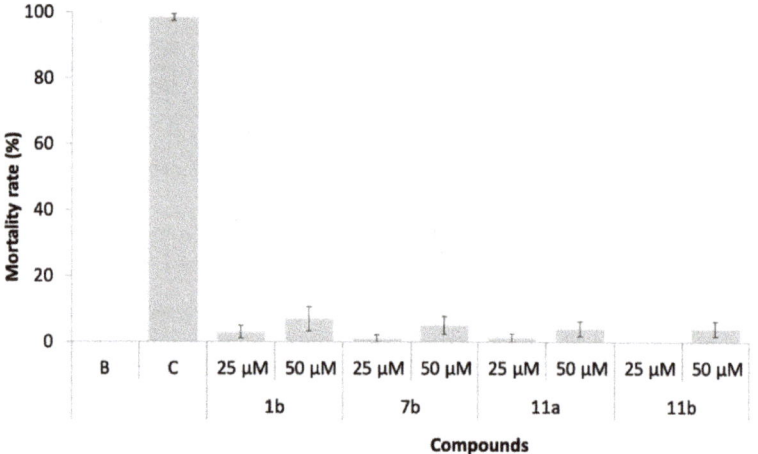

Figure 6. Mortality rate of *Artemia salina* nauplii after 48 h of exposure to compounds **1b**, **7b**, **11a** and **11b**, B: DMSO (1% in filtered seawater). C: $K_2Cr_2O_7$ (13.6 µM, filtered seawater).

3. Materials and Methods

3.1. Synthesis and Structure Elucidation of Chalcones and Flavones

MW reactions were performed using a glassware setup for atmospheric pressure reactions and a 100 mL Teflon reactor (internal reaction temperature measurements with a fiber-optic probe sensor) and were carried out using an Ethos MicroSYNTH 1600 Microwave Labstation from Milestone (Thermo Unicam, Oeiras, Portugal). The reactions were monitored by analytical thin-layer chromatography (TLC) Macherey-Nagel Silica gel 60 F254 (Macherey-Nagel, Dueren, Germany), Purifications of compounds were carried out by flash chromatography using Macherey-Nagel silica gel 60 (0.04–0.063 mm) (Macherey-Nagel, Dueren, Germany), preparative TLC using Macherey-Nagel silica gel 60 (GF254) (Macherey-Nagel, Dueren, Germany) plates and crystallization. Melting points were obtained in a Köfler microscope (Wagner and Munz, Munich, Germany) and are uncorrected. ^{1}H and ^{13}C NMR spectra were taken in CDCl$_3$ or DMSO-d$_6$ at room temperature, on Bruker Avance 300 and 500 instruments (Bruker Biosciences Corporation, Billerica, MA, USA) (300.13 MHz or 500 MHz for ^{1}H and 75.47 or 120 MHz for ^{13}C). Chemical shifts are expressed in δ (ppm) values relative to tetramethylsilane (TMS) as an internal reference; ^{13}C NMR assignments were made by 2D (HSQC and HMBC) NMR experiments (long-range ^{13}C-^{1}H coupling constants were optimized to 7 Hz). HRMS mass spectra of compounds **2a**, **2b**, **3a**, **3b**, **4a**, **4b**, **7a**, **7b** and **8b** were performed on an APEXQe FT-ICR MS (Bruker Daltonics, Billerica, MA) equipped with a 7T actively shielded magnet, at C.A.C.T.I.—University of Vigo, Spain. Ions were generated using a Combi MALDI-electrospray ionization (ESI) source. HRMS mass spectrometry of compound **8a** was performed on an LTQ Orbitrap™ XL hybrid mass spectrometer (Thermo Fischer Scientific, Bremen, Germany) controlled by LTQ Tune Plus 2.5.5 and Xcalibur 2.1.0. at CEMUP—University of Porto, Portugal. Phloroglucinol, ethyl 3,4-dimethoxybenzoylacetate, ethyl 3,4,5-trimethoxybenzoylacetate, 2,4-dihydroxyacetophenone and 2,3,4,6-tetra-O-acetyl-α-D-glucopyranosyl bromide were purchased from Sigma Aldrich (St. Louis, MO, USA). 3,4-Dimethoxybenzaldehyde and 3,4,5-trimethoxybenzaldehyde were purchased from Acros Organics (Janssen Pharmaceuticalaan, Geel, Belgium). 2-Azidoethyl-2,3,4,6-tetra-O-acetyl-β-D-glucopyranoside was purchased from Synthose (Concord, ON, Canada).

3.1.1. Synthesis of Flavones **1a** and **1b**

A mixture of phloroglucinol (0.175 g, 1.39 mmol) and ethyl 3,4-dimethoxybenzoylacetate (0.700 g, 2.78 mmol) or ethyl 3,4,5-trimethoxybenzoylacetate (0.739 g, 2.78 mmol) was heated at 240 °C in muffle furnace (Thermo Fisher Scientific, Oeiras, Portugal) for 60–100 min. Afterwards, the crude mixture was dissolved in 10% NaOH (20 mL) and washed with diethyl ether (2 × 20 mL), and the product was precipitated by adding 37% HCl. The solid was filtered and washed with water, and the flavones **1a** and **1b** were obtained with 74% and 77% yields, respectively. The structure elucidation of compounds **1a** and **2b** was established by ^{1}H and ^{13}C NMR techniques and data were in accordance with previously reported results [19].

3.1.2. Synthesis of 7-O-Propargylflavones **2a** and **2b**

To a solution of **1a** (0.200 g, 0.64 mmol) or **1b** (0.200 g, 0.58 mmol), cesium carbonate (0.207 g, 0.64 mmol or 0.189 g, 0.58 mmol), tetrabutylammonium bromide (TBAB) (0.205 g, 0.64 mmol or 0.187 g, 0.58 mmol) in anhydrous acetone (20 mL), and propargyl bromide solution, 80 wt.% in toluene (0.071 mL, 0.64 mmol or 0.065 mL, 0.58 mmol), were added. The mixture was refluxed at 60 °C during 6 h and filtered. The filtrate was evaporated under reduced pressure and purification was carried out by flash column chromatography (SiO$_2$; n-hexane: ethyl acetate), 8:2) followed by crystallization in acetone.

2-(3,4-dimethoxyphenyl)-5-hydroxy-7-(prop-2-yn-1-yloxy)-4H-chromen-4-one (**2a**). Light yellow solid; Yield: 66%; m.p.: 222–224 °C (acetone); ^{1}H NMR (DMSO-d$_6$, 500 MHz), δ: 12.93 (1H, s, OH-5), 7.71 (1H, dd, J = 8.5 and 2.2 Hz, H-6′), 7.57 (1H, d, J = 2.2 Hz, H-2′), 7.14 (1H, d, J = 8.7 Hz, H-5′), 7.03 (1H, s, H-3), 6.87 (1H, d, J = 2.2 Hz, H-8), 6.44 (1H, d,

J = 2.3 Hz, H-6), 4.94 (2H, d, J = 2.5 Hz, H-1″), 3.88 (3H, s, 3′-OCH$_3$), 3.85 (3H, s, 4′-OCH$_3$), 3.66 (1H, t, J = 2.4 Hz, H-3″). ^{13}C NMR (DMSO-d$_6$, 120 MHz) δ: 182.3 (C4), 164.0 (C2), 163.2 (C7), 161.3 (C5), 157.3 (C8a), 152.5 (C4′), 149.2 (C3′), 122.9 (C1′), 120.5 (C6′), 111.9 (C5′), 109.6 (C2′), 105.3 (C4a), 104.3 (C3), 98.8 (C6), 94.0 (C8), 79.2 (C3″), 78.6 (C2″), 56.4 (C1″), 56.1, 56.0 (3′-OCH$_3$ and 4′-OCH$_3$). HRMS (ESI$^+$) m/z calcd for C$_{20}$H$_{17}$O$_6$ [M + H$^+$] 353.10196, found 353.10174.

5-hydroxy-7-(prop-2-yn-1-yloxy)-2-(3,4,5-trimethoxyphenyl)-4H-chromen-4-one (**2b**). Light yellow solid; Yield: 55%; m.p.: 211–213 °C (acetone); ^{1}H NMR (DMSO-d$_6$, 300.13 MHz), δ: 12.87 (1H, s, OH-5), 7.36 (2H, s, H-2′ and H-6′), 7.16 (1H, s, H-3), 6.91 (1H, d, J = 2.3 Hz, H-8), 6.46 (1H, d, J = 2.3 Hz, H-6), 4.96 (2H, d, J = 2.4 Hz, H-1″), 3.91 (6H, s, 3′-OCH$_3$ and 5′-OCH$_3$), 3.76 (3H, s, 4′- OCH$_3$), 3.70 (1H, t, J = 2.4 Hz, H-3″). ^{13}C NMR (DMSO-d$_6$, 75.47 MHz) δ: 182.2 (C4), 163.4 (C2), 163.1 (C7), 161.2 (C5), 157.1 (C8a), 153.3 (C3′ and C5′), 140.9 (C4′), 125.8 (C1′), 105.3 (C3), 105.2 (C4a), 104.2 (C2′ and C6′), 98.7 (C6), 93.9 (C8), 79.1 (C2″), 78.4 (C3″), 60.3 (4′-OCH$_3$), 56.4 (C1″, 3′-OCH$_3$ and 5′-OCH$_3$). HRMS (ESI$^+$) m/z calcd for C$_{21}$H$_{19}$O$_7$ [M + H$^+$] 383.11253, found 383.11233.

3.1.3. Synthesis of Flavone-Triazolyl-Glycosides **3a** and **3b**

To a solution of **2a** (0.100 g, 0.28 mmol) or **2b** (0.100 g, 0.27 mmol) and 2,3,4,6-tetra-O-acetyl-β-D-glucopyranosyl azide (0.106 g, 0.28 mmol or 0.102 g, 0.27 mmol) in THF/water solvent mixture (2:1; 30 mL), sodium ascorbate (0.225 g, 1.14 mmol or 0.216 g, 1.09 mmol) and copper(II) sulphate pentahydrate (0.142 g, 0.57 mmol or 0.136 g, 0.54 mmol) were added. The reaction vessel was sealed and the mixture was kept stirring and heated for 30 min at 70 °C under MW irradiation of 500 W. After cooling, the reaction mixture was filtered and concentrated under reduced pressure. The water suspension was extracted with ethyl acetate (2 × 20 mL), and the combined organic layers were dried over anhydrous sodium sulphate, evaporated under reduced pressure, and then purified by crystallization in acetone.

(2R,3R,4S,5R,6R)-2-(acetoxymethyl)-6-(4-(((2-(3,4-dimethoxyphenyl)-5-hydroxy-4-oxo-4H-chromen-7-yl)oxy)methyl)-1H-1,2,3-triazol-1-yl)tetrahydro-2H-pyran-3,4,5-triyl triacetate (**3a**). Light yellow solid; Yield: 82%; m.p.: 143–145 °C (acetone); ^{1}H NMR (DMSO-d$_6$, 500 MHz), δ: 12.93 (1H, s, OH-5), 8.61 (1H, s, H-3″), 7.71 (1H, dd, J = 8.5 and 2.1 Hz, H-6′), 7.60 (1H, d, J = 2.2 Hz, H-2′), 7.15 (1H, d, J = 8.7 Hz, H-5′), 7.05 (1H, s, H-3), 6.94 (1H, d, J = 2.2 Hz, H-8), 6.47 (1H, d, J = 2.2 Hz, H-6), 6.39 (1H, d, J = 9.2 Hz, H-1‴), 5.68 (1H, t, J = 9.4 Hz), 5.56 (1H, t, J = 9.5 Hz), 5.19 (1H, t, J = 9.8 Hz) (H-2‴, H-3‴, H-4‴), 5.32 (2H, s, H-1″), 4.39–4.36 (1H, m, H-5‴), 4.15–4.07 (2H, m, H-6‴), 3.86 (3H, s, 4′-OCH$_3$), 3.83 (3H, s, 3′-OCH$_3$), 2.03, 1.99, 1.96, 1.77 (12H, s, 2‴, 3‴, 4‴, -COCH$_3$). ^{13}C NMR (DMSO-d$_6$, 120 MHz) δ: 182.1 (C4), 170.1, 169.6, 169.4, 168.5 (2‴, 3‴, 4‴, 6‴-COCH$_3$), 163.7 (C2 and C7), 161.2 (C5), 158.0 (C8a), 152.3 (C4′), 149.1 (C3′), 142.7 (C2″), 124.0 (C3″), 122.7 (C1′), 120.2 (C6′), 111.7 (C5′), 109.5 (C2′), 105.0 (C3), 104.1 (C4a), 98.7 (C6), 93.7 (C8), 83.9 (C1‴), 73.3 (C5‴), 72.1, 70.1, 67.5 (C2‴, C3‴, C4‴), 61.8 (C6‴), 61.7 (C1″), 55.9, 55.8 (3′-OCH$_3$ and 4′-OCH$_3$), 20.5, 20.4, 20.3, 19.9 (2‴, 3‴, 4‴, 6‴-COCH$_3$). HRMS (ESI$^+$) m/z calcd for C$_{34}$H$_{36}$N$_3$O$_{15}$ [M + H$^+$] 726.21409, found 726.21380.

(2R,3R,4S,5R,6R)-2-(acetoxymethyl)-6-(4-(((5-hydroxy-4-oxo-2-(3,4,5-trimethoxyphenyl)-4H-chromen-7-yl)oxy)methyl)-1H-1,2,3-triazol-1-yl)tetrahydro-2H-pyran-3,4,5-triyl triacetate (**3b**). Yellow solid; Yield: 79%; m.p.: 169–171 °C (acetone); ^{1}H NMR (DMSO-d$_6$, 300.13 MHz), δ: 12.85 (1H, s, OH-5), 8.61 (1H, s, H-3″), 7.38 (2H, s, H-2′ and H-6′), 7.17 (1H, s, H-3), 7.00 (1H, d, J = 2.2 Hz, H-8), 6.49 (1H, d, J = 2.2 Hz, H-6), 6.39 (1H, d, J = 9.1 Hz, H-1‴), 5.68 (1H, t, J = 9.3 Hz), 5.56 (1H, t, J = 9.4 Hz), 5.19 (1H, t, J = 9.7 Hz) (H-2‴, H-3‴, H-4‴), 5.33 (2H, s, H-1″), 4.40–4.36 (1H, m, H-5‴), 4.17–4.06 (2H, m, H-6‴), 3.91 (6H, s, 3′-OCH$_3$ and 5′-OCH$_3$), 3.76 (3H, s, 4′-OCH$_3$), 2.03, 2.00, 1.96, 1.77 (12H, s, 2‴, 3‴, 4‴, 6‴-COCH$_3$). ^{13}C NMR (DMSO-d$_6$, 75.47 MHz) δ: 182.2 (C4), 170.1, 169.6, 169.4, 168.5 (2‴, 3‴, 4‴, 6‴-COCH$_3$), 163.8 (C7), 163.4 (C2), 161.2 (C5), 157.3 (C8a), 153.3 (C3′ and C5′), 142.7 (C2″), 140.9 (C4′), 125.8 (C1′), 123.9 (C3″), 105.1 (C3 and C4a), 104.2 (C2′ and C6′), 98.7 (C6),

93.9 (C8), 83.9 (C1''''), 73.3 (C5''''), 72.1, 70.1, 67.5 (C2'''', C3'''', C4''''), 61.8 (C1'' and C6''''), 60.3 (4'-OCH$_3$), 56.3 (3'-OCH$_3$ and 5'-OCH$_3$), 20.5, 20.4, 20.3, 19.9 (2'''', 3'''', 4'''', 6''''-COC̲H$_3$). HRMS (ESI$^+$) m/z calcd for C$_{35}$H$_{38}$N$_3$O$_{16}$ [M + H$^+$] 756.22466, found 756.22445.

3.1.4. Synthesis of Flavone-Triazolyl-Glycosides 4a and 4b

To a solution of 2a (0.090 g, 0.26 mmol) or 2b (0.100 g, 0.26 mmol) and 2-azidoethyl-2,3,4,6-tetra-O-acetyl-β-D-glucopyranoside (0.109 g, 0.26 mmol) in tetrahydrofuran/water solvent mixture (2:1; 30 mL), sodium ascorbate (0.207 g, 1.05 mmol) and copper(II) sulphate pentahydrate (0.131 g, 0.52 mmol) were added. The reaction vessel was sealed and the mixture was kept stirring and heated for 30 min at 70 °C under MW irradiation of 500 W. After cooling, the reaction mixture was filtered and concentrated under reduced pressure. The water suspension was extracted with ethyl acetate (2 × 20 mL), and the combined organic layers were dried over anhydrous sodium sulphate, evaporated under reduced pressure, and then purified by crystallization in ethyl acetate/n-hexane (4a) or by flash column chromatography (SiO$_2$; n-hexane: ethyl acetate, 3:7) (4b).

(2R,3R,4S,5R,6R)-2-(acetoxymethyl)-6-(2-(4-(((2-(3,4-dimethoxyphenyl)-5-hydroxy-4-oxo-4H-chromen-7-yl)oxy)methyl)-1H-1,2,3-triazol-1-yl)ethoxy)tetrahydro-2H-pyran-3,4,5-triyl triacetate (4a). Light brown solid; Yield: 60%; m.p.: 99–100 °C (n-hexane: ethyl acetate); ^{1}H NMR (DMSO-d$_6$, 300.13 MHz), δ: 12.94 (1H, s, OH-5), 8.15 (1H, s, H-3''), 7.72 (1H, dd, J = 8.5, 1.8 Hz, H-6'), 7.59 (1H, d, J = 1.9 Hz, H-2'), 7.14 (1H, d, J = 8.6 Hz, H-5'), 7.05 (1H, s, H-3), 6.96 (1H, d, J = 2.1 Hz, H-8), 6.47 (1H, d, J = 2.1 Hz, H-6), 5.28 (2H, s, H-1''), 5.23 (1H, t, J = 9.6 Hz), 4.90 (1H, t, J = 9.7 Hz), 4.77–4.71 (1H, m) (H-2'''', H-3'''', H-4''''), 4.72 (1H, d, J = 8.1 Hz, H-1''''), 4.60–4.57 (2H, m, H-6''''), 4.19–4.01 (5H, m, H-1''', H-2''', H-5'''), 3.89 (3H, s, 3'-OCH$_3$), 3.86 (3H, s, 4'-OCH$_3$), 2.02, 1.98, 1.92, 1.89 (12H, s, 2'''', 3'''', 4'''', 6''''-COCH$_3$). ^{13}C NMR (DMSO-d$_6$, 75.47 MHz) δ: 182.1 (C4), 170.1, 169.6, 169.3, 169.0 (2'''', 3'''', 4'''', 6''''-C̲OCH$_3$), 163.9 (C7), 163.7 (C2), 161.2 (C5), 157.2 (C8a), 152.3 (C4'), 149.0 (C3'), 141.7 (C2''), 125.2 (C3''), 122.8 (C1'), 120.2 (C6'), 111.7 (C5'), 109.5 (C2'), 105.0 (C4a), 104.1 (C3), 99.2 (C1''''), 98.6 (C6), 93.5 (C8), 71.9, 70.7, 68.1 (C2'''', C3'''', C4''''), 70.6, 67.4, 61.7 (C1''', C2''', C5''''), 61.9 (C1''), 55.9, 55.8 (3'-OCH$_3$ and 4'-OCH$_3$), 49.4 (C6''''), 20.5, 20.4, 20.3, 20.3 (2'''', 3'''', 4'''', 6''''-COC̲H$_3$). HRMS (ESI$^+$) m/z calcd for C$_{36}$H$_{40}$N$_3$O$_{16}$ [M + H$^+$] 770.24031, found 770. 23792.

(2R,3R,4S,5R,6R)-2-(acetoxymethyl)-6-(2-(4-(((5-hydroxy-4-oxo-2-(3,4,5-trimethoxyphenyl)-4H-chromen-7-yl)oxy)methyl)-1H-1,2,3-triazol-1-yl)ethoxy)tetrahydro-2H-pyran-3,4,5-triyl triacetate (4b). Light yellow solid; Yield: 49%; m.p.: 96–98 °C (n-hexane: ethyl acetate); ^{1}H NMR (DMSO-d$_6$, 300.13 MHz), δ: 12.86 (1H, s, OH-5), 8.15 (1H, s, H-3''), 7.38 (2H, s, H-2' and H-6'), 7.17 (1H, s, H-3), 7.02 (1H, d, J = 2.2 Hz, H-8), 6.49 (1H, d, J = 2.2 Hz, H-6), 5.29 (2H, s, H-1''), 5.23 (1H, t, J = 9.5 Hz), 4.90 (1H, t, J = 9.7 Hz), 4.74 (1H, t, J = 8.8 Hz) (H-2'''', H-3'''', H-4''''), 4.84 (1H, d, J = 8.0, H-1''''), 4.60–4.56 (2H, m, H-6''''), 4.21–4.01 (5H, m, H-5'''', H-1''' and H-2'''), 3.91 (6H, s, 3'-OCH$_3$ and 5'-OCH$_3$), 3.76 (3H, s, 4'-OCH$_3$), 2.02, 1.98, 1.92, 1.89 (12H, s, 2'''', 3'''', 4'''', 6''''-COCH$_3$). ^{13}C NMR (DMSO-d$_6$, 75.47 MHz) δ: 182.2 (C4), 170.1, 169.6, 169.3, 169.0 (2'''', 3'''', 4'''', 6''''-C̲OCH$_3$), 164.0 (C7), 163.4 (C2), 161.1 (C5), 157.3 (C8a), 153.3 (C3' and C5'), 141.6 (C2''), 140.9 (C4'), 125.8 (C1'), 125.2 (C3''), 105.3 (C4a), 105.1 (C3), 104.2 (C2' and C6'), 99.2 (C1''''), 98.7 (C6), 93.7 (C8), 71.9, 70.7, 70.6, 68.1 (C2'''', C3'''', C4'''' and C5''''), 67.4, 61.7 (C1''', C2'''), 62.0 (C1''), 60.3 (4'-OCH$_3$), 56.4 (3' and 5'-OCH$_3$), 49.4 (C6''''), 20.5, 20.4, 20.3, 20.3 (2'''', 3'''', 4'''', 6''''-COC̲H$_3$). HRMS (ESI$^+$) m/z calcd for C$_{37}$H$_{42}$N$_3$O$_{17}$ [M + H$^+$] 800.25087, found 800.24829.

3.1.5. Synthesis of Propargyloxyacetophenone 5

To a solution of 2,4-dihydroxyacetophenone (1.00 g, 6.57 mmol) and potassium carbonate (0.91 g, 6.57 mmol) in anhydrous acetone (20 mL), propargyl bromide solution, 80 wt.% in toluene (0.73 mL, 6.57 mmol) was added. The mixture was refluxed at 60 °C during 3 h. Then, the reaction mixture was filtered, evaporated under reduced pressure and purified by flash column chromatography (SiO$_2$; n-hexane: ethyl acetate), 9:1), giving rise to 5 with

76% yield. The structure elucidation of compound **5** was established by ^{1}H and ^{13}C NMR techniques and data were in accordance with previously reported results [23].

3.1.6. Synthesis of Propargyloxychalcones **6a** and **6b**

To a solution of **5** (0.350 g, 1.84 mmol) in methanol (20 mL) was added a solution of 40% NaOH in methanol, until pH 14, under stirring. Afterwards, 3,4-dimethoxybenzaldehyde (0.612 g, 3.68 mmol) or 3,4,5-trimethoxybenzaldehyde (0.772 g, 3.68 mmol) was slowly added to the reaction mixture. The reaction was submitted to MW irradiation at 180 W at 70 °C for 4 h. After, a solution of 10% HCl was added until pH 5, and the obtained solid was filtered, washed with water, and purified by crystallization with methanol, giving rise to chalcone **6a** and **6b** with 41% and 43% yield, respectively. The structure elucidation of compounds **6a** and **6b** was established by ^{1}H and ^{13}C NMR techniques and data were in accordance with previously reported results [23].

3.1.7. Synthesis of Chalcone-Triazolyl-Glycosides **7a** and **7b**

To a solution of **6a** (0.140 g, 0.41 mmol) or **6b** (0.200 g, 0.54 mmol) and 2,3,4,6-tetra-*O*-acetyl-β-D-glucopyranosyl azide (0.309 g, 0.82 mmol or 0.405 g, 1.09 mmol) in tetrahydrofuran (THF)/water solvent mixture (2:1; 30 mL), sodium ascorbate (0.328 g, 1.66 mmol or 0.430 g, 2.17 mmol) and copper(II) sulphate pentahydrate (0.207 g, 0.83 mmol or 0.271 g, 1.09 mmol) were added. The reaction mixture was heated for 1 h at 70 °C under MW irradiation of 250 W with agitation. After cooling, the reaction mixture was filtered and concentrated under reduced pressure. The water suspension was extracted with ethyl acetate (2 × 20 mL) and the combined organic layers were washed with water (1 × 20 mL), dried over anhydrous sodium sulphate, evaporated under reduced pressure, and then purified by crystallization with methanol.

(2*R*,3*R*,4*S*,5*R*,6*R*)-2-(acetoxymethyl)-6-(4-((4-(€-3-(3,4-dimethoxyphenyl)acryloyl)-3- hydroxyphenoxy)methyl)-1H-1,2,3-triazol-1-yl)tetrahydro-2H-pyran-3,4,5-triyl triacetate (**7a**). Yellow solid; yield: 51%; m.p.: 169–171 °C (methanol); ^{1}H NMR (CDCl$_3$, 300.13 MHz), δ: 13.49 (1H, s, OH-2′), 7.89 (1H, s, H-3″), 7.86 (1H, d, *J* = 9.3 Hz, H-6′), 7.84 (1H, d, *J* = 15.5 Hz, H-β), 7.43 (1H, d, *J* = 15.5 Hz, H-α), 7.26–7.22 (1H, m, H-6), 7.16 (1H, d, *J*= 1.9 Hz, H-2), 6.90 (1H, d, *J*= 8.3 Hz, H-5), 6.58–6.55 (2H, m, H-3′ and H-5′), 5.90 (1H, d, *J*= 9.2 Hz, H-1‴), 5.48–5.38 (2H, m), 5.27–5.18 (1H, m) (H-2‴, H-3‴,H-4‴), 5.24 (2H, s, H-1″), 4.33–4.11 (2H, m, H-6‴), 4.04–3.98 (1H, m, H-5‴), 3.96 (3H, s, 3-OCH$_3$), 3.93 (3H, s, 4-OCH$_3$), 2.07, 2.06, 2.02, 1.86 (12H, s, 2‴, 3‴, 4‴, 6‴-COCH$_3$). ^{13}C NMR (CDCl$_3$, 75.47 MHz) δ: 192.0 (CO), 170.6, 170.0, 169.5, 169.1 (2‴, 3‴, 4‴, 6‴-COCH$_3$), 166.6 (C2′), 164.5 (C4′), 151.8 (C3), 149.4 (C4) 145.0 (Cβ), 144.1 (C2″), 131.4 (C6′), 127.8 (C1), 123.6 (C6), 121.5 (C3″), 118.0 (Cα), 114.7 (C1′), 111.3 (C5), 110.3 (C2), 107.9 (C5′), 102.3 (C3′), 85.9 (C1‴), 75.3 (C5‴), 72.7, 70.4, 67.8 (C2‴, C3‴, C4‴), 62.0 (C1″), 61.6 (C6‴), 56.2 (3-OCH$_3$), 56.1 (4-OCH$_3$), 20.8, 20.7, 20.6, 20.3 (2‴, 3‴, 4‴, 6‴-COCH$_3$). HRMS (ESI$^+$) *m/z* calcd for C$_{34}$H$_{38}$N$_3$O$_{14}$ [M + H$^+$] 712.23483, found 712.23337.

(2*R*,3*R*,4*S*,5*R*,6*R*)-2-(acetoxymethyl)-6-(4-((3-hydroxy-4-((*E*)-3-(3,4,5-trimethoxyphenyl) acryloyl)phenoxy)methyl)-1H-1,2,3-triazol-1-yl)tetrahydro-2H-pyran-3,4,5-triyl triacetate (**7b**). Yellow solid; yield: 57%; m.p.: 127–128 °C (quamarnol); ^{1}H NMR (CDCl$_3$, 300.13 MHz), δ: 13.41 (1H, s, OH-2′), 7.89 (1H, s, H-3″), 7.87 (1H, d, *J* = 8.8 Hz, H-6′), 7.81 (1H, d, *J* = 15.4 Hz, H-β), 7.45 (1H, d, *J* = 15.4 Hz, H-α), 6.87 (2H, s, H-2 and H-6), 6.60–6.56 (2H, m, H-3′ and H-5′), 5.91–5.88 (1H, m, H-1‴), 5.48–5.39 (2H, m), 5.27–5.21 (1H, m) (H-2‴, H-3‴, H-4‴), 5.25 (2H, s, H-1″), 4.34–4.13 (2H, m, H-6‴), 4.03–4.00 (1H, m, H-5‴), 3.93 (6H, s, 3-OCH$_3$ and 5-OCH$_3$), 3.91 (3H, s, 4-OCH$_3$), 2.08, 2.07, 2.02, 1.87 (12H, s, 2‴, 3‴, 4‴, 6‴-COCH$_3$). ^{13}C NMR (CDCl$_3$, 75.47 MHz) δ: 191.9 (CO), 170.6, 170.0, 169.5, 169.1 (2‴, 3‴, 4‴, 6‴-COCH$_3$), 166.6 (C2′), 164.6 (C4′), 153.7 (C3 and C5), 145.0 (Cβ), 144.1 (C2″), 140.8 (C4), 131.5 (C6′), 130.3 (C1), 121.5 (C3″), 119.5 (Cα), 114.7 (C1′), 108.0 (C5′), 105.9 (C2 and C6), 102.3 (C3′), 86.0 (C1‴), 75.4 (C5‴), 72.7, 70.4, 67.8 (C2‴, C3‴, C4‴), 62.1 (C1″), 61.6 (C6‴),

61.2 (4-OCH$_3$), 56.4 (3-OCH$_3$ and 5-OCH$_3$), 20.8, 20.7, 20.6, 20.3 (2''', 3''', 4''', 6'''-CO$\underline{\text{C}}$H$_3$). HRMS (ESI$^+$) m/z calcd for C$_{35}$H$_{40}$N$_3$O$_{15}$ [M + H$^+$] 742.24539, found 742.24366.

3.1.8. Synthesis of Chalcone-Triazolyl-Glycosides 8a and 8b

To a solution of **6a** (0.050 g, 0.15 mmol) or **6b** (0.2500 g, 0.68 mmol) and 2-azidoethyl-2,3,4,6-tetra-O-acetyl-β-D-glucopyranoside (0.123 g, 0.30 mmol or 0.566 g, 1.36 mmol) in THF/water solvent mixture (2:1; 30 mL), sodium ascorbate (0.117 g, 0.59 mmol or 0.538 g, 2.71 mmol) and copper(II) sulphate pentahydrate (0.074 g, 0.30 mmol or 0.339 g, 1.36 mmol) were added. The reaction mixture was heated for 1 h at 70 °C under MW irradiation of 250 W with agitation. After cooling, the reaction mixture was filtered and the THF in the filtrate was evaporated under reduced pressure. Then, the water suspension was extracted with ethyl acetate (2 × 20 mL) and the combined organic layers were washed with water (1 × 20 mL), dried over anhydrous sodium sulphate, concentrated under reduced pressure, and then purified by preparative TLC (SiO$_2$; n-hexane: ethyl acetate, 2:8) (**8a**) or flash column chromatography (SiO$_2$; n-hexane: ethyl acetate, 5:5) (**8b**).

(2R,3R,4S,5R,6R)-2-(acetoxymethyl)-6-(2-(4-((4-((E)-3-(3,4-dimethoxyphenyl)acryloyl)-3-hydroxyphenoxy)methyl)-1H-1,2,3-triazol-1-yl)ethoxy)tetrahydro-2H-pyran-3,4,5-triyl triacetate (**8a**). Yellow solid; yield: 65%; m.p.: 77–79 °C (n-hexane: ethyl acetate); ^{1}H NMR (CDCl$_3$, 300.13 MHz), δ: 13.49 (1H, s, OH-2'), 7.87 (1H, d, J = 9.7 Hz, H-6'), 7.85 (1H, d, J = 15.4 Hz, H-β), 7.73 (1H, s, H-3''), 7.44 (1H, d, J = 15.4 Hz, H-α), 7.25 (1H, dd, J = 8.1, 1.8, H-6), 7.16 (1H, d, J = 1.8, H-2), 6.91 (1H, d, J = 8.4, H-5), 6.60–6.56 (2H, m, H-3' and H-5'), 5.23 (2H, s, H-1''), 5.18 (1H, t, J = 9.4), 5.06 (1H, t, J = 9.6), 5.03–4.97 (1H, m) (H-2'''', H-3'''', H-4''''), 4.68–4.52 (2H, m, H-6''''), 4.48 (1H, d, J = 7.9, H-1''''), 4.27–4.21 (2H, m), 4.15–4.10 (1H, m), 3.90–3.81 (1H, m) (H-1''', H-2'''), 3.96 (3H, s, 3-OCH$_3$), 3.94 (3H, s, 4-OCH$_3$), 3.72–3.66 (1H, m, H-5''''), 2.08, 2.01, 1.99, 1.95 (12H, s, 2'''', 3'''', 4'''', 6''''-COCH$_3$). ^{13}C NMR (CDCl$_3$, 75.47 MHz) δ: 192.0 (CO), 170.7, 170.3, 169.6, 169.5 (2'''', 3'''', 4'''', 6''''-$\underline{\text{C}}$OCH$_3$), 166.6 (C2'), 164.6 (C4'), 151.8 (C4), 149.4 (C3) 144.9 (Cβ), 143.1 (C2''), 131.5 (C6'), 127.9 (C1), 124.6 (C3''), 123.6 (C6), 118.1 (Cα), 114.7 (C1'), 111.3 (C5), 110.3 (C2), 107.9 (C5'), 102.3 (C3'), 100.6 (C1''''), 72.1 (C5''''), 72.6, 71.1, 68.3 (C2'''', C3'''' and C4''''), 67.8, 61.8 (C1''' and C2'''), 62.1 (C1''), 56.2 (3'-OCH$_3$), 56.1 (4'-OCH$_3$), 50.3 (C6''''), 20.9, 20.7, 20.7, 20.7 (2'''', 3'''', 4'''', 6''''-CO$\underline{\text{C}}$H$_3$). HRMS (ESI$^+$) m/z calcd for C$_{36}$H$_{42}$N$_3$O$_{15}$ [M + H$^+$] 756.261044, found 756.26373.

(2R,3R,4S,5S,6S)-2-(acetoxymethyl)-6-(2-(4-((3-hydroxy-4-((E)-3-(3,4,5-trimethoxyphenyl)acryloyl)phenoxy)methyl)-1H-1,2,3-triazol-1-yl)ethoxy)tetrahydro-2H-pyran-3,4,5-triyl triacetate (**8b**). Yellow solid; yield: 45%; m.p.: 78–81 °C (n-hexane: ethyl acetate); ^{1}H NMR (CDCl$_3$, 300.13 MHz), δ: 13.41 (1H, s, OH-2'), 7.87 (1H, d, J = 9.8 Hz, H-6'), 7.81 (1H, d, J = 15.4 Hz, H-β), 7.74 (1H, s, H-3''), 7.46 (1H, d, J = 15.4 Hz, H-α), 6.87 (2H, s, H-2 and H-6), 6.61–6.57 (2H, m, H-3' and H-5'), 5.24 (2H, s, H-1''), 5.18 (1H, t, J= 9.4), 5.07 (1H, t, J = 9.6), 4.99 (1H, t, J = 8.7) (H-2'''', H-3'''', H-4''''), 4.68–4.52 (2H, m, H-6''''), 4.48 (1H, d, J = 7.9, H-1''''), 4.28–4.21 (2H, m), 4.13–4.08 (2H, m) (H-1''' and H-2'''), 3.93 (3H, s, 4-OCH$_3$), 3.91 (6H, s, 3-OCH$_3$ and 5-OCH$_3$), 3.72–3.66 (1H, m, H-5''''), 2.04, 2.02, 1.99, 1.95 (12H, s, 2'''', 3'''', 4'''', 6''''-COCH$_3$). ^{13}C NMR (CDCl$_3$, 75.47 MHz) δ: 191.9 (CO), 170.7, 170.3, 169.6, 169.5 (2'''', 3'''', 4'''', 6''''-$\underline{\text{C}}$OCH$_3$), 166.7 (C2'), 164.8 (C4'), 153.6 (C3 and C5), 144.9 (Cβ), 143.0 (C2''), 140.7 (C4), 131.5 (C6'), 130.4 (C1), 124.7 (C3''), 119.6 (Cα), 114.6 (C1'), 108.0 (C5'), 105.9 (C2 and C6), 102.3 (C3'), 100.6 (C1''''), 72.1 (C5''''), 72.6, 71.1, 68.3 (C2'''', C3'''' and C4''''), 67.8, 61.9 (C1''' and C2'''), 62.1 (C1''), 60.5 (4-OCH$_3$), 56.4 (3-OCH$_3$ and 5-OCH$_3$), 50.3 (C6''''), 21.2, 20.9, 20.7, 20.7 (2'''', 3'''', 4'''', 6''''-CO$\underline{\text{C}}$H$_3$). HRMS (ESI$^+$) m/z calcd for C$_{37}$H$_{44}$N$_3$O$_{16}$ [M + H$^+$] 786.27161, found 786.26915.

3.1.9. Synthesis of Acetophenone 9

To a solution of 2,4-dihydroxyacetophenone (1.00 g, 6.57 mmol) and potassium carbonate (2.73 g, 19.72 mmol) in anhydrous acetone (20 mL), chloromethyl methyl ether (0.749 mL, 9.86 mmol) was added and the mixture refluxed for 1 h at 60 °C. Then, the reaction mixture was filtered, evaporated under reduced pressure and purified by flash column chromatography (SiO$_2$; n-hexane: ethyl acetate, 9:1), giving rise to **9** with 84% yield. The structure elucidation of compound **9** was established by ^{1}H and ^{13}C NMR techniques and data were in accordance with previously reported results [55].

3.1.10. Synthesis of Chalcones **10a** and **10b**

To a solution of **9** (0.500 g, 2.55 mmol) in methanol (20 mL) a solution of 40% NaOH in methanol was added until pH 14, under stirring. Then, a solution of 3,4-dimethoxybenzaldehyde (0.847 g, 5.10 mmol) or 3,4,5-trimethoxybenzaldehyde (1.00 g, 5.10 mmol) in methanol was slowly added to the reaction mixture. The reaction was submitted to MW irradiation at 180 W at 70 °C for 4 h. Then, a solution of 10% HCl was added until pH 5, and the obtained solid was filtered and washed with water and purified by crystallization with methanol, giving rise to **10a** and **10b** with 33% and 47% yield, respectively. The structure elucidation of both compounds was established by ^{1}H and ^{13}C NMR techniques and data of **10a** were in accordance with previously reported results [24]. Although the synthesis of compound **10b** has been previously reported [25], the NMR data are described here for the first time (E)-1-(2-hydroxy-4-(methoxymethoxy)phenyl)-3-(3,4,5-trimethoxyphenyl)prop-2-en-1-one (**10b**). Yellow solid; yield: 47%; m.p.: 132–134 °C (methanol); ^{1}H NMR (CDCl$_3$, 500 MHz), δ: 13.29 (1H, s, OH-2′), 7.85 (1H, d, J = 9.1 Hz, H-6′), 7.81 (1H, d, J = 15.4 Hz, H-β), 7.45 (1H, d, J = 15.4 Hz, H- α) 6.87 (2H, s, H-2 and H-6), 6.65 (1H, d, J = 2.4 Hz, H-3′), 6.60 (1H, dd, J = 9.0,2.5 Hz, H-5′), 5.23 (2H, s, H-1″), 3.93 (6H, s, 3-OCH$_3$ and 5-OCH$_3$), 3.91 (3H, s, 4-OCH$_3$), 3.49 (3H, s, H-2″). ^{13}C NMR (CDCl$_3$, 120 MHz) δ: 192.0 (CO), 166.4 (C2′), 163.8 (C4′), 153.6 (C3 and C5), 144.9 (Cβ), 140.7 (C4), 131.4 (C6′), 130.4 (C1), 119.5 (Cα), 115.0 (C1′), 108.4 (C5′), 105.9 (C2 and C6), 104.1 (C3′), 94.2 (C1″), 61.2 (4-OCH$_3$), 56.6 (C2″), 56.4 (3-OCH$_3$ and 5-OCH$_3$).

3.1.11. Synthesis of Chalcones **11a** and **11b**

To a solution of **10a** (0.200 g, 0.58 mmol) or **10b** (0.250 g, 0.67 mmol) in methanol (10 mL), p-toluenesulfonic acid monohydrate (0.110 g, 0.58 mmol or 0.127 g, 0.67 mmol) was added. The reaction was submitted to conventional heating at 50 °C for 5 h. After the addiction of 10 mL of water, methanol was evaporated, and the aqueous solution was extracted with ethyl acetate (2 × 20 mL). The organic phase was washed with water (1 × 20 mL), dried over anhydrous sodium sulphate and concentrated under reduced pressure, giving rise to an orange solid. The crude product was purified by flash column chromatography (n-hexane: ethyl acetate, 8:2) (**11a**) or crystallization with chloroform (**11b**), giving rise to chalcone **11a** and **11b** with 24% and 31% yield, respectively. The structure elucidation of compounds **11a** and **11b** was established by ^{1}H and ^{13}C NMR techniques and data were in accordance with previously reported results [56,57].

3.1.12. Synthesis of 2,3,4,6-Tetra-O-Acetyl-β-D-Glucopyranosyl Azide (**12**)

To a solution of 2,3,4,6-tetra-O-acetyl-α-D-glucopyranosyl bromide (1.00 g, 2.43 mmol) in acetone: water (9 mL, 2:1), sodium azide (0.197 g, 3.04 mmol) was added and the reaction mixture stirred at room temperature for 3 h. After, the acetone was evaporated under reduced pressure and a white solid was filtered. Crystallization of the solid with ethanol afforded 2,3,4,6-tetra-O-acetyl-α-D-glucopyranosyl azide **12** with 72% yield. The structure elucidation was established by ^{1}H and ^{13}C NMR techniques and data were in accordance with previously reported results [27].

3.2. Mussel (Mytilus galloprovincialis) Larvae Anti-Settlement Activity

Mussel (*Mytilus galloprovincialis*) plantigrades were collected in juvenile aggregates during low neap tides at Memória beach, Matosinhos, Portugal (41°13′59″ N; 8°43′28″ W). In laboratory, mussel plantigrade larvae (0.5–2 mm) were isolated in a binocular magnifier (Olympus SZX2-ILLT, Tokyo, Japan) to a petri dish with filtered seawater, and those with functional foot and competent exploring behaviour were selected for the bioassays.

The flavonoids were screened at 50 µM in 24-well microplates with 4 well replicates per condition and 5 larvae per well, for 15 h, in the darkness at 18 ± 1 °C, following Almeida et al. (2015) [58]. Test solutions were obtained by dilution of the compounds stock solutions (50 mM) in DMSO and prepared with filtered seawater. All bioassays included a negative control with DMSO and a positive control with $CuSO_4$, a potent AF agent. After the exposure period, the anti-settlement activity was determined by the presence/absence of attached byssal threads produced by each individual larvae.

All compounds that caused more than 60% of settlement inhibition (≤40% of settlement) in the screening bioassay were considered active and selected for the determination of the semi-maximum response concentration that inhibited 50% of larval settlement (EC_{50}), at compounds concentrations of 3.12, 6.25, 12.5, 25, 50, 100, 200 µM.

3.3. Quantitative Structure–Activity Relationship

The eighteen flavonoid derivatives (**1a**, **1b**, **2a**, **2b**, **3a**, **3b**, **4a**, **4b** from Scheme 1; **6a**, **6b**, **7a**, **7b**, **8a**, **8b** from Scheme 2; and **10a**, **10b**, **11a**, **11b** from Scheme 3) were used to build a QSAR model using the experimental data obtained from the mussel (*Mytilus galloprovincialis*) larvae anti-settlement activity in vivo bioassay (AF activity = log(100/%settlement). AF activity was selected as a dependent variable in the QSAR analysis. The 18 molecules were randomly distributed into a training set (15 molecules) and a test set (3 molecules). CODESSA software (version 2.7.10, University of Florida, Gainesville, FL, USA) was used to calculate more than 500 constitutional, topological, geometrical, electrostatic, quantum-chemical and thermodynamical molecular descriptors [59]. The heuristic multilinear regression methodology was chosen to perform a complete search for the best multilinear correlations with a multitude of descriptors of the training set [60]. The 2D-QSAR model with the best square of the correlation coefficient (R^2), F-test (F), and squared standard error (S^2) was selected. The final model was further validated using the test set and leave-one-out (LOO) internal validation.

3.4. Inhibitory Activity against Biofilm-Forming Marine Bacteria Growth

For anti-bacterial screening, five strains of marine biofilm-forming bacteria from the Spanish Type Culture Collection (CECT): *Cobetia marina* CECT 4278, *Vibrio harveyi* CECT 525, *Halomonas aquamarina* CECT 5000, *Pseudoalteromonas atlantica* CECT 570, and *Roseobacter litoralis* CECT 5395 were used. Bacteria were inoculated and incubated for 24 h at 26 °C in marine broth (Difco) at an initial density of 0.1 (OD600) in 96 well flat-bottom microtiter plates and exposed to the test compounds at 15 µM. Test solutions were obtained by dilution of the compounds stock solutions (50 mM) in DMSO. Bacterial growth inhibition in the presence of the compounds was determined in quadruplicate at 600 nm using a microplate reader (Biotek Synergy HT, Vermont, USA). Negative and positive controls used were a solution of marine broth with DMSO, and a solution of marine broth with penicillin–streptomycin–neomycin, respectively. Compounds exerting a significant anti-bacterial activity (Dunnet test, $p < 0.05$) in the screening bioassays were selected for the determination of the effective inhibitory concentration (EC_{50}).

3.5. Inhibitory Activity against Biofilm-Forming Marine Diatom Growth

The anti-microalgal activity of the most promising compounds was also evaluated against a benthic marine diatom, *Navicula* sp., purchased from the (Telde, Gran Canaria) Spanish Collection of Algae (BEA). Diatom cells were inoculated in f/2 medium (Sigma) at an initial concentration of 2–4 × 106 cells mL^{-1} and grown in 96-well flat-bottom microtiter plates for 10 days at 20 °C. *Navicula* growth inhibition in the presence of each compound at 15 µM was determined in quadruplicate and quantified based on the difference in cell densities among the treatments, and cells were counted using a Neubauer counting chamber. A positive control with cycloheximide (3.55 µM) and a negative control with f/2 medium 0.1% DMSO were included. Compounds that showed significant inhibitory activity in the screening assay (Dunnet test, $p < 0.05$) were selected for further determination of their effective inhibitory concentrations (EC_{50}).

3.6. In Vitro Acetylcholinesterase (AChE) and Tyrosinase (Tyr) Activities

The ability of the most promising compounds to inhibit AChE and Tyr was tested to assess their potential mode of action related with neurotransmission disruption or impairment of adhesive metabolism pathways, respectively.

AChE activity was evaluated using Electrophorus electric AChE Type V-S (SIGMA C2888, E.C. 3.1.1.7), according to Ellman et al. (1961) [61] with some modifications [58,62]. Reaction solution containing 1 M phosphate buffer pH 7.2, 10 mM dithiobisnitrobenzoate (DTNB) (acid dithiobisnitrobenzoate and sodium hydrogen carbonate in phosphate buffer) and 0.075 M acetylcholine iodide was added to pure AChE enzyme (0.25 U/mL) and each test compound (final concentration of 25, 50 and 100 µM, 1% DMSO) in quadruplicate. All tests included a positive control with eserine (200 µM, water) and a negative control with 1% DMSO in water. The optical density was measured at 412 nm in a microplate reader (Biotek Synergy HT, Winooski, Vermont, USA) during 5 min at 25 °C.

Tyr inhibition assay was performed using *Agaricus bisporus* Tyr (EC1.14.18.1) according to Adhikari et al. (2008) [63] with some modifications [8]. The enzymatic reaction follows the catalytic conversion of L-Dopa to dopaquinone and the formation of dopachrome by measuring the absorbance at 475 nm. Briefly, Tyr (25 U/mL) was added to 50 mM phosphate buffer pH 6.5 and the tested compounds at 25, 50 and 100 µM (final concentrations, 1% DMSO). The enzymatic activity was triggered by the addition of L-dopa (25 mM). Kojic acid (1.4 mM, water) was included as positive control and 1% DMSO in water as negative control.

3.7. Environmental Fate Parameters: Artemia Salina Ecotoxicity Bioassay

The brine shrimp (*Artemia salina*) nauplii lethality test was used to determine the toxicity of promising AF compounds to non-target organisms [64]. *Artemia salina* eggs were allowed to hatch in seawater for 48 h at 25 °C. Bioassays were performed in 96-wells microplates with 15–20 nauplii per well and 200 µL of the compounds test solution. Compounds were tested at final concentrations of 25 and 50 µM (filtered seawater with 1% DMSO). All tests included $K_2Cr_2O_7$ (13.6 µM) as positive control and DMSO (1%) as negative control. Bioassays were run in the dark at 25 °C, and the percentage of mortality was determined after 48 h of exposure.

3.8. Statistical Analysis

Datasets from anti-settlement, antibacterial and anti-microalgal bioassay, and determination of AChE and Tyr activities, were analysed by one-way analysis of variance (ANOVA) followed by a multi-comparisons Dunnett's test against negative control ($p < 0.05$). For the AF bioassays, the half maximum response concentration (EC_{50}) values for each compound, when applicable, were calculated using Probit regression analysis. Significance was considered at $p < 0.01$, and 95% lower and upper confidence limits (95%LCL; UCL). The software IBM SPSS Statistics 26 (Armonk, New York, USA) was used for statistical analysis.

4. Conclusions

In this study, eight new triazole-flavonoid hybrids were synthesized using the click chemistry approach. From the series of synthesized compounds, flavone **1b** and chalcones **7b**, **11a** and **11b** showed significant anti-settlement activity towards the macrofouling species *Mytilus galloprovincialis* adhesive larvae. Regarding the compounds' structures, HACA1 was the most significant descriptor for the obtained QSAR model, contributing positively to the AF activity. Particularly, triazolyl glycosylated chalcone **7b**, with a high number of hydrogen-bonding acceptors, showed the most effective anti-settlement activity ($EC_{50} = 3.28$ µM; 2.43 µg·mL^{-1}) with the highest therapeutic ratio ($LC_{50}/EC_{50} > 60.98$), exhibiting also a significant inhibitory activity against the marine diatom *Navicula* sp.

(EC_{50} = 41.76 µM; 30.94 µg·mL^{-1}), suggesting potential in the suppression of biofouling colonization succession. Flavone **1b**, which was effective against the settlement of mussel larvae, also showed capacity to inhibit the activity of Tyr, which might explain the specific AF activity against mussel larvae. Ecotoxicity studies on the non-target species *Artemia salina* revealed that the flavonoids **1b**, **7b**, **11a** and **11b** did not show ecotoxicity to the nauplii of this sensitive crustacean, even at 50 µM, a concentration much higher than their EC_{50}. These results disclosed synthetic flavonoids, particularly a new chalcone incorporating a 1,2,3- triazole ring (**7b**), with potential to be a good environmentally compatible alternative to the majority of the antifoulants in use. Flavonoids are ubiquitous in Nature and, therefore, they come with the advantage that they have been selected during evolution to have high specificity, high efficiency and some might be potential nontoxic inhibitors of fouling. Natural compounds are usually biodegradable, not leaving residue in the environment, and are thus considered one of the most promising alternatives to the biocides in use. However, the yields of natural compounds from marine organisms are generally poor, hindering their development as AF agents. Moreover, optimizing a micro-organism for enhanced production of antifoulant is generally laborious and time consuming. Synthesis of nature-like antifoulants seems to be a more sustainable way to create an opportunity to produce commercial supplies for the antifouling industry.

Author Contributions: Conceptualization, H.C.; methodology, J.R.A.; M.C.-d.-S.; and H.C.; compounds synthesis, D.P.; B.T.M.; compounds structure elucidation, D.P.; quantitative structure-activity relationship studies, A.P.; in vivo AF bioassays, enzymatic determinations and ecotoxicological bioassays, C.G.; J.R.A.; resources, M.P.; V.V.; writing—original draft preparation, D.P.; C.G.; writing—review and editing, D.P.; C.G.; J.R.A.; M.C.-d.-S.; H.C.; M.P.; V.V.; supervision, J.R.A.; M.C.-d.-S.; H.C.; project administration, J.R.A. and M.C.-d.-S.; funding acquisition, V.V., J.R.A. and M.C.-d.-S. All authors have read and agreed to the published version of the manuscript.

Funding: This research was supported by national funds through the FCT—Foundation for Science and Technology within the scope of UIDB/04423/2020 and UIDP/04423/2020 and under the projects: NASCEM-PTDC/BTA-BTA/31422/2017 (POCI-01-0145-FEDER-031422), and PTDC/AAG-TEC/0739/2014 (POCI-01-0145-FEDER-016793; Project 9471-RIDTI) co-financed by FCT, PORTUGAL2020 COMPETE 2020, through the European Regional Development Fund (ERDF); and by the structured program of R&D&I ATLANTIDA (reference NORTE-01-0145-FEDER-000040), supported by the North Portugal Regional Operational Programme (NORTE2020), through the ERDF. D. P. and C. G. acknowledge the grants they received (SFRH/BD/147207/2019 and NASCEM/BI-Lic/2019-53, respectively).

Institutional Review Board Statement: Not applicable.

Informed Consent Statement: Not applicable.

Data Availability Statement: Data is contained within the article.

Acknowledgments: The authors thank Sara Cravo for all the technical and scientific support.

Conflicts of Interest: The authors declare no conflict of interest.

References

1. Amara, I.; Miled, W.; Slama, R.B.; Ladhari, N. Antifouling processes and toxicity effects of antifouling paints on marine environment. A review. *Environ. Toxicol. Pharmacol.* **2018**, *57*, 115–130. [CrossRef] [PubMed]
2. Wang, K.-L.; Wu, Z.-H.; Wang, Y.; Wang, C.-Y.; Xu, Y. Mini-Review: Antifouling Natural Products from Marine Microorganisms and Their Synthetic Analogs. *Mar. Drugs* **2017**, *15*, 266. [CrossRef] [PubMed]
3. Dubalska, K.; Rutkowska, M.; Bajger-Nowak, G.; Konieczka, P.; Namieśnik, J. Organotin Compounds: Environmental Fate and Analytics. *Crit. Rev. Anal. Chem.* **2013**, *43*, 35–54. [CrossRef]
4. Bao, V.W.W.; Leung, K.M.Y.; Lui, G.C.S.; Lam, M.H.W. Acute and chronic toxicities of Irgarol alone and in combination with copper to the marine copepod Tigriopus japonicus. *Chemosphere* **2013**, *90*, 1140–1148. [CrossRef]
5. Kyei, S.K.; Darko, G.; Akaranta, O. Chemistry and application of emerging ecofriendly antifouling paints: A review. *J. Coat. Technol. Res.* **2020**, *17*, 315–332. [CrossRef]
6. Rossini, P.; Napolano, L.; Matteucci, G. Biotoxicity and life cycle assessment of two commercial antifouling coatings in marine systems. *Chemosphere* **2019**, *237*, 124475. [CrossRef]

7. Martins, B.T.; Correia da Silva, M.; Pinto, M.; Cidade, H.; Kijjoa, A. Marine natural flavonoids: Chemistry and biological activities. *Nat. Prod. Res.* **2019**, *33*, 3260–3272. [CrossRef]
8. Almeida, J.R.; Correia-da-Silva, M.; Sousa, E.; Antunes, J.; Pinto, M.; Vasconcelos, V.; Cunha, I. Antifouling potential of Nature-inspired sulfated compounds. *Sci. Rep.* **2017**, *7*, 42424. [CrossRef]
9. Almeida, J.R.; Moreira, J.; Pereira, D.; Pereira, S.; Antunes, J.; Palmeira, A.; Vasconcelos, V.; Pinto, M.; Correia-da-Silva, M.; Cidade, H. Potential of synthetic chalcone derivatives to prevent marine biofouling. *Sci. Total Environ.* **2018**, *643*, 98–106. [CrossRef]
10. Trojer, M.A.; Movahedi, A.; Blanck, H.; Nydén, M. Imidazole and Triazole Coordination Chemistry for Antifouling Coatings. *J. Chem.* **2013**, *2013*, 23.
11. Hou, J.; Liu, X.; Shen, J.; Zhao, G.; Wang, P.G. The impact of click chemistry in medicinal chemistry. *Expert Opin. Drug Discov.* **2012**, *7*, 489–501. [CrossRef] [PubMed]
12. Totobenazara, J.; Burke, A.J. New click-chemistry methods for 1,2,3-triazoles synthesis: Recent advances and applications. *Tetrahedron Lett.* **2015**, *56*, 2853–2859. [CrossRef]
13. Agalave, S.G.; Maujan, S.R.; Pore, V.S. Click chemistry: 1,2,3-triazoles as pharmacophores. *Chem Asian J.* **2011**, *6*, 2696–2718. [CrossRef] [PubMed]
14. Kolb, H.C.; Sharpless, K.B. The growing impact of click chemistry on drug discovery. *Drug Discov. Today* **2003**, *8*, 1128–1137. [CrossRef]
15. Ma, N.; Wang, Y.; Zhao, B.X.; Ye, W.C.; Jiang, S. The application of click chemistry in the synthesis of agents with anticancer activity. *Drug Des. Devel Ther.* **2015**, *9*, 1585–1599.
16. Tron, G.C.; Pirali, T.; Billington, R.A.; Canonico, P.L.; Sorba, G.; Genazzani, A.A. Click chemistry reactions in medicinal chemistry: Applications of the 1,3-dipolar cycloaddition between azides and alkynes. *Med. Res. Rev.* **2008**, *28*, 278–308. [CrossRef]
17. Andjouh, S.; Blache, Y. Screening of bromotyramine analogues as antifouling compounds against marine bacteria. *Biofouling* **2016**, *32*, 871–881. [CrossRef]
18. Kantheti, S.; Narayan, R.; Raju, K.V.S.N. The impact of 1,2,3-triazoles in the design of functional coatings. *RSC Adv.* **2015**, *5*, 3687–3708. [CrossRef]
19. Seijas, J.A.; Vazquez-Tato, M.P.; Carballido-Reboredo, R. Solvent-free synthesis of functionalized flavones under microwave irradiation. *J. Org. Chem* **2005**, *70*, 2855–2858. [CrossRef]
20. Rostovtsev, V.V.; Green, L.G.; Fokin, V.V.; Sharpless, K.B. A stepwise huisgen cycloaddition process: Copper(I)-catalyzed regioselective "ligation" of azides and terminal alkynes. *Angew. Chem. Int. Ed.* **2002**, *41*, 2596–2599. [CrossRef]
21. Tornøe, C.W.; Christensen, C.; Meldal, M. Peptidotriazoles on solid phase: [1,2,3]-Triazoles by regiospecific copper(I)-catalyzed 1,3-dipolar cycloadditions of terminal alkynes to azides. *J. Org. Chem.* **2002**, *67*, 3057–3064. [CrossRef] [PubMed]
22. Liang, L.; Astruc, D. The copper(I)-catalyzed alkyne-azide cycloaddition (CuAAC) "click" reaction and its applications. An overview. *Coord Chem Rev.* **2011**, *255*, 2933–2945. [CrossRef]
23. Zhao, L.; Mao, L.; Hong, G.; Yang, X.; Liu, T. Design, synthesis and anticancer activity of matrine-1H-1,2,3-triazole-chalcone conjugates. *Bioorg. Med. Chem. Lett.* **2015**, *25*, 2540–2544. [CrossRef] [PubMed]
24. Park, J.; Khloya, P.; Seo, Y.; Kumar, S.; Lee, H.K.; Jeon, D.-K.; Jo, S.; Sharma, P.K.; Namkung, W. Potentiation of ΔF508- and G551D-CFTR-Mediated Cl- Current by Novel Hydroxypyrazolines. *PLoS ONE* **2016**, *11*, e0149131. [CrossRef]
25. Zhang, X.; Fu, X.L.; Yang, N.; Wang, Q.A. Synthesis and cytotoxicity of chalcones and 5-deoxyflavonoids. *Sci. World J.* **2013**, *2013*. [CrossRef]
26. Loureiro, D.R.P.; Magalhães, Á.F.; Soares, J.X.; Pinto, J.; Azevedo, C.M.G.; Vieira, S.; Henriques, A.; Ferreira, H.; Neves, N.; Bousbaa, H.; et al. Yicathins B and C and Analogues: Total Synthesis, Lipophilicity and Biological Activities. *ChemMedChem* **2020**, *15*, 749–755. [CrossRef]
27. Adesoye, O.G.; Mills, I.N.; Temelkoff, D.P.; Jackson, J.A.; Norris, P. Synthesis of a d-Glucopyranosyl Azide: Spectroscopic Evidence for Stereochemical Inversion in the SN2 Reaction. *J. Chem. Educ.* **2012**, *89*, 943–945. [CrossRef]
28. Briand, J.F. Marine antifouling laboratory bioassays: An overview of their diversity. *Biofouling* **2009**, *25*, 297–311. [CrossRef]
29. Kojima, R.; Kobayashi, S.; Satuito, C.G.P.; Katsuyama, I.; Ando, H.; Seki, Y.; Senda, T. A Method for Evaluating the Efficacy of Antifouling Paints Using Mytilus galloprovincialis in the Laboratory in a Flow-Through System. *PLoS ONE* **2016**, *11*, e0168172. [CrossRef]
30. Aldred, N.; Ista, L.K.; Callow, M.E.; Callow, J.A.; Lopez, G.P.; Clare, A.S. Mussel (Mytilus edulis) byssus deposition in response to variations in surface wettability. *J. R Soc. Interface* **2006**, *3*, 37–43. [CrossRef]
31. Qian, P.Y.; Xu, Y.; Fusetani, N. Natural products as antifouling compounds: Recent progress and future perspectives. *Biofouling* **2010**, *26*, 223–234. [CrossRef] [PubMed]
32. Dudek, A.Z.; Arodz, T.; Gálvez, J. Computational methods in developing quantitative structure-activity relationships (QSAR): A review. *Comb. Chem. High. Throughput Screen.* **2006**, *9*, 213–228. [CrossRef] [PubMed]
33. Dunn, W.J.; Hopfinger, A.J. *3D QSAR of Flexible Molecules Using Tensor Representation*; Kluwer Academic Publishers: NewYork, NY, USA, 2002; Volume 3.
34. Kubinyi, H. *QSAR: Hansch Analysis and Related Approaches*; Wiley-VCH: Weinheim, Germany, 1993; Volume 1.
35. Veerasamy, R.; Rajak, H.; Jain, A.; Sivadasan, S.; Christopher, P.V.; Agrawal, R. Validation of QSAR Models-Strategies and Importance. *Int. J. Drug Design Discov.* **2011**, *2*, 511–519.
36. Alexander, D.L.J.; Tropsha, A.; Winkler, D.A. Beware of R(2): Simple, Unambiguous Assessment of the Prediction Accuracy of QSAR and QSPR Models. *J. Chem. Inf. Model.* **2015**, *55*, 1316–1322. [CrossRef] [PubMed]

37. Liu, P.; Long, W. Current Mathematical Methods Used in QSAR/QSPR Studies. *Int. J. Mol. Sci.* **2009**, *10*, 1978–1998. [CrossRef] [PubMed]
38. Gramatica, P. On the Development and Validation of QSAR Models. In *Computational Toxicology: Volume II*; Reisfeld, B., Mayeno, A.N., Eds.; Humana Press: Totowa, NJ, USA, 2013; pp. 499–526.
39. Golbraikh, A.; Shen, M.; Xiao, Z.; Xiao, Y.-D.; Lee, K.-H.; Tropsha, A. Rational selection of training and test sets for the development of validated QSAR models. *J. Comput.-Aided Mol. Des.* **2003**, *17*, 241–253. [CrossRef]
40. OECD. *Guidance Document on the Validation of (Quantitative) Structure-Activity Relationships [(Q)SAR] Models*; OECD: Paris, France, 2007.
41. Todeschini, R.; Consonni, V. *Molecular Descriptors for Chemoinformatics*; Wiley-VCH: Weinheim, Germany, 2009; Volume I.
42. Dunn, W.J. Handbook of Molecular Descriptors. Methods and Principles in Medicinal Chemistry Series. Volume 11 By Roberto Todeschini and Viviana Consonni (Universita degli Studi di Milano-Bicocca). Edited by R. Mannold, H. Kubinyi, and H. Timmerman. Wiley-VCH: Weinheim and New York. 2000. xxi + 668 pp. 498 DM. ISBN 3-527-29913-O. *J. Am. Chem. Soc.* **2001**, *123*, 7198.
43. Roy, K.; Kar, S.; Das, R.N. *Understanding the Basics of QSAR for Applications in Pharmaceutical Sciences and Risk Assessment*; Academic Press: Boston, MA, USA, 2015.
44. Almeida, J.R.; Vasconcelos, V. Natural antifouling compounds: Effectiveness in preventing invertebrate settlement and adhesion. *Biotechnol. Adv.* **2015**, *33*, 343–357. [CrossRef]
45. Qian, P.Y.; Chen, L.; Xu, Y. Mini-review: Molecular mechanisms of antifouling compounds. *Biofouling* **2013**, *29*, 381–400. [CrossRef]
46. Chen, L.; Qian, P.Y. Review on Molecular Mechanisms of Antifouling Compounds: An Update since 2012. *Mar. Drugs* **2017**, *15*, 264. [CrossRef]
47. Chen, L.; Au, D.W.; Hu, C.; Peterson, D.R.; Zhou, B.; Qian, P.Y. Identification of Molecular Targets for 4,5-Dichloro-2-n-octyl-4-isothiazolin-3-one (DCOIT) in Teleosts: New Insight into Mechanism of Toxicity. *Environ. Sci. Technol.* **2017**, *51*, 1840–1847. [CrossRef] [PubMed]
48. Chen, L.; Zhang, H.; Sun, J.; Wong, Y.H.; Han, Z.; Au, D.W.; Bajic, V.B.; Qian, P.Y. Proteomic changes in brain tissues of marine medaka (Oryzias melastigma) after chronic exposure to two antifouling compounds: Butenolide and 4,5-dichloro-2-n-octyl-4-isothiazolin-3-one (DCOIT). *Aquat. Toxicol. (Amst. Neth.)* **2014**, *157*, 47–56. [CrossRef] [PubMed]
49. Nong, X.H.; Wang, Y.F.; Zhang, X.Y.; Zhou, M.P.; Xu, X.Y.; Qi, S.H. Territrem and butyrolactone derivatives from a marine-derived fungus Aspergillus terreus. *Mar. Drugs* **2014**, *12*, 6113–6124. [CrossRef] [PubMed]
50. Tadesse, M.; Svenson, J.; Sepcic, K.; Trembleau, L.; Engqvist, M.; Andersen, J.H.; Jaspars, M.; Stensvag, K.; Haug, T. Isolation and synthesis of pulmonarins A and B, acetylcholinesterase inhibitors from the colonial ascidian Synoicum pulmonaria. *J. Nat. Prod.* **2014**, *77*, 364–369. [CrossRef] [PubMed]
51. Jiang, W.; Duysen, E.G.; Lockridge, O. Induction of plasma acetylcholinesterase activity and apoptosis in mice treated with the organophosphorus toxicant, tri-o-cresyl phosphate. *Toxicol. Res.* **2012**, *1*, 55–61. [CrossRef]
52. Martin-Rodriguez, A.J.; Babarro, J.M.; Lahoz, F.; Sanson, M.; Martin, V.S.; Norte, M.; Fernandez, J.J. From broad-spectrum biocides to quorum sensing disruptors and mussel repellents: Antifouling profile of alkyl triphenylphosphonium salts. *PLoS ONE* **2015**, *10*, e0123652. [CrossRef]
53. Katranitsas, A.; Castritsi-Catharios, J.; Persoone, G. The effects of a copper-based antifouling paint on mortality and enzymatic activity of a non-target marine organism. *Mar. Pollut. Bull.* **2003**, *46*, 1491–1494. [CrossRef]
54. Koutsaftis, A.; Aoyama, I. Toxicity of four antifouling biocides and their mixtures on the brine shrimp Artemia salina. *Sci. Total Environ.* **2007**, *387*, 166–174. [CrossRef]
55. Sugamoto, K.; Matsusita, Y.-i.; Matsui, K.; Kurogi, C.; Matsui, T. Synthesis and antibacterial activity of chalcones bearing prenyl or geranyl groups from Angelica keiskei. *Tetrahedron* **2011**, *67*, 5346–5359. [CrossRef]
56. Lim, S.S.; Jung, S.H.; Ji, J.; Shin, K.H.; Keum, S.R. Synthesis of flavonoids and their effects on aldose reductase and sorbitol accumulation in streptozotocin-induced diabetic rat tissues. *J. Pharm. Pharmacol.* **2001**, *53*, 653–668. [CrossRef]
57. Neves, M.P.; Cravo, S.; Lima, R.T.; Vasconcelos, M.H.; Nascimento, M.S.J.; Silva, A.M.S.; Pinto, M.; Cidade, H.; Corrêa, A.G. Solid-phase synthesis of 2′-hydroxychalcones. Effects on cell growth inhibition, cell cycle and apoptosis of human tumor cell lines. *Bioorg. Med. Chem.* **2012**, *20*, 25–33. [CrossRef] [PubMed]
58. Almeida, J.R.; Freitas, M.; Cruz, S.; Leão, P.N.; Vasconcelos, V.; Cunha, I. Acetylcholinesterase in Biofouling Species: Characterization and Mode of Action of Cyanobacteria-Derived Antifouling Agents. *Toxins* **2015**, *7*, 2739–2756. [CrossRef] [PubMed]
59. Katritsky, A.; Karelson, M.; Lobanov, V.S.; Dennington, R.; Keith, T. *CODESSA 2.7.10*; Semichem, Inc.: Shawnee, KS, USA, 2004.
60. Ćwik, J.; Koronacki, J. A Heuristic Method of Model Choice for Nonlinear Regression. In Proceedings of the Rough Sets and Current Trends in Computing, Berlin, Heidelberg, 22–26 June 1998; pp. 68–74.
61. Ellman, G.L.; Courtney, K.D.; Andres, V.; Featherstone, R.M. A new and rapid colorimetric determination of acetylcholinesterase activity. *Biochem. Pharmacol.* **1961**, *7*, 88–95. [CrossRef]
62. Cunha, I.; Garcia, L.M.; Guilhermino, L. Sea-urchin (Paracentrotus lividus) glutathione S-transferases and cholinesterase activities as biomarkers of environmental contamination. *J. Environ. Monit* **2005**, *7*, 288–294. [CrossRef]
63. Adhikari, A.; Devkota, H.P.; Takano, A.; Masuda, K.; Nakane, T.; Basnet, P.; Skalko-Basnet, N. Screening of Nepalese crude drugs traditionally used to treat hyperpigmentation: In vitro tyrosinase inhibition. *Int. J. Cosmet. Sci.* **2008**, *30*, 353–360. [CrossRef]
64. Meyer, B.N.; Ferrigni, N.R.; Putnam, J.E.; Jacobsen, L.B.; Nichols, D.E.; McLaughlin, J.L. Brine shrimp: A convenient general bioassay for active plant constituents. *Planta Med.* **1982**, *45*, 31–34. [CrossRef]

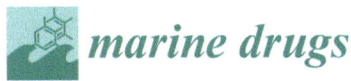

Article

Natural Cyanobacterial Polymer-Based Coating as a Preventive Strategy to Avoid Catheter-Associated Urinary Tract Infections

Bruna Costa [1,2], Rita Mota [1,3], Paula Tamagnini [1,3,4], M. Cristina L. Martins [1,2,5] and Fabíola Costa [1,2,*]

1. i3S—Instituto de Investigação e Inovação em Saúde, Universidade do Porto, Rua Alfredo Allen, 208, 4200-135 Porto, Portugal; bruna.costa@i3s.up.pt (B.C.); rita.mota@ibmc.up.pt (R.M.); pmtamagn@ibmc.up.pt (P.T.); cmartins@ineb.up.pt (M.C.L.M.)
2. INEB—Instituto de Engenharia Biomédica, Universidade do Porto, Rua Alfredo Allen, 208, 4200-135 Porto, Portugal
3. IBMC—Instituto de Biologia Molecular e Celular, Universidade do Porto, Rua Alfredo Allen, 208, 4200-135 Porto, Portugal
4. Faculdade de Ciências, Departamento de Biologia, Universidade do Porto, Rua do Campo Alegre, Edifício FC4, 4169-007 Porto, Portugal
5. ICBAS—Instituto de Ciências Biomédicas Abel Salazar, Universidade do Porto, Rua Jorge de Viterbo Ferreira 228, 4050-313 Porto, Portugal
* Correspondence: fabiolamoutinho@ineb.up.pt; Tel.: +351-220-408-800

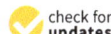

Received: 17 April 2020; Accepted: 24 May 2020; Published: 26 May 2020

Abstract: Catheter-associated urinary tract infections (CAUTIs) represent about 40% of all healthcare-associated infections. Herein, the authors report the further development of an infection preventive anti-adhesive coating (CyanoCoating) meant for urinary catheters, and based on a natural polymer released by a marine cyanobacterium. CyanoCoating performance was assessed against relevant CAUTI etiological agents, namely *Escherichia coli*, *Proteus mirabilis*, *Klebsiella pneumoniae*, methicillin resistant *Staphylococcus aureus* (MRSA), and *Candida albicans* in the presence of culture medium or artificial urine, and under biofilm promoting settings. CyanoCoating displayed a broad anti-adhesive efficiency against all the uropathogens tested (68–95%), even in the presence of artificial urine (58–100%) with exception of *P. mirabilis* in the latter condition. Under biofilm-promoting settings, CyanoCoating reduced biofilm formation by *E. coli*, *P. mirabilis,* and *C. albicans* (30–60%). In addition, CyanoCoating prevented large crystals encrustation, and its sterilization with ethylene oxide did not impact the coating stability. Therefore, CyanoCoating constitutes a step forward for the implementation of antibiotic-free alternative strategies to fight CAUTIs.

Keywords: cyanobacteria; uropathogens; anti-adhesive coating; urinary catheters; surface modification; catheter-associated urinary tract infections

1. Introduction

Urinary catheters are the most common indwelling device, with 15–25% of hospitalized patients undergoing catheterization [1]. More than 30 million urinary catheters are used per year to manage urinary incontinence and urinary retention, during and/or after surgical practices in the USA only [2]. Infection is the main concern associated with the use of catheters (either long- or short-term). Catheter-associated urinary tract infections (CAUTIs) account for approximately 40% of all healthcare-associated infections; therefore, are associated to major economic burden ($1000 per treatment of CAUTI in USA) [3]. This problem is rising together with bacterial antibiotic resistance, which is considered by the World Health Organization (WHO) as one of the most severe health threats around the world [4]. CAUTI establishment is related with the impairment of the natural defense systems of the healthy urological mucosa. When the use of a catheter is required, the natural flush of bacteria by micturition is hampered [5]. Moreover, damage to the inner walls of the urinary system breaches the natural protection against bacterial adhesion, which, adding to the presence of a foreign material and a compromised immune system, contributes to the establishment of CAUTIs. CAUTIs arise from cross contamination derived from the patient's normal fecal flora or from the healthcare personnel handling [6]. These infections are always associated with the occurrence of microbial biofilms, being the most prevalent Gram-negative bacteria, such as *Escherichia coli*, *Klebsiella pneumoniae*, *Proteus mirabilis*, and *Pseudomonas aeruginosa*, Gram-positive *Staphylococcus aureus* (including methicillin-resistant strains), and yeasts—particularly *Candida* species, etiological agents that are particularly well adapted to the urinary tract microenvironment [7].

CAUTIs are a major cause of catheter encrustation, which is promoted by urease-positive pathogens, such as *P. mirabilis*, *P. aeruginosa*, and *K. pneumoniae* [8]. Urease catalyzes the hydrolysis of urea into ammonia and carbamate, which in turn increases the urine pH promoting the formation of crystals [9]. The formation of biofilm itself may also promote catheter occlusion by the large amount of mucoid material produced (e.g., by *P. aeruginosa*, *K. pneumoniae*) or by the emergence of hyphae (e.g., *C. albicans*). Other CAUTI associated complications include bladder stones, septicemia, endotoxic shock, and pyelonephritis contributing to patients' suffering, and frequently worsening other concomitant chronic pathologies [10]. In this way, new strategies are needed to optimize patient safety, control costs, and to reduce bacterial resistance. The current materials used to produce catheters include polyurethanes (PUs), silicone, polytetrafluoroethylene (PTFE), polyvinylchloride (PVC), and latex rubber [8]. PUs are among the best choices for biomedical applications due to their mechanical properties, namely durability, elasticity, fatigue resistance, and compliance [8]. The advantage of using PUs instead of silicone for urinary catheters is that PUs originate catheters with larger internal diameters (due to thinner walls) that are less prone to occlusion, and soften within the patient's body, becoming more comfortable [8,11].

The most promising approach to improve urinary catheter safety is to alter its surface to avoid biofilm formation preventing the consequent infection [12–15]. For the development of anti-adhesive surfaces, natural polymers, such as hyaluronic acid and heparin, can be used [15–17]. Polysaccharides from marine sources, such as alginate, ulvan, agarose, and carrageenans have also been reported as possible alternatives [16,18,19]. Previously, Costa et al. [20] developed CyanoCoating, a coating based on a well-characterized extracellular polymer produced by a marine cyanobacterium [21]. These authors demonstrated that CyanoCoating has anti-adhesive properties against *S. aureus*, *S. epidermidis*, *P. aeruginosa*, and *E. coli*, and is biocompatible, having the potential to be applied to a wide range of medical devices, including blood contacting materials [20].

The present study is aimed at evaluating CyanoCoating capability to endure urinary catheter specifications (urine, uropathogens, and sterilization). Moreover, the absence of contaminants in the raw biological material was confirmed. Overall, the results obtained highlight the translational potential of CyanoCoating to mitigate challenges imposed by CAUTIs.

2. Results

2.1. Biopolymer Regulatory Compliance Assessment: Metal and Microbial Contamination

The extracellular cyanobacterial polymer, mainly of heteropolysaccharidic nature, used to prepare the CyanoCoating is a new material not yet described on pharmacopeia, thus, metal and microbial contamination was addressed. The Inductively Coupled Plasma–Atomic Emission Spectrometry (ICP–AES) results showed that the isolated biopolymer was not contaminated with arsenic (As), cadmium (Cd), lead (Pb), or mercury (Hg) (Supplementary Table S1). Moreover, the microbiological assays showed that the biopolymer was not contaminated with bacteria or fungi, even before the autoclave sterilization process, as no colony-forming units (CFUs) where observed up to 5 days.

2.2. CyanoCoating Surface Characterization

CyanoCoating was previously characterized in terms of thickness and wettability [20]. However, since surface topography is known to impact biofilm development, this parameter was evaluated by atomic force microscopy (AFM). CyanoCoating and medical grade polyurethane (PU) were covalently bound through a polydopamine (pDA) layer to gold (Au) substrates, as previously described [20]. The deposition of either the pDA + CyanoCoating or the control pDA + PU increased significantly surface roughness of Au substrates, as depicted in Figure 1A. CyanoCoating exhibited a smoother surface in comparison with PU, as demonstrated by the decrease of the average roughness (Ra) (Figure 1A$_1$) and the root mean square roughness (Rq) (Figure 1A$_2$). Representative AFM three-dimensional (3D) images of the threes surfaces can be observed in Figure 1B.

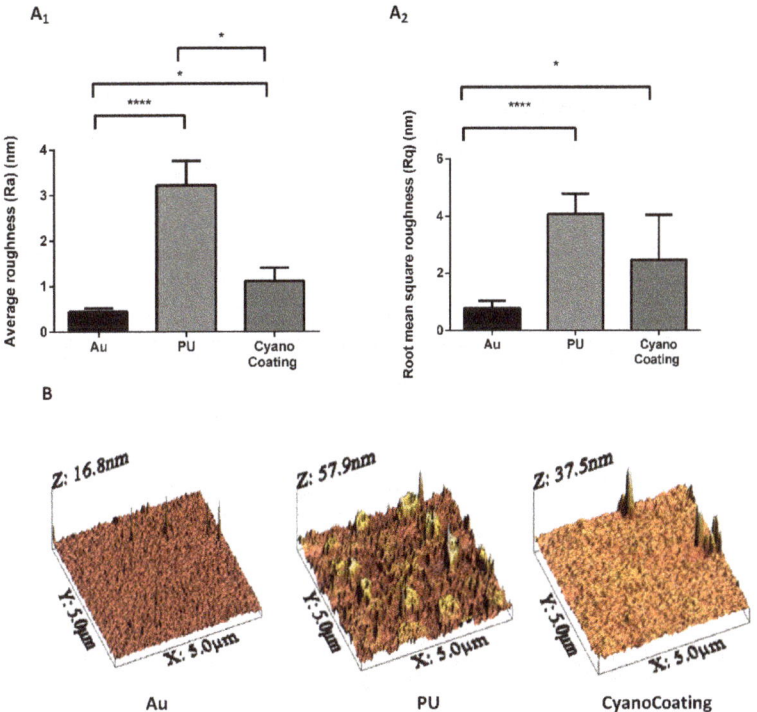

Figure 1. Characterization, by atomic force microscopy (AFM), of the surface roughness of gold substrates (Au), Au substrates coated with a polydopamine (pDA) layer plus polyurethane (PU), or Au substrates coated with a pDA layer plus CyanoCoating. (**A$_1$**) Average roughness (Ra), (**A$_2$**) Root mean square roughness (Rq) and (**B**) AFM three-dimensional (3D) surface images. Statistical analysis was performed by non-parametric Kruskal–Wallis analysis and statistical differences are indicated with * ($p < 0.05$) and **** ($p < 0.001$).

2.3. CyanoCoating Biological Performance

2.3.1. Microbial Adhesion Assays

As the anti-adhesive performance of CyanoCoating was previously evaluated against *Escherichia coli* and *Pseudomonas aeruginosa* [20], herein, we focused on other relevant uropathogens for catheter-associated urinary tract infections (CAUTIs): *Proteus mirabilis*, *Klebsiella pneumoniae*, methicillin resistant *Staphylococcus aureus* (MRSA), and *Candida albicans* [22], according to ISO 22196:2007 [23]. Overall, the results obtained (Figure 2 and Figure S1) showed that microbial adhesion to CyanoCoating was significantly lower than the adhesion to medical grade PU, ranging from 68 ± 28% (*P. mirabilis*) to 95 ± 48% (*K. pneumoniae*). Importantly, CyanoCoating was efficient in preventing *S. aureus* (MRSA) adhesion (80 ± 27%), a microorganism that is very difficult to eradicate. Moreover, CyanoCoating could also reduce in 69 ± 19% the adhesion of the yeast *C. albicans* (responsible for 10–15% of CAUTIs [24]).

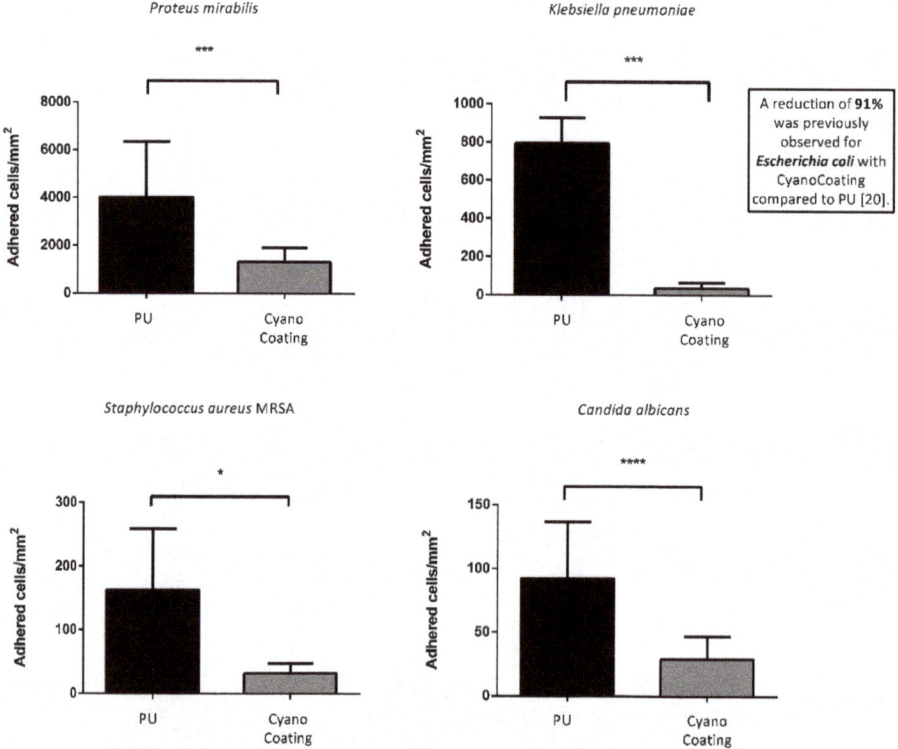

Figure 2. CyanoCoating anti-adhesive performance compared to medical grade polyurethane (PU). The coatings were tested against the uropathogens mentioned above each graph using the respective growth medium; see Materials and Methods. Data represent mean ± Standard deviation (n = 9). The assay was performed according to ISO 22196. Statistical analysis was performed by non-parametric Kruskal–Wallis analysis and statistical differences are indicated with * ($p < 0.05$), *** ($p < 0.005$) and **** ($p < 0.001$).

2.3.2. Microbial Adhesion Assays with Artificial Urine

The anti-adhesive performance of CyanoCoating was subsequently assessed with artificial urine medium (AUM) against *E. coli*, *P. mirabilis*, *K. pneumoniae*, *S. aureus* (MRSA) and *C. albicans*, also according to ISO 22196:2007. In the presence of AUM, CyanoCoating significantly reduced the adhesion of most of the uropathogens compared to PU. For the Gram-negative *E. coli* and *K. pneumoniae* a reduction of 65 ± 28% and 98 ± 54%, respectively, was observed, while for the Gram-positive *S. aureus* (MRSA) and the yeast *C. albicans*, a striking 95 ± 34% and 100% reduction, respectively, was observed (Figure 3 and Figure S2).

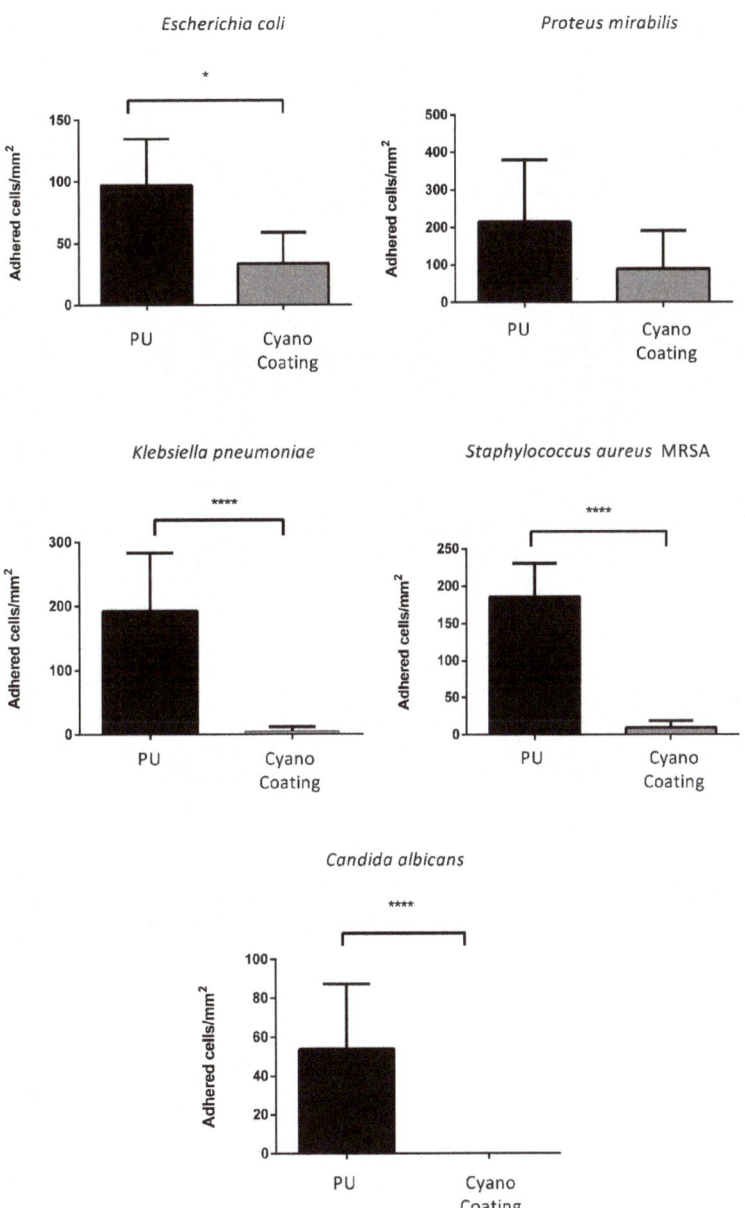

Figure 3. CyanoCoating anti-adhesive performance compared to medical grade polyurethane (PU) with artificial urine medium. The coating was tested against the uropathogens mentioned above each graph. Data represent mean ± Standard deviation (n = 9). The assay was performed according to ISO 22196. Statistical analysis was performed by non-parametric Kruskal–Wallis analysis and statistical differences are indicated with * ($p < 0.05$) and **** ($p < 0.001$).

2.3.3. Biofilm Formation

In order to evaluate CyanoCoating effectiveness in preventing biofilm formation, a biofilm assay was performed according to Costa et al., [25]. After 24 h, the number of CFUs detached from the surfaces by sonication were determined. The efficiency of the sonication process was verified by observing the surfaces using inverted fluorescence microscopy. A reduction trend on biofilm formation was observed for *E. coli* (39 ± 10%), *P. mirabilis* (39 ± 15%) and *C. albicans* (60 ± 30%) on CyanoCoating samples compared to the control PU, while for *K. pneumoniae* and *S. aureus* MRSA no significant differences were observed (Figure 4).

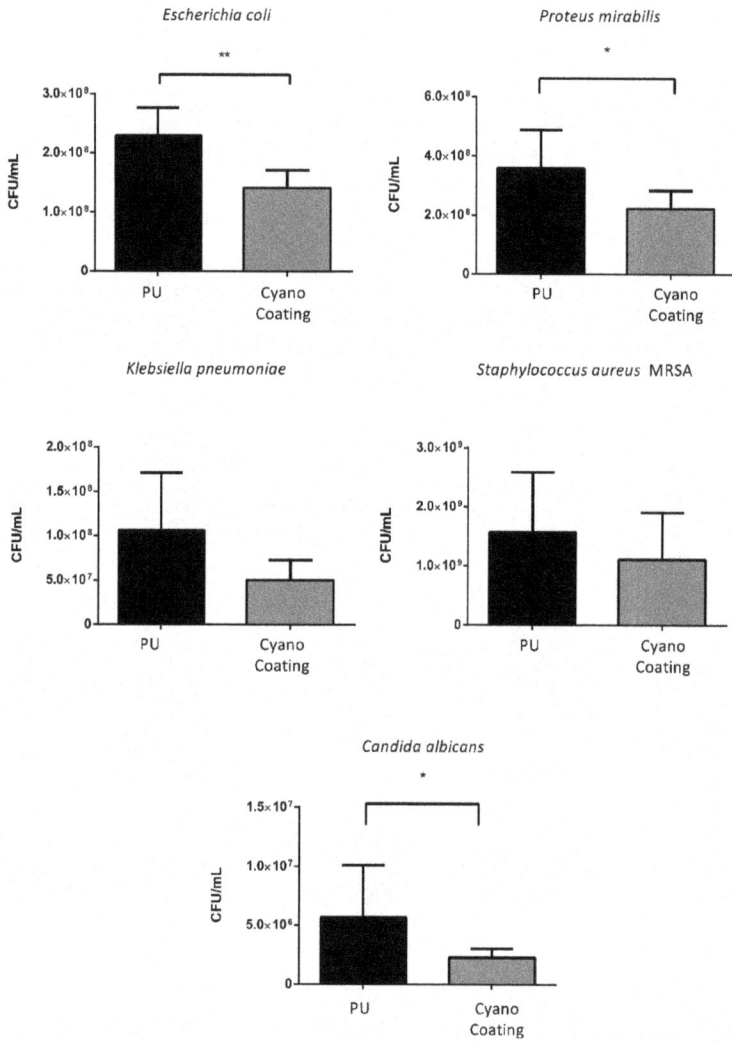

Figure 4. Effect of CyanoCoating on the prevention of biofilm formation compared to medical grade polyurethane (PU), by measuring the bacteria detached from the surfaces. Data represent mean ± Standard deviation (n = 9). Statistical analysis was performed by Mann–Whitney test (*t*-test) analysis and statistical differences are indicated with * ($p < 0.05$) and ** ($p < 0.01$).

2.4. Encrustation Development

Salts deposition on top of CyanoCoating, was evaluated by scanning electron microscopy (SEM) and energy-dispersive X-ray spectroscopy (EDS), after incubation with supplemented artificial urine medium (AUS). This urine is supplemented with urease and ovalbumine to promote an encrustation environment [26,27]. SEM micrographs (Figure 5A, left panel) show the clean surfaces of the CyanoCoating and the control PU at the initial time points (before the immersion in AUS). Seven days after the immersion, it was possible to observe salt deposition on top of the samples (Figure 5A, right panel), particularly in the PU surface where agglomerates of larger crystals are clearly visible. The EDS spectra (Figure 5B) indicate the presence of elements that could suggest the formation of struvite ($NH_4MgPO_4 \cdot 6H_2O$), brushite ($CaHPO_4 \cdot 2H_2O$), or hydroxyapatite ($Ca_5(PO_4)_3(OH)$) in the surface of the samples immersed in AUS (Figure 5B, lower panel). Higher amounts of magnesium (Mg) and phosphorus (P) were found on PU samples suggesting accumulation of struvite, whereas the presence of calcium (Ca) and P on CyanoCoating suggests accumulation of brushite or hydroxyapatite. Before immersion in AUS, EDS spectra of PU and CyanoCoating samples only present silicon (Si), gold (Au) and carbon (C), the expected elements of the substrates, and palladium (Pd) from the SEM analysis sputtering.

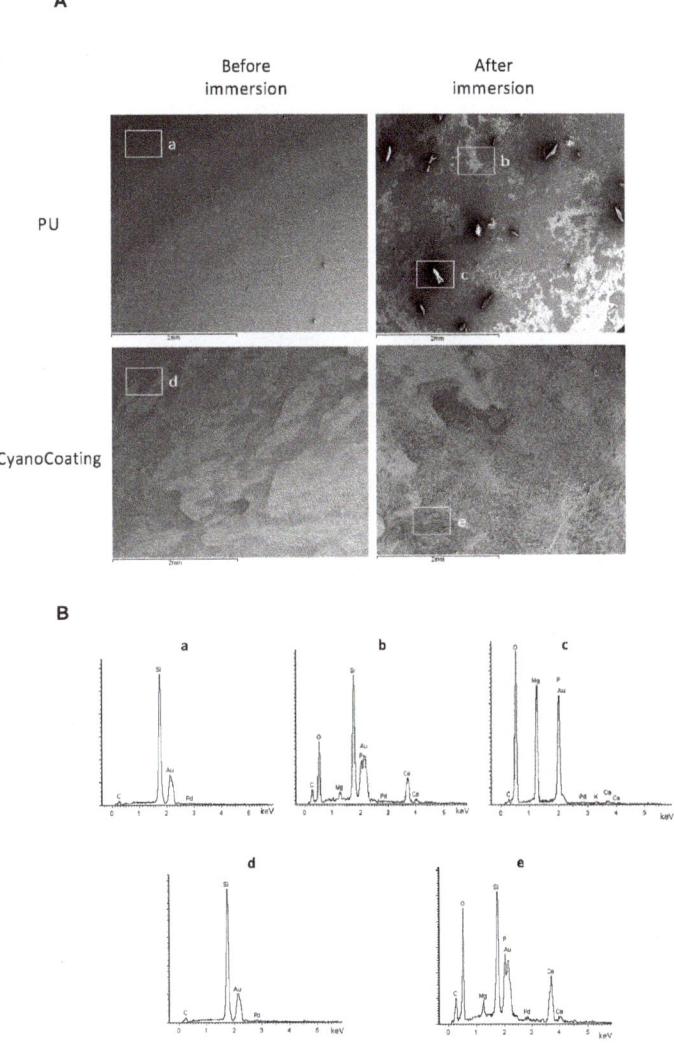

Figure 5. Encrustation development on CyanoCoating compared to medical grade polyurethane (PU).

(**A**) SEM micrographs of the coatings before and after 7 days immersion in supplemented artificial urine medium (AUS). Magnification 30×. (**B**) Energy-dispersive X-ray spectroscopy (EDS) spectra of the selected areas on each coating surfaces before and after 7 days of immersion in AUS. **a** to **e** correspond to the areas highlighted in the SEM micrographs above.

2.5. CyanoCoating Stability After Sterilization

To evaluate the stability of CyanoCoating after sterilization by ethylene oxide (EO), the most common industrial sterilization technique for medical devices [28] and compatible with most of the biomaterials used in their manufacture, samples were characterized both physically (water contact angle measurements) and biologically (anti-adhesive performance). Our results revealed that EO sterilization did not significantly alter CyanoCoating wettability, compared to unsterilized samples, and samples submitted to the regular laboratorial ethanol-based disinfection protocol (Figure 6). Similarly, the anti-adhesive performance of CyanoCoating after EO sterilization was not altered, compared to samples submitted to the ethanol-based disinfection protocol, using *E. coli* or *P. mirabilis* as model bacteria (Figure 7).

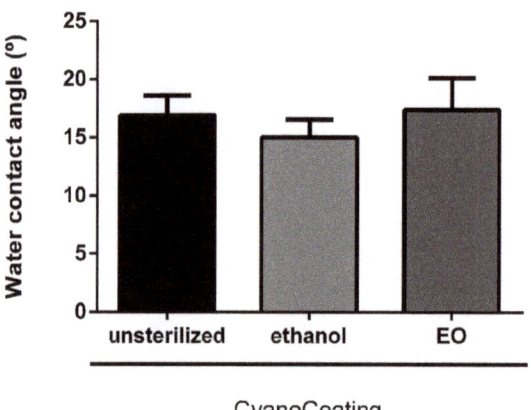

Figure 6. Surface characterization, by water contact angle (captive bubble method), of CyanoCoating samples without sterilization, after sterilization with ethanol 70% (*v/v*) or with ethylene oxide (EO). Data represent mean ± Standard deviation (n = 9).

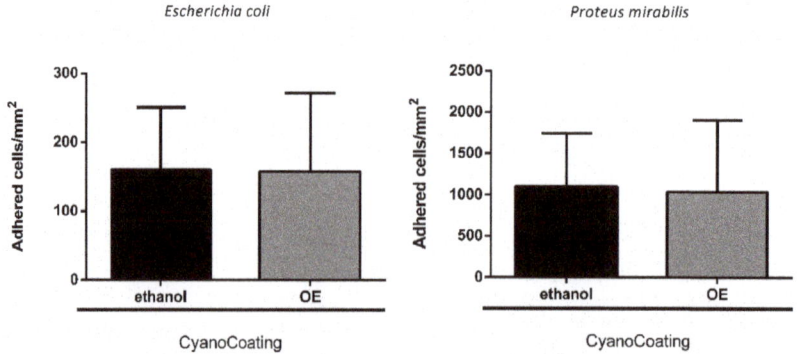

Figure 7. CyanoCoating anti-adhesive performance after sterilization with ethanol 70% (*v/v*) or ethylene oxide (EO). Data represent mean ± Standard deviation (n = 9). Adhesion of *Escherichia coli* and *Proteus mirabilis* in Tryptic Soy Broth (TSB). The assay was performed according to ISO 22196.

3. Discussion

Among all healthcare-associated infections, catheter-associated urinary tract infections (CAUTIs) are recognized as the most prevalent worldwide [29]. In this work, we explore the possibility of a previously developed anti-adhesive coating, CyanoCoating [20], to endure urinary catheters specifications.

Concerning the quality of the raw material (cyanobacterial extracellular polymer) used to produce CyanoCoating, the absence of fungi and bacteria indicate that all steps performed from the cell cultures to the polymer extraction ensured a high purity level of the product, fulfilling the quality requirements suggested by pharmacopeia, and the regulations imposed by healthcare authorities.

In the previous work, the broad-spectrum activity of CyanoCoating was assessed against relevant etiological agents responsible for medical devices-associated infections, including the uropathogens *Escherichia coli* and *Pseudomonas aeruginosa* (reducing bacterial adhesion by at least 80%) [20]. Here, the potential of CyanoCoating for CAUTIs mitigation was assessed against other relevant uropathogens, namely *Proteus mirabilis*, *Klebsiella pneumoniae*, methicillin-resistant *Staphylococcus aureus* (MRSA), and the yeast *Candida albicans* [30–32]. Overall, CyanoCoating greatly impaired the adhesion of the tested microorganisms (ranging from $68 \pm 28\%$ to $95 \pm 48\%$). Considering that CyanoCoating is highly hydrophilic and exhibits a smoother topography compared to polyurethane (as visible in the AFM images) the hypothesis of an anti-adhesive mechanism of action is the most plausible. It is known that highly hydrophilic surfaces prevent the adsorption of proteins/cells due to the establishment of a hydration layer formed by well-structured water molecules linked to the surface by hydrogen bonds that works as a physical barrier [33]. In addition, the lack of bactericidal activity previously reported [20] reinforce our hypothesis. Similar results were obtained by other authors, using poly(ethylene glycol) (PEG) [34] or sulfobetaine methacrylate (SBMA) [35] anti-adhesive synthetic coatings onto PU or silicone surfaces, with *E. coli* and *S. epidermidis* or *P. aeruginosa* and *S. aureus* only. Our results demonstrate that CyanoCoating is effective against a broader range of microorganisms, including urease-positive bacteria and yeasts (this work and [20]).

To better mimic the in vivo environment that bacteria encounter in the urinary tract [32,36], artificial urine medium was used for the in vitro adhesion assays. The microorganisms were chosen since *E. coli* is the most prevalent in CAUTIs, *P. mirabilis* is responsible for the most severe cases, *C. albicans* causes 10–15% of these infections and the other bacteria are also relevant [22,37]. In the presence of artificial urine medium, the overall microbial adhesion to CyanoCoating and PU surfaces was significantly lower than with culture medium, in particular for the Gram-negative bacteria *E. coli*, *P. mirabilis*, and *K. pneumoniae*. This result can be associated to the media composition; culture media promote bacterial growth and biofilm formation mechanisms since they contain glucose as a carbon source, in contrast with the artificial urine medium. Nevertheless, CyanoCoating performance was much better than PU against all the microorganisms tested, in particular for *K. pneumoniae* and *C. albicans*. In addition, we demonstrated that the efficiency of CyanoCoating was not negatively affected by clinically relevant sterilization procedures such as ethylene oxide (EO).

The efficiency of CyanoCoating on preventing biofilm formation was assessed against all uropathogens mentioned above. This method counts the CFUs originated after detachment of the biofilm by sonication instead of other indirect methods commonly used, e.g. the resazurin assay that assess the metabolic activity of bacteria in biofilms [38] or the canonical crystal violet assay that stains the extracellular matrix [38]. This last method cannot be used here due to the heteropolysaccharidic nature of the polymer used to generate the CyanoCoating [21]. Biofilm formation was significantly impaired for *E. coli*, *P. mirabilis*, and *C. albicans* ranging from $39 \pm 10\%$ to $60 \pm 30\%$, suggesting that CyanoCoating hinders biofilm formation against a broad-spectrum of microorganisms, even for the difficult to eradicate fungi *C. albicans* [39]. Our results reinforce the strategy of using natural polymers to prevent biofilm formation, as reported by others, e.g., the use of carboxymethyl chitosan to coat medical grade silicone and that reduced biofilm formation by Gram-negative bacteria [37], or the low-molecular weight chitosan hydrogels used to coat polystyrene microplates that avoid biofilm formation by

Candida spp. [39]. Current technologies in the market are based on the release of antimicrobial agents by the coating, such as antiseptics or antibiotics, to inhibit the colonization of the catheters. However, in spite of the broad-spectrum activity, these coatings exhaust their antimicrobial activities over long periods, are associated with toxicity and contribute for the development of antimicrobial resistance [2,40]. Having in mind the goal of developing an antibiotic-free coating, CyanoCoating may be combined with bactericidal compounds, such as antimicrobial peptides, that can be either immobilized or delivered [41,42].

Another critical aspect on indwelling urinary catheters is the mineral deposition on their surfaces. Frequently urinary catheters become blocked by hard mineral deposits, resulting in urine leakage, discomfort to the patient, and even catheter encrustation. In the worst-case scenario, the encrustation can only be solved by removing the catheter, which may cause trauma to the urethra [26,43]. The encrustation is exacerbated by the presence of urease positive pathogens, such as *P. mirabilis* [26]. Therefore, we challenge CyanoCoating with artificial urine medium supplemented with urease, which also contains albumin that mimics the bacterial and cellular debris that infected urine frequently contains [26]. The energy-dispersive X-ray spectroscopy (EDS) results clearly indicated the presence of Ca, P, Mg, and O that could suggest struvite ($NH_4MgPO_4 \cdot 6H_2O$), brushite ($CaHPO_4 \cdot 2H_2O$) or hydroxyapatite ($Ca_5(PO_4)_3(OH)$) formation. However, while on the control PU surface big rectangular shaped crystals protruded from the surface suggesting the formation of struvite [44], on the CyanoCoating individual crystallites with powdery appearance and smaller in size were formed, which is consistent with brushite or hydroxyapatite [45,46]. All together, these results show that CyanoCoating is less prone to encrustation, and therefore less prone to promote catheter blockage.

4. Materials and Methods

4.1. Cyanobacterium Growth Conditions and Biopolymer Isolation

The unicellular cyanobacterium *Crocosphaera chwakensis* CCY0110 [47] (previously identified as *Cyanothece* sp. CCY 0110; Culture Collection of Yerseke, The Netherlands; kindly provided by Lucas Stal) was grown in 2 L bioreactors with ASNIII medium, at conditions previously described [20,21]. Cells were grown until an optical density at 730 nm of approximately 2.5–3.5 and the extracellular biopolymer was isolated as previously described [20].

4.2. Biopolymer Contaminants

4.2.1. Assessment of Metal Contaminants

To assess the putative contamination of the cyanobacterial polymer with heavy metals, the presence of arsenic (As), cadmium (Cd), lead (Pb), and mercury (Hg) was evaluated. For this purpose, aqueous polymer solutions 0.5% (*w/v*) were prepared and mineralized using 5% HNO_3 (*v/v*). Then, an Inductively Coupled Plasma–Atomic Emission Spectrometer (ICP–AES) (Ultima, Jobin Yvon), equipped with a 40.68 MHz RF generator and a Czerny-Turner monochromator with 1.00 m) was used for metals quantification.

4.2.2. Polymer Microbiological Control

To assess the microbiological quality of the raw material, polymer bioburden (contamination with bacteria or fungi) was evaluated by microbiological assays as recommended by Portuguese Pharmacopeia [48]. To perform the assays, 10 mL of polymer solution 1% (*w/v*) were filtered by a 0.45 µm filter (Merck). Then, the filter was cut into halves and each part was placed on top of either Tryptic Soy Agar (TSA) plates or Sabouraud Dextrose Agar (SDA). After 24 h incubation period at 37 °C, the number of colonies-forming units (CFUs) were counted. Two replicates of each condition were performed.

4.3. CyanoCoating Development

CyanoCoating was prepared as previously reported by [20]. Briefly, gold substrates (Au) were cleaned for 5 min, with "piranha" solution (7 parts of sulfuric acid (95%, *v/v* (BDH Prolabo): 3 parts of hydrogen peroxide (Merck), (CAUTION: this solution reacts violently with organic solvents and should be handled with care). Then, substrates were immersed in freshly prepared dopamine solution (2-(3,4-Dihydroxyphenyl)ethylamine hydrochloride, Sigma-Aldrich) (2 mg/mL in 10 mM TrisHCl pH 8.5) to allow formation of a polydopamine (pDA) layer on top of the Au substrate [20]. Subsequently, the polymer solution at 0.5% (*w/v*) was spin-coated (model WS-650-23, Laurell Technologies Corporation, North Wales, PA, USA) at 9000 rpm for 1 min on top of pDA-coated Au substrate. As control samples, medical grade polyurethane (PU) surfaces were prepared by similarly spin-coating the PU (Pellethane 2363 80 AE; Velox) solution at 0.1% (*w/v*) in tetrahydrofuran (Merck), on top of pDA-coated Au substrate [20].

4.4. CyanoCoating Surface Characterization by Atomic Force Microscopy (AFM)

Atomic Force Microscopy (AFM) images were obtained using a PicoPlus 5500 controller (Keysight Technologies, Santa Rosa, CA, USA). The images of gold substrate were performed in Tapping Mode, in air using a bar-shaped cantilever with a spring constant (k) in the range of 1–5 N/m (AppNano, Mountain View, CA, USA). The images on polyurethane (PU) and CyanoCoating were obtained in Contact Mode, in air, using a triangular shape cantilever V-shaped cantilever with a spring constant k = 0.085 N/m (Hydra-All-G, AppNano, Mountain View, CA, USA). The scan speed was set at 1.0 l/s, for both AFM modes. The scan size was 5×5 μm^2. The software used to obtain the images was the PicoView 1.2 (Keysight Technologies, Santa Rosa, CA, USA). The WSxM5.0 software (Nanotec Electronica, Feldkirchen, Germany) was used to perform the roughness surface measurements [49].

4.5. CyanoCoating Biological Performance Evaluation

4.5.1. Microbial Strains, Media, and Growth Conditions

P. mirabilis (clinical isolate provided by Faculdade de Medicina Dentária, Universidade do Porto) was grown on cystine-lactose-lectrolyte-deficient agar (CLED agar) (Merck) and tryptic soya broth (TSB) (Merck). *E. coli* (ATCC 25922) and *S. aureus* MRSA (ATCC 33591), obtained from the American Type Culture Collection (ATCC), were grown on tryptic soya agar (TSA) (Merck) and TSB (Merck). *K. pneumoniae* (clinical isolate provided by Centro Hospitalar do Porto) was grown on TSA and Todd Hewitt Broth (THB). *C. albicans* (DSM 1386), obtained from the German Collection of Microorganisms and Cell Cultures GmbH (DSM), was grown on Sabouraud Dextrose Agar (SDA) (Merck) and Sabouraud Dextrose Broth (SDB) (Merck). The initial microbial inoculum was adjusted in TSB for *E. coli* and *S. aureus*, in THB for *K. pneumoniae*, or in SDB for *C. albicans*, according to OD$_{600nm}$ measurement and subsequently confirmed by count of CFUs.

4.5.2. Microbial Adhesion Assays

Microbial adhesion assays were performed using *P. mirabilis*, *K. pneumoniae*, *S. aureus* MRSA and *C. albicans* according to ISO 22196:2007 (Plastics—Measurement of antibacterial activity on plastics surfaces) [23]. For CyanoCoating and PU disinfection, samples were immersed subsequently for 15 min, twice in ethanol 70% (Merck) and twice in filtered type II water (0.22 μm syringe filter), being dried with argon stream in a flow hood, and then transferred to a 24-well plate. Then, a 5 μL inoculum drop (1.8×10^6 CFUs/mL) was placed on top of the samples and then covered with a previously sterilized polypropylene (PP) coverslip (Ø 9 mm), using the method described above. Samples were incubated for 24 h at 37 °C in moisturized condition. After 24 h, samples were rinsed with Phosphate Buffered Saline (PBS) three times. Adhered bacteria or fungi were fixed with paraformaldehyde 4% (*v/v*) in PBS, for 30 min at room temperature (RT). After rinsing with PBS three times, samples were stained with 4′,6-diamidino-2-phenylindole (DAPI) (0.1 μg/mL) for 30 min at RT, protected from light.

Afterwards, samples were rinsed with PBS and transferred to an uncoated 24-well μ-plate (#82406, IBIDI, Gräfelfing, Germany) with the surface facing the bottom. Results represent average of three independent assays, with three replicates per sample.

High-content screening microscope (IN Cell Analyzer 2000, GE Healthcare, Chicago, IL, USA) with a Nikon 20× / 0.95 NA Plan Apo objective (binning 1 × 1), using a charge-coupled device (CCD) Camera (CoolSNAP K4) was used to observe samples from microbial adhesion assays. Image field of view (FOV) x-y for this objective is 0.8 × 0.8 cm. Moreover, 9 FOV per sample were acquired spanning an area of 5.76 cm^2. The excitation and emission filters used were DAPI (excitation: 365 nm; emission: 420 nm). On-the-fly deconvolution was performed. The number of adherent bacteria were quantified using the ImageJ software, and values were converted to bacteria per mm^2.

Adhesion reduction percentages were calculated according to the formula: [number of adhered bacteria per mm^2 on CyanoCoating × 100]/[number of adhered bacteria per mm^2 on PU]. The standard deviations were calculated considering error propagation of the measurements uncertainties.

4.5.3. Antimicrobial Adhesion Assays in the Presence of Artificial Urine Medium

To better simulate the conditions of microbial adhesion inside urinary tract, the anti-adhesive performance of CyanoCoating against *E. coli, P. mirabilis, K. pneumoniae, S. aureus* MRSA, and *C. albicans* was performed as explained previously (see Section 4.5.2.), but using artificial urine medium prepared according to Brooks et al. [32] (composition: Supplementary Table S2) to adjust initial inoculum. After 24 h incubation period, samples were processed, as described in Section 4.5.2., the number of adherent bacteria were quantified using the ImageJ software, and values were converted to bacteria per mm^2. Results represent average of three independent assays, with three replicates per sample. The adhesion reduction percentages and respective standard deviations were calculated, as described in Section 4.5.2.

4.5.4. Biofilm Formation Assessment

E. coli, P. mirabilis, K. pneumoniae, S. aureus MRSA, and *C. albicans* were grown overnight in respective culture media, described in Section 4.5.1. PU and CyanoCoating samples were disinfected, as described in Section 4.5.2., being then dried with argon stream in a flow hood and transferred to a 24-well tissue culture polystyrene plates (TCPS, Sarstedt, Nümbrecht, Germany). Then, 100 μL of inoculum (1.0 × 10^7 CFUs/mL) were added to each well containing samples pre-hydrated in 900 μL of TSB for 30 min. After a 2 h incubation period at 37 °C, surfaces were rinsed three times with sterile PBS and re-incubated with 1000 μL of TSB during 24 h. After incubation, samples were rinsed five times with PBS to remove planktonic and loosely bound bacteria. Then, surfaces were transferred to 5 mL SARSTEDT tubes containing 1 mL of 0.5% Tween 80 in PBS and placed on ice, then sonicated using BactoSonicR (BANDELIN, Heinrichstraße, Berlin, Germany) at 160 W for 15 min, placed on ice for 5 min, sonicated again for 15 min and put on ice. As a control, the adjusted inoculum was submitted to the same sonication protocol to verify if the sonication applied interferes with microorganism viability. After, serial dilutions were done and plated for CFU counting. Results are the average of three replicates of three independent assays.

To ensure that after sonication all bacteria were removed from the surfaces, PU and CyanoCoating samples were transferred to a 24-well plate and fixed with paraformaldehyde 4% (*v/v*) in PBS, for 30 min at RT. After rinsing with PBS three times, samples were stained with 4′,6-diamidino-2-phenylindole (DAPI) (0.1 μg/mL) for 30 min at RT, protected from light. Afterwards, samples were rinsed with PBS and transferred to an uncoated 24-well μ-plate (#82406, IBIDI) with the surface facing the bottom. The image acquisition and analysis were performed, described in Section 4.5.2. The adhesion reduction percentages and respective standard deviations were calculated, as described in Section 4.5.2.

4.6. Encrustation Assay

The evaluation of the deposition of crystals on the surface of samples was performed using supplemented artificial urine medium, prepared as described by Cox and collaborators [26] (composition: Supplementary Table S3). Samples were immersed in 2 mL of AUS and incubated at 37 °C, 60 rpm for 7 days. These experiments were executed in triplicate. After 7 days, the samples were washed gently using distilled water to remove any salts that may be loosely deposited on the surface of the materials. Then, samples were dried in vacuum oven (Trade Raypa, Barcelona, Spain) overnight. The samples conductivity was enhanced by sputtering with Au/Pd for 60 s and 15 mA current using the SPI Module Sputter Coater equipment (Structure Probe, Inc., West Chester, PA, USA). The SEM / EDS analysis was performed using a High resolution (Schottky) Environmental Scanning Electron Microscope with X-Ray Microanalysis and Electron Backscattered Diffraction analysis (JEOL JSM 6301F / Oxford INCA Energy 350, Jeol, Peabody, MA, USA). Micrographs of the surfaces were taken using an electron beam intensity of 5 kV (accelerating voltage) and a magnification of 30×, at CEMUP (University of Porto, Porto, Portugal).

4.7. Assessment of CyanoCoating Stability after Ethylene Oxide Sterilization

4.7.1. Water Contact Angle (WCA)

To assess the performance of CyanoCoating after clinically relevant sterilization procedure, samples were submitted to ethylene oxide (EO) sterilization (kindly performed at sterilization service of Hospital de São João, Porto, Portugal) and compared to samples disinfected with the protocol described in Section 4.5.2. (control samples). The ethylene oxide sterilization was performed using a sterilizer cabinet EOGas series 3 plus with ampoules system (Andersen Products, Essex, UK) during 16 h (4 h of sterilization plus 12 h of aeration) at 50 °C.

Water contact angle measurements were performed using captive bubble method with a goniometer model OCA 15, equipped with a video CCD-camera and SCA 20 software (Data Physics, Filderstadt, Germany). Samples were tape glued to a microscope slide and placed with the surface facing the bottom in a quartz chamber filled with type I water. Subsequently, 10 µL bubbles of room air were introduced using a J-shaped syringe at a dose rate of 2 µL/s. Bubble profiles were fitted using tangent formula, to obtain the contact angle. Results are the average of two measurements of three replicates of three independent assays.

4.7.2. Microbial Assays

In order to understand if EO sterilization process compromises bacterial adhesion in CyanoCoating surface, anti-adhesive assays performance was also evaluated, as described in Section 4.5 using *P. mirabilis* and *E. coli*.

4.8. Statistical Analysis

Statistical analysis was performed using Mann–Whitney test (*t*-test) and non-parametric Kruskal–Wallis test using the GraphPad Prism program version 6 (GraphPad Software, San Diego, CA, USA). Data is expressed as the mean ± standard deviation (SD) and p values of < 0.05 were considered significant.

5. Conclusions

Cyanobacteria are a prolific source of extracellular polymeric substances with particular characteristics that represent an untapped source of natural polymers for industrial applications, namely biomedicine. The evaluation of the cyanobacterial polymer-based CyanoCoating demonstrated that this coating is highly efficient in preventing the adhesion of most relevant uropathogens tested here, both in the presence of culture medium or artificial urine, when compared to medical grade PU.

Moreover, a significant biofilm formation reduction was observed for three of these uropathogens, namely *E. coli*, *P. mirabilis*, and *C. albicans*. In addition, CyanoCoating is also promising on encrustation mitigation, and is rather stable after being subjected to an industrial sterilization technique (ethylene oxide). In the post-antibiotic era, strategies similar to the one reported here will play an important role as effective and non-cytotoxic solutions in the battle against CAUTIs.

Supplementary Materials: The following are available online at http://www.mdpi.com/1660-3397/18/6/279/s1, Table S1: Metal contaminants assessment by Inductively Coupled Plasma–Atomic Emission Spectroscopy (ICP–AES). Table S2: Composition of the artificial urine medium according to Brooks et al., 1997 [32]. Table S3: Composition of the supplemented artificial urine medium according to Cox et al., 1987 [26]. Figure S1: Micrographs of *Proteus mirabilis*, *Klebsiella pneumoniae*, *Staphylococcus aureus* MRSA and *Candida albicans* cells adhered to polyurethane (PU) and CyanoCoating after 24 h incubation at 37 °C and stained with Draq5 and propidium iodide (PI) (scale bars—60 µm). Figure S2: Micrographs of *Escherichia coli*, *Proteus mirabilis*, *Klebsiella pneumoniae*, *Staphylococcus aureus* MRSA and *Candida albicans* cells adhered to polyurethane (PU) and CyanoCoating after 24 h incubation at 37 °C, in the presence of artificial urine medium (AUM), and stained with Draq5 and propidium iodide (PI) (scale bars—60 µm).

Author Contributions: Conceptualization, R.M., and F.C.; Data curation, B.C., R.M., and F.C.; Funding acquisition, R.M., P.T., M.C.L.M., and F.C.; Investigation, B.C., R.M., and F.C.; Methodology, B.C., R.M., and F.C.; Validation, R.M., P.T., M.C.L.M., and F.C.; Writing—original draft, B.C. and F.C.; Writing—review and editing, B.C., R.M., P.T., M.C.L.M., and F.C. All authors have read and agreed to the published version of the manuscript.

Funding: This project has received funding from "la Caixa" Foundation (ID 100010434), under the agreement LCF/TR/CI18/50030020". Additionally, this work was financed by FEDER - Fundo Europeu de Desenvolvimento Regional funds through the COMPETE 2020 - Operacional Programme for Competitiveness and Internationalisation (POCI), Portugal 2020, and by Portuguese funds through FCT - Fundação para a Ciência e a Tecnologia/Ministério da Ciência, Tecnologia e Ensino Superior in the framework of the project POCI-01-0145-FEDER-028779 (PTDC/BIA-MIC/28779/2017) and in the framework of the project "Institute for Research and Innovation in Health Sciences" (UID/BIM/04293/2020). Fabíola Costa also thanks FCT/MCTES for her contract under Stimulus of Scientific Employment 2017 (CEECIND/01921/2017/CP1392/CT0002). The authors acknowledge the support of the i3S Scientific Platform BioSciences Screening (BS), member of the national infrastructure PPBI - Portuguese Platform of Bioimaging (PPBI-POCI-01-0145-FEDER- 022122) and i3S Scientific Platform Biointerfaces and Nanotechnology (BN).

Acknowledgments: The authors acknowledge the support of the Biosciences Screening (André Maia) & Biointerfaces and Nanotechnology (Manuela Brás) i3S Scientific Platforms. The authors would like to thank to sterilization unit of Centro Hospitalar de São João, Porto, Portugal, to Daniela Silva for technical assistance with SEM/EDS from Centro de Materiais da Universidade do Porto (CEMUP), Porto, Portugal, and to Laboratório de Análises - REQUIMTE, Faculdade de Ciências e Tecnologia da Universidade Nova de Lisboa, Lisboa, Portugal.

Conflicts of Interest: The authors declare no conflict of interest.

References

1. Trautner, B.W. Management of catheter-associated urinary tract infection. *Curr. Opin. Infect. Dis.* **2010**, *23*, 76–82. [CrossRef] [PubMed]
2. Andersen, M.J.; Flores-Mireles, A.L. Urinary Catheter Coating Modifications: The Race against Catheter-Associated Infections. *Coatings* **2020**, *10*, 23. [CrossRef]
3. Hollenbeak, C.S.; Schilling, A.L. The attributable cost of catheter-associated urinary tract infections in the United States: A systematic review. *Am. J. Infect. Control* **2018**, *46*, 751–757. [CrossRef] [PubMed]
4. World Health Organization. *Global Action Plan on Antimicrobial Resistance*; WHO Library: Geneva, Switzerland, 2015; ISBN 9789241509763.
5. Feneley, R.C.; Hopley, I.B.; Wells, P.N. Urinary catheters: History, current status, adverse events and research agenda. *J. Med. Eng. Technol.* **2015**, *39*, 459–470. [CrossRef]
6. Assadi, F. Strategies for Preventing Catheter-associated Urinary Tract Infections. *Int. J. Prev. Med.* **2018**, *9*, 50. [CrossRef]
7. Ramstedt, M.; Ribeiro, I.A.C.; Bujdakova, H.; Mergulhao, F.J.M.; Jordao, L.; Thomsen, P.; Alm, M.; Burmolle, M.; Vladkova, T.; Can, F.; et al. Evaluating Efficacy of Antimicrobial and Antifouling Materials for Urinary Tract Medical Devices: Challenges and Recommendations. *Macromol. Biosci.* **2019**, *19*, e1800384. [CrossRef]
8. Singha, P.; Locklin, J.; Handa, H. A review of the recent advances in antimicrobial coatings for urinary catheters. *Acta Biomater.* **2017**, *50*, 20–40. [CrossRef]

9. Torzewska, A.; Rozalski, A. Inhibition of crystallization caused by *Proteus mirabilis* during the development of infectious urolithiasis by various phenolic substances. *Microbiol. Res.* **2014**, *169*, 579–584. [CrossRef]
10. Cortese, Y.J.; Wagner, V.E.; Tierney, M.; Devine, D.; Fogarty, A. Review of Catheter-Associated Urinary Tract Infections and In Vitro Urinary Tract Models. *J. Healthc. Eng.* **2018**, *2018*, 2986742. [CrossRef]
11. Desrousseaux, C.; Sautou, V.; Descamps, S.; Traore, O. Modification of the surfaces of medical devices to prevent microbial adhesion and biofilm formation. *J. Hosp. Infect.* **2013**, *85*, 87–93. [CrossRef]
12. Bjarnsholt, T.; Ciofu, O.; Molin, S.; Givskov, M.; Høiby, N. Applying insights from biofilm biology to drug development—Can a new approach be developed? *Nat. Rev. Drug Discov.* **2013**, *12*, 791–808. [CrossRef] [PubMed]
13. Bazaka, K.; Jacob, M.V.; Crawford, R.J.; Ivanova, E.P. Efficient surface modification of biomaterial to prevent biofilm formation and the attachment of microorganisms. *Appl. Microbiol. Biotechnol.* **2012**, *95*, 299–311. [CrossRef]
14. Tenke, P.; Mezei, T.; Bőde, I.; Köves, B. Catheter-associated Urinary Tract Infections. *Eur. Urol. Suppl.* **2017**, *16*, 138–143. [CrossRef]
15. Campoccia, D.; Montanaro, L.; Arciola, C.R. A review of the biomaterials technologies for infection-resistant surfaces. *Biomaterials* **2013**, *34*, 8533–8554. [CrossRef] [PubMed]
16. Junter, G.A.; Thebault, P.; Lebrun, L. Polysaccharide-based antibiofilm surfaces. *Acta Biomater.* **2016**, *30*, 13–25. [CrossRef] [PubMed]
17. Romano, C.L.; Scarponi, S.; Gallazzi, E.; Romano, D.; Drago, L. Antibacterial coating of implants in orthopaedics and trauma: A classification proposal in an evolving panorama. *J. Orthop. Surg. Res.* **2015**, *10*, 157. [CrossRef] [PubMed]
18. Elsabee, M.Z.; Abdou, E.S.; Nagy, K.S.A.; Eweis, M. Surface modification of polypropylene films by chitosan and chitosan/pectin multilayer. *Carbohydr. Polym.* **2008**, *71*, 187–195. [CrossRef]
19. Gadenne, V.; Lebrun, L.; Jouenne, T.; Thebault, P. Antiadhesive activity of ulvan polysaccharides covalently immobilized onto titanium surface. *Colloids Surf. B Biointerfaces* **2013**, *112*, 229–236. [CrossRef]
20. Costa, B.; Mota, R.; Parreira, P.; Tamagnini, P.; Martins, L.; Cristina, M.; Costa, F. Broad-Spectrum Anti-Adhesive Coating Based on an Extracellular Polymer from a Marine Cyanobacterium. *Mar. Drugs* **2019**, *17*, 243. [CrossRef]
21. Mota, R.; Guimaraes, R.; Buttel, Z.; Rossi, F.; Colica, G.; Silva, C.J.; Santos, C.; Gales, L.; Zille, A.; De Philippis, R.; et al. Production and characterization of extracellular carbohydrate polymer from *Cyanothece* sp. CCY 0110. *Carbohydr. Polym.* **2013**, *92*, 1408–1415. [CrossRef]
22. Maharjan, G.; Khadka, P.; Siddhi Shilpakar, G.; Chapagain, G.; Dhungana, G.R. Catheter-Associated Urinary Tract Infection and Obstinate Biofilm Producers. *Can. J. Infect. Dis. Med. Microbiol.* **2018**, *2018*, 7624857. [CrossRef] [PubMed]
23. International Organization of Standardization. *ISO 22196:2007(E)—Plastics: Measurement of Antibacterial Activity on Plastic Surfaces*; ISO: Geneva, Switzerland, 2007.
24. Kojic, E.M.; Darouiche, R.O. *Candida* infections of medical devices. *Clin. Microbiol. Rev.* **2004**, *17*, 255–267. [CrossRef] [PubMed]
25. Costa, F.; Sousa, D.M.; Parreira, P.; Lamghari, M.; Gomes, P.; Martins, M.C.L. N-acetylcysteine-functionalized coating avoids bacterial adhesion and biofilm formation. *Sci. Rep.* **2017**, *7*, 17374. [CrossRef] [PubMed]
26. Cox, A.J.; Hukins, D.W.L.; Davies, K.E.; Irlam, J.C.; Sutton, T.M. An Automated Technique for In Vitro Assessment of the Susceptibility of Urinary Catheter Materials to Encrustation. *Eng. Med.* **1987**, *16*, 37–41. [CrossRef] [PubMed]
27. Tunney, M.M.; Keane, P.F.; Jones, D.S.; Gonnan, S.P. Comparative assessment of ureteral stent biomaterial encrustation. *Biomaterials* **1996**, *17*, 1541–1546. [CrossRef]
28. Mendes, G.C.; Brandao, T.R.; Silva, C.L. Ethylene oxide sterilization of medical devices: A review. *Am. J. Infect. Control* **2007**, *35*, 574–581. [CrossRef]
29. Percival, S.L.; Suleman, L.; Vuotto, C.; Donelli, G. Healthcare-associated infections, medical devices and biofilms: Risk, tolerance and control. *J. Med. Microbiol.* **2015**, *64*, 323–334. [CrossRef]
30. Wazait, H.D.; Patel, H.R.; Veer, V.; Kelsey, M.; Van Der Meulen, J.H.; Miller, R.A.; Emberton, M. Catheter-associated urinary tract infections: Prevalence of uropathogens and pattern of antimicrobial resistance in a UK hospital (1996–2001). *BJU Int.* **2003**, *91*, 806–809. [CrossRef] [PubMed]

31. Prashamsa, K.; Dhital, D.; Madhup, S.K.; Sherchan, J.B. Catheter Associated Urinary Tract Infection: Prevalence, Microbiological Profile and Antibiogram at a Tertiary Care Hospital. *Clin. Chem. Lab. Med.* **2018**, *3*, 3–10.
32. Brooks, T.; Keevil, C.W. A simple artificial urine for the growth of urinary pathogens. *Lett. Appl. Microbiol.* **1997**, *24*, 203–206. [CrossRef]
33. Damodaran, V.B.; Murthy, N.S. Bio-inspired strategies for designing antifouling biomaterials. *Biomater. Res.* **2016**, *20*, 18. [CrossRef] [PubMed]
34. Park, K.D.; Kim, Y.S.; Han, D.K.; Kim, Y.H.; Lee, E.H.; Suh, H.; Choi, K.S. Bacterial adhesion on PEG modified polyurethane surfaces. *Biomaterials* **1998**, *19*, 851–859. [CrossRef]
35. Diaz Blanco, C.; Ortner, A.; Dimitrov, R.; Navarro, A.; Mendoza, E.; Tzanov, T. Building an Antifouling Zwitterionic Coating on Urinary Catheters Using an Enzymatically Triggered Bottom-Up Approach. *ACS Appl. Mater. Interfaces* **2014**, *6*, 11385–11393. [CrossRef] [PubMed]
36. Ipe, D.S.; Ulett, G.C. Evaluation of the In Vitro growth of urinary tract infection-causing gram-negative and gram-positive bacteria in a proposed synthetic human urine (SHU) medium. *J. Microbiol. Methods* **2016**, *127*, 164–171. [CrossRef]
37. Wang, R.; Neoh, K.G.; Shi, Z.; Kang, E.T.; Tambyah, P.A.; Chiong, E. Inhibition of *Escherichia coli* and *Proteus mirabilis* adhesion and biofilm formation on medical grade silicone surface. *Biotechnol. Bioeng.* **2012**, *109*, 336–345. [CrossRef]
38. Catto, C.; Cappitelli, F. Testing Anti-Biofilm Polymeric Surfaces: Where to Start? *Int. J. Mol. Sci.* **2019**, *20*, 3794. [CrossRef]
39. Cavalheiro, M.; Teixeira, M.C. *Candida* Biofilms: Threats, Challenges, and Promising Strategies. *Front. Med.* **2018**, *5*, 28. [CrossRef]
40. Al-Qahtani, M.; Safan, A.; Jassim, G.; Abadla, S. Efficacy of anti-microbial catheters in preventing catheter associated urinary tract infections in hospitalized patients: A review on recent updates. *J. Infect. Public Health* **2019**, *12*, 760–766. [CrossRef]
41. Grassi, L.; Maisetta, G.; Esin, S.; Batoni, G. Combination Strategies to Enhance the Efficacy of Antimicrobial Peptides against Bacterial Biofilms. *Front. Microbiol.* **2017**, *8*, 2409. [CrossRef]
42. Monteiro, C.; Costa, F.; Pirttila, A.M.; Tejesvi, M.V.; Martins, M.C.L. Prevention of urinary catheter-associated infections by coating antimicrobial peptides from crowberry endophytes. *Sci. Rep.* **2019**, *9*, 10753. [CrossRef]
43. Barros, A.A.; Rita, A.; Duarte, C.; Pires, R.A.; Sampaio-Marques, B.; Ludovico, P.; Lima, E.; Mano, J.F.; Reis, R.L. Bioresorbable ureteral stents from natural origin polymers. *J. Biomed. Mater. Res. B Appl. Biomater.* **2015**, *103*, 608–617. [CrossRef]
44. Prywer, J.; Torzewska, A.; Plocinski, T. Unique surface and internal structure of struvite crystals formed by *Proteus mirabilis*. *Urol. Res.* **2012**, *40*, 699–707. [CrossRef] [PubMed]
45. Tang, R.; Nancollas, G.H.; Giocondi, J.L.; Hoyer, J.R.; Orme, C.A. Dual roles of brushite crystals in calcium oxalate crystallization provide physicochemical mechanisms underlying renal stone formation. *Kidney Int.* **2006**, *70*, 71–78. [CrossRef] [PubMed]
46. Grover, P.K.; Kim, D.-S.; Ryall, R.L. The effect of seed crystals of hydroxyapatite and brushite on the crystallization of calcium oxalate in undiluted human urine In Vitro: Implications for urinary stone pathogenesis. *Mol. Med.* **2002**, *8*, 200–209. [CrossRef] [PubMed]
47. Mares, J.; Johansen, J.R.; Hauer, T.; Zima, J., Jr.; Ventura, S.; Cuzman, O.; Tiribilli, B.; Kastovsky, J. Taxonomic resolution of the genus *Cyanothece* (Chroococcales, Cyanobacteria), with a treatment on *Gloeothece* and three new genera, *Crocosphaera*, *Rippkaea*, and *Zehria*. *J. Phycol.* **2019**, *55*, 578–610. [CrossRef] [PubMed]
48. *Farmacopeia Portuguesa 9*; Ministério da Saúde, Infarmed: Lisboa, Portugal, 2008.
49. Horcas, I.; Fernandez, R.; Gomez-Rodriguez, J.M.; Colchero, J.; Gomez-Herrero, J.; Baro, A.M. WSXM: A software for scanning probe microscopy and a tool for nanotechnology. *Rev. Sci. Instrum.* **2007**, *78*, 013705. [CrossRef]

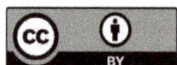

© 2020 by the authors. Licensee MDPI, Basel, Switzerland. This article is an open access article distributed under the terms and conditions of the Creative Commons Attribution (CC BY) license (http://creativecommons.org/licenses/by/4.0/).

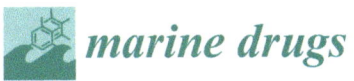

Article

The Effect of Molecular Weight on the Antimicrobial Activity of Chitosan from *Loligo opalescens* for Food Packaging Applications

Luciana C. Gomes [1], Sara I. Faria [1], Jesus Valcarcel [2], José A. Vázquez [2], Miguel A. Cerqueira [3], Lorenzo Pastrana [3], Ana I. Bourbon [3] and Filipe J. Mergulhão [1,*]

1. LEPABE—Laboratory for Process Engineering, Environment, Biotechnology and Energy, Faculty of Engineering, University of Porto, Rua Dr. Roberto Frias, 4200-465 Porto, Portugal; luciana.gomes@fe.up.pt (L.C.G.); sisf@fe.up.pt (S.I.F.)
2. Grupo de Reciclado y Valorización de Materiales Residuales (REVAL), Instituto de Investigaciones Marinas (IIM-CSIC), C/Eduardo Cabello, 6, CP36208 Vigo, Spain; jvalcarcel@iim.csic.es (J.V.); jvazquez@iim.csic.es (J.A.V.)
3. International Iberian Nanotechnology Laboratory, Department of Life Sciences, Av. Mestre José Veiga s/n, 4715-330 Braga, Portugal; miguel.cerqueira@inl.int (M.A.C.); lorenzo.pastrana@inl.int (L.P.); ana.bourbon@inl.int (A.I.B.)
* Correspondence: filipem@fe.up.pt; Tel.: +351-225-081-668

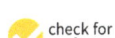

Citation: Gomes, L.C.; Faria, S.I.; Valcarcel, J.; Vázquez, J.A.; Cerqueira, M.A.; Pastrana, L.; Bourbon, A.I.; Mergulhão, F.J. The Effect of Molecular Weight on the Antimicrobial Activity of Chitosan from *Loligo opalescens* for Food Packaging Applications. *Mar. Drugs* **2021**, *19*, 384. https://doi.org/10.3390/md19070384

Academic Editors: Tom Turk and Joana Reis Almeida

Received: 31 May 2021
Accepted: 28 June 2021
Published: 2 July 2021

Publisher's Note: MDPI stays neutral with regard to jurisdictional claims in published maps and institutional affiliations.

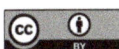

Copyright: © 2021 by the authors. Licensee MDPI, Basel, Switzerland. This article is an open access article distributed under the terms and conditions of the Creative Commons Attribution (CC BY) license (https://creativecommons.org/licenses/by/4.0/).

Abstract: The growing requirement for sustainable processes has boosted the development of biodegradable plastic-based materials incorporating bioactive compounds obtained from waste, adding value to these products. Chitosan (Ch) is a biopolymer that can be obtained by deacetylation of chitin (found abundantly in waste from the fishery industry) and has valuable properties such as biocompatibility, biodegradability, antimicrobial activity, and easy film-forming ability. This study aimed to produce and characterize poly(lactic acid) (PLA) surfaces coated with β-chitosan and β-chitooligosaccharides from a *Loligo opalescens* pen with different molecular weights for application in the food industry. The PLA films with native and depolymerized Ch were functionalized through plasma oxygen treatment followed by dip-coating, and their physicochemical properties were assessed by Fourier-transform infrared spectroscopy, X-ray diffraction, water contact angle, and scanning electron microscopy. Their antimicrobial properties were assessed against *Escherichia coli* and *Pseudomonas putida*, where Ch-based surfaces reduced the number of biofilm viable, viable but nonculturable, and culturable cells by up to 73%, 74%, and 87%, respectively, compared to PLA. Biofilm growth inhibition was confirmed by confocal laser scanning microscopy. Results suggest that Ch films of higher molecular weight had higher antibiofilm activity under the food storage conditions mimicked in this work, contributing simultaneously to the reuse of marine waste.

Keywords: chitin; chitosan; marine waste; antimicrobial activity; poly(lactic acid); active packaging

1. Introduction

One of the major growth segments in the food industry is minimally processed, preservative-free, and ready-to-eat meals and food products [1,2]. As a consequence, the waste from traditional plastic packaging is also increasing (around 4.2% per year) [3] and is considered one of the main factors responsible for short- and long-term environmental pollution [3–5]. Another problem facing the food industry is microbial contamination since microorganisms can attach to food and packaging surfaces and form biofilms in a complex and multifaceted process, causing food spoilage, illness, and shelf-life reduction of food products [1,6]. Biofilms are organized communities of microorganisms that attach to a surface and produce extracellular polymeric substances (EPS), which protect them from adverse environmental conditions [6]. These two factors are putting increasing pressure on the food industry to develop new types of antimicrobial packaging materials, mainly based on natural and renewable sources, in order to ensure food safety, quality maintenance, and shelf-life enhancement, as well as to reduce environmental issues caused by non-biodegradable packaging materials [7–9].

Among different biopolymers, chitosan (Ch) has received substantial attention from academics and industry for food packaging applications due to its particular physicochemical features, biodegradability, non-toxicity, biocompatibility, good film-forming properties, chemical stability, high reactivity, low cost, and availability in nature [10–12]. Chitosan also has intrinsic antioxidant and antimicrobial activities against fungi, molds, yeasts, and Gram-negative and Gram-positive bacteria [13]. As a result of these properties, chitosan was classified as Generally Recognized as Safe by the US FDA in 2001 [14]. However, inherent drawbacks of Ch, including low mechanical and thermal stability and high sensitivity to humidity, have been restricting its industrial application [15]. One strategy to overcome these disadvantages is to combine chitosan with other biopolymers [16] such as the poly(lactic acid) (PLA) used in the present work. PLA is a commonly used polymer for packaging because it has mechanical, thermal, and barrier properties comparable to the most used synthetic plastics, having the advantage of being biodegradable and obtained from renewable sources [17]. Particularly in the last decade, different research groups have focused on the development of PLA/Ch materials [18–22]. Sébastien et al. [18] and Grande and Carvalho [19] obtained composite films by solution mixing and film casting processes. Although the Ch-PLA films produced by Sébastien et al. [18] showed interesting antifungal activity, their heterogeneity and high water sensitivity restrict their usage as food packaging materials [18]. Later, Soares et al. [20] synthesized biodegradable sheets of PLA and coated them with cross-linked chitosan by both spraying and immersion techniques. Nevertheless, the antimicrobial performance of these films was not further evaluated [20]. Bonilla et al. [21] and Chang et al. [22] prepared chitosan–PLA films containing various amounts of chitosan by extrusion and demonstrated their antibacterial activity in refrigerated meat and fish samples, respectively.

The main source of commercial chitosan is chitin, which is the second most abundant polysaccharide on Earth, only preceded by cellulose. Chitin is formed by N-acetylglucosamine units linked by β-(1→4) glycosidic bonds and is commonly sourced from crustacean shells [23], although some molluscs, such as squid, insects [24], and fungi [25], also incorporate this polysaccharide. The disposition of the chitin chains depends on the source; in the case of a squid pen, the source of the chitosan tested in this work, this is parallel (β-chitin), leading to weaker inter- and intra-molecular forces and, as a result, increased solubility and water-absorbing capacity [26]. Weaker forces also carry advantages for the partial deacetylation of N-acetylglucosamine to glucosamine units in chitin to produce chitosan. A sufficient number of glucosamine units enables dissolution in dilute acids due to the protonation of the free amino groups. Furthermore, deacetylation of squid pen β-chitin by alkaline hydrolysis produces more homogeneous chitosan as acetyl groups are more easily accessible than in other sources [27].

In addition to the chemical potential of the chitin/chitosan extracted from the squid pens, their use can help to solve disposal problems for the processing industry and potential environmental impacts. In fact, global squid captures have risen in the last few decades, reaching almost 4 million tonnes in 2015 [28]. Although only representing 5% of all fish, molluscs, and crustaceans captured, squid processing produces a substantial amount of waste. Considering that the yield of edible flesh in squid ranges from 60 to 80% [29], the annual waste generation can be estimated at 0.8 to 1.6 million tonnes and the disposal can be costly in developed countries [30]. Despite the huge potential of chitin and chitosan, currently, they are only employed in a few areas of industrial chemistry, such as cosmetics, textiles, water treatment, and biomedicine [30]. Therefore, a novel concept of shell biorefinery has been suggested on account of the massive potential of chitin valorization. Shell biorefinery consists of the sustainable conversion of chitin into several nitrogen-rich chemicals for pharmaceuticals, cosmetics, textiles, water treatment, household cleansers, soaps, and carbon dioxide sequestration, which benefits both the economy and the environment [30–32].

Variations in chitosan's antibacterial efficacy arise from numerous parameters, including intrinsic factors of chitosan, such as positive charge density, molecular weight (Mw), concentration, and hydrophilic/hydrophobic characteristics [33,34]. In the present work, the effect of Mw on the antimicrobial activity of chitosan is addressed. Although several studies have focused on this parameter, they have generated contradictory results concerning the relation between bactericidal activity and chitosan Mw. Some studies reported that increasing chitosan Mw leads to decreasing chitosan activity against *Escherichia coli*, while others suggested that high Mw chitosan displays greater activity than low Mw chitosan [34].

This study was undertaken to (1) produce β-chitosan and β-chitooligosaccharides from the *Loligo opalescens* pen, (2) develop and characterize PLA surfaces coated with β-chitosan and its derivatives of different Mw, and (3) evaluate the antimicrobial activity of PLA/Ch composite films against *Escherichia coli* and *Pseudomonas putida*, which are bacterial strains present in food processing environments [35,36] and may be responsible for the spoilage of chilled food products [37,38]. This work encompasses the crucial steps for the synthesis and characterization of PLA/Ch films for application in food contact surfaces, from the extraction of chitin and production of chitosan from marine by-products to antimicrobial tests, using innovative combinations of PLA and chitosan and its derivatives.

2. Results

2.1. Production and Characterization of Chitosan and Derivatives

Endoskeleton (pen) by-products of the squid species *Loligo opalescens* were initially processed to obtain chitosan by a combination of enzymatic and alkaline treatments, following the optimal conditions defined in a previous work [39]. Alcalase was the enzyme selected for the first step of pen deproteinization to produce chitin, and NaOH was the alkali utilized for the subsequent conversion of chitin into chitosan (Figure 1a). A highly purified β-chitosan (β-Ch) with a 92% of deacetylation degree (Figure 1b) and molecular weights of Mn (number average molecular weight) = 206 kDa/Mw (weight average molecular weight) = 294 kDa was finally recovered (Figure 1c). Based on the protocol of sodium nitrite depolymerization (see Section 4.1), three β-chitooligosaccharides (β-Cho) were produced: (1) a Ch of Mn = 138 kDa/Mw = 186 kDa (β-ChoA, Figure 2a), (2) a Ch of Mn = 84 kDa/Mw = 129 kDa (β-ChoB, Figure 2b), and (3) a Ch of Mn = 37 kDa/Mw = 61 kDa (β-ChoC, Figure 2c).

The rheological behavior of 1% (w/v) β-Ch and β-Cho solutions was assessed by evaluating their flow curves at 25 °C (Figure 3). All chitosan solutions revealed a Newtonian behavior, i.e., the viscosity was not dependent on the shear rate. However, it was possible to observe that the β-Ch solution was approximately 10 times more viscous than the three β-Cho samples (β-ChoA, β-ChoB, and β-ChoC).

2.2. Characterization of Functionalized Poly(lactic acid) (PLA) Films

2.2.1. Water Contact Angle

Oxygen plasma was applied on the PLA surface to enhance its wettability, adhesion, and biocompatibility [40]. Figure 4 shows the effect of oxygen plasma treatment on the water contact angle of the film. The value of the water contact angle obtained for the PLA before treatment was 79.2 ± 1.1°. A surface with a water contact angle between 0° and 30° can be considered hydrophilic, while a hydrophobic surface is characterized by contact angles over 90° [41]. Therefore, the PLA surface was quite hydrophobic as the initial contact angle for the untreated surface was close to 90°. After the plasma treatment, a significant reduction in the contact angle value was observed. Figure 4 also presents the water contact angles after the deposition of chitosan samples on the PLA surface. PLA films were functionalized with the 1% (w/v) β-Ch and β-Cho solutions described above by the dip-coating method. After chitosan deposition, a decrease of approximately 45% in the contact angle of the surfaces was observed compared to the non-functionalized PLA after plasma treatment. This result indicates that chitosan was successfully deposited on the PLA films. Moreover, the type of immobilized chitosan did not influence the wettability of the surfaces since their water contact angles were very similar (around 38°).

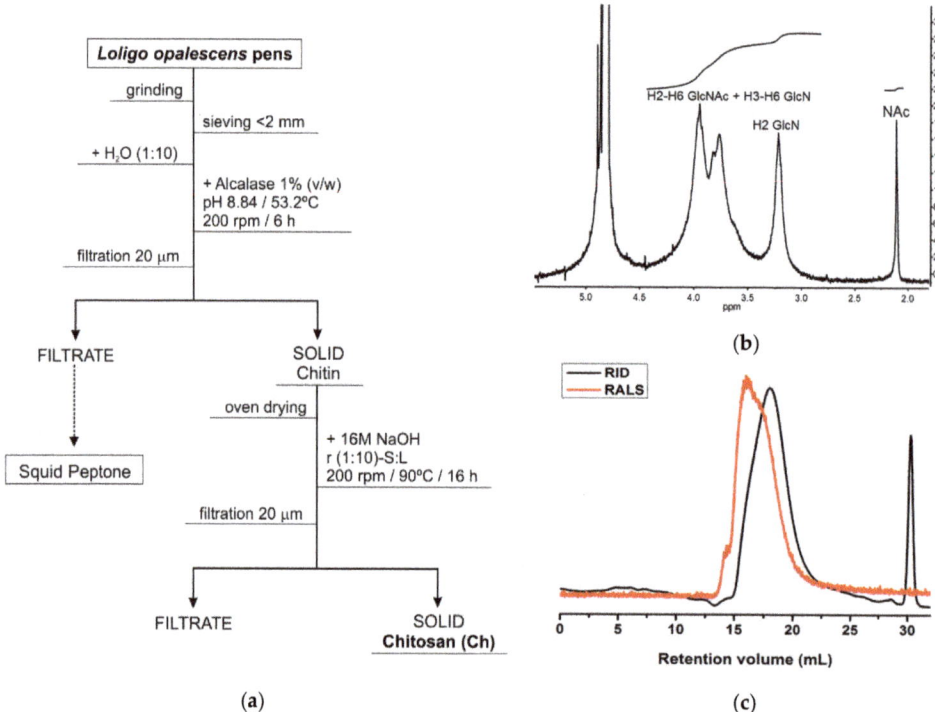

Figure 1. (a) Flowchart of chitosan (Ch) production from *Loligo opalescens* squid; (b) analysis of Ch by nuclear magnetic resonance (NMR) to calculate the purity and degree of deacetylation; (c) eluogram of Ch analyzed by gel permeation chromatography (GPC) for molecular weight determination (RID—refractive index signal, RALS—right angle light scattering signal).

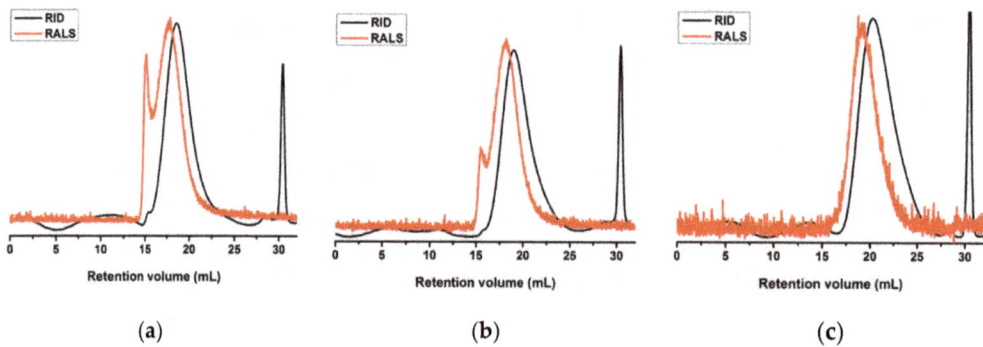

Figure 2. Eluograms of (a) β-ChoA, (b) β-ChoB, and (c) β-ChoC analyzed by gel permeation chromatography (GPC) for molecular weight determination (RID—refractive index signal, RALS—right angle light scattering signal).

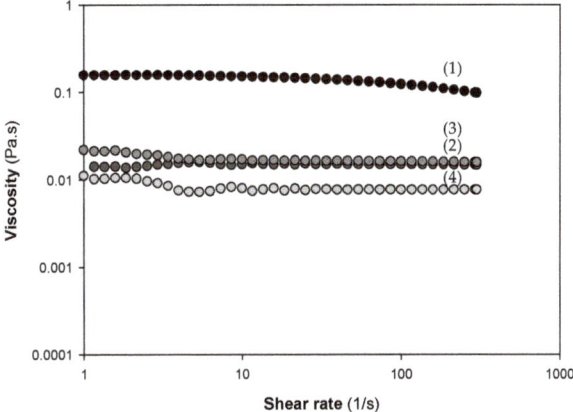

Figure 3. Flow curves of 1% (*w/v*) solutions of chitosan and derivatives used for surface preparation: β-Ch (1), β-ChoA (2), β-ChoB (3), and β-ChoC (4).

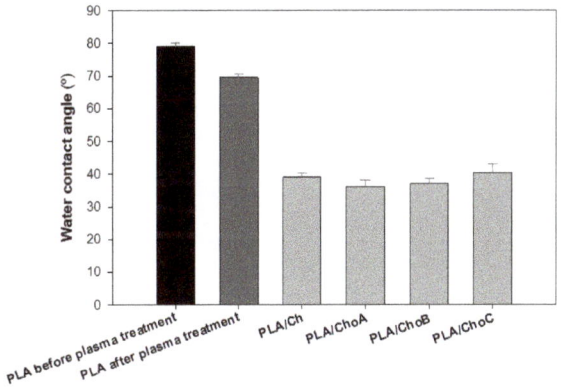

Figure 4. Water contact angles ± standard deviations (SDs) for PLA films before and after oxygen plasma treatment, and PLA/Ch films created by dip-coating method (PLA/Ch, PLA/ChoA, PLA/ChoB, and PLA/ChoC).

2.2.2. Fourier-Transform Infrared Spectroscopy (FTIR) Analysis

FTIR spectra of different types of chitosan immobilized onto the PLA surface are shown in Figure 5. The different types of chitosan deposited onto PLA did not reveal significant differences in FTIR results (Figure 5a). Characteristic bands of chitosan were covered by the presence of bands from the PLA film. The broad _OH stretching absorption band between 3680 and 2750 cm^{-1} and one between 2980 and 2750 cm^{-1} assigned to aliphatic C-H stretching indicated the presence of chitosan on PLA films [42]. Furthermore, a characteristic NH stretching band of chitosan with a maximum at 3350 cm^{-1} was identified on the functionalized PLA/Ch films (Figure 5a).

The FTIR spectrum of PLA films is included in Figure 5b. Results show that characteristic bands of PLA with high-intensity peaks were represented at 1750 cm^{-1} corresponding to CO, at 1188–1090 cm^{-1} corresponding to CO, at 1452–1368 cm^{-1} corresponding to COH, and at 3000 cm^{-1} corresponding to CH. These results are in accordance with those reported by Stoleru et al. [43]. In general, FTIR spectra revealed that surface immobilization of chitosan onto PLA films was successfully achieved.

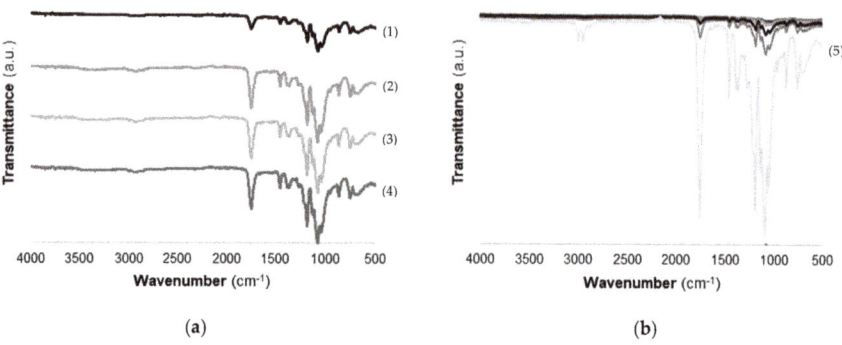

Figure 5. FTIR spectrum of (**a**) different types of chitosan immobilized onto PLA (β-Ch (1), β-ChoA (2), β-ChoB (3), β-ChoC (4)) and (**b**) PLA films (PLA (5)).

2.2.3. X-ray Diffraction (XRD)

The diffraction patterns of PLA films and the effect of different types of chitosan immobilized on PLA are shown in Figure 6. In the case of PLA film, diffraction peaks at 2θ = 16.5°, 20°, and 22° were observed, which corresponded to the characteristic peaks of PLA, indicating a crystalline PLA matrix [44]. An accentuated band at 2θ = 28° suggested the presence of calcium carbonate on PLA films, as described in the literature [45]. The immobilization of chitosan solutions caused a decrease in the intensity peaks at 2θ = 16.5°, 20°, and 22° [46], which confirmed the deposition of chitosan. This modification could indicate a decrease in the crystalline part of PLA/Ch films. It is also possible to conclude that different types of chitosan did not affect the XRD pattern.

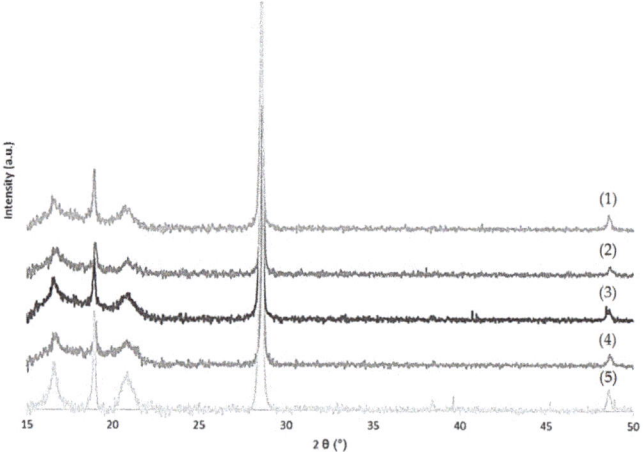

Figure 6. X-ray diffraction (XRD) patterns of different types of chitosan immobilized onto PLA surface (β-ChoC (1), β-ChoB (2), β-ChoA (3), and β-Ch (4)) and of PLA film (5).

2.2.4. Morphological Studies

For determination of the surface morphology of the control PLA and Ch-based films, scanning electron microscopy (SEM) analysis was performed. The SEM image corresponding to the PLA film (Figure 7a) reveals a homogeneous surface with a uniform appearance. After the deposition of chitosan onto PLA surfaces, the presence of small particles, which could be unsoluble materials of chitosan, was detected (Figure 7b–e). Although the functionalized surfaces were heterogeneous (Figure 7b–e), no significant differences in PLA/Ch appearance were observed for the different types of chitosan tested.

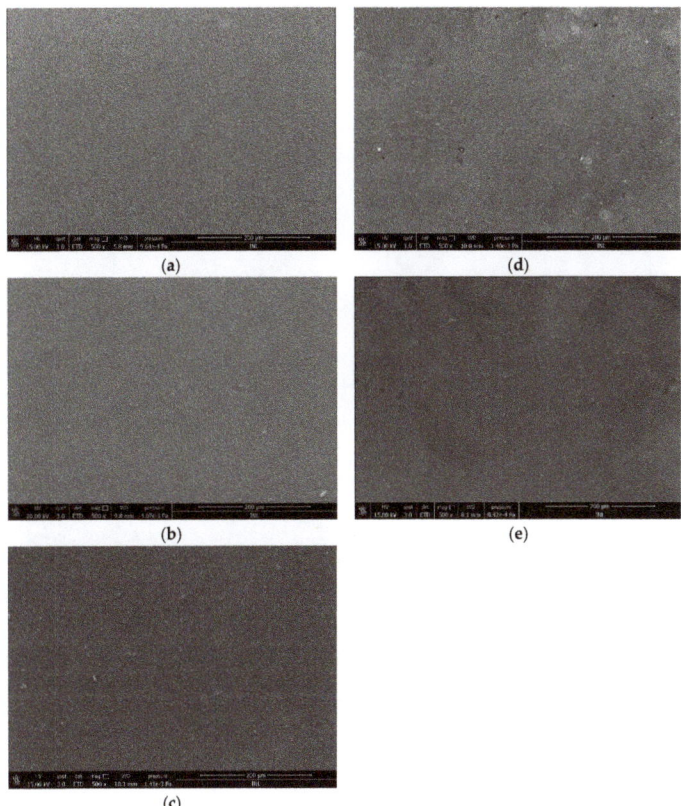

Figure 7. Scanning electron micrographs of (**a**) PLA surface and (**b–e**) Ch-based surfaces: (**b**) β-Ch, (**c**) β-ChoA, (**d**) β-ChoB, and (**e**) β-ChoC.

2.3. Antimicrobial Activity of Functionalized PLA Films

The antimicrobial properties of PLA and PLA/Ch surfaces were evaluated in conditions mimicking the storage conditions of packaged food products, namely a short incubation period (1 day), refrigeration temperature (5 °C), and static conditions. Furthermore, two different biofilm-forming bacteria typically associated with the food environment were used: *Escherichia coli* (a model pathogen) and *Pseudomonas putida* (isolated from a salad processing industry) [35,36].

The cellular composition of *E. coli* and *P. putida* single-species biofilms formed on the control PLA and PLA/Ch films was evaluated by counting viable, viable but non-culturable (VBNC), and culturable cells (Figure 8), whereas the spatial distribution of the biofilms developed by both bacterial strains on the surfaces was analyzed by confocal laser scanning microscopy (CLSM; Figures 9 and 10).

The analysis of *E. coli* biofilm cells (Figure 8a) indicated that there was a significant decrease in the number of all cell types considered (viable, VBNC, and culturable cells) on the chitosan-coated PLA surfaces compared to PLA, except in the case of PLA/ChoB (i.e., the PLA coated by the β-chitooligosaccharide of intermediate molecular weights derived from β-chitosan). Indeed, the biofilms formed on PLA/Ch, PLA/ChoA, and PLA/ChoC surfaces exhibited, on average, 70%, 74%, and 63% fewer *E. coli* viable, VBNC, and culturable cells, respectively, than PLA ($p < 0.001$, Figure 8a). When comparing the antimicrobial efficacy of immobilized native chitosan (PLA/Ch) with its derivatives (PLA/ChoA, PLA/ChoB, and PLA/ChoC, in descending order of molecular weight), it was observed that PLA films coated with depolymerized chitosan had bactericidal behavior similar to PLA films coated with native chitosan (Figure 8a), except for PLA/ChoB.

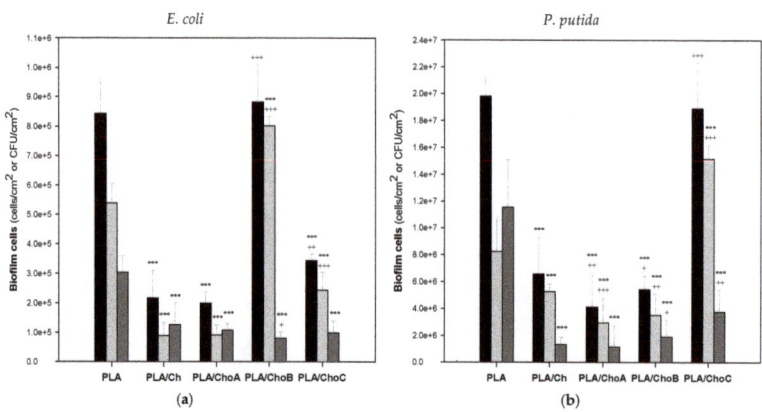

Figure 8. Cellular composition of (**a**) *E. coli* and (**b**) *P. putida* biofilms on PLA and Ch-based surfaces: viable (■), viable but non-culturable (VBNC) (■), and culturable cells (■). Inferential statistics were performed using unpaired *t*-tests or Mann–Whitney tests according to the normality of the variables' distributions. The means ± SDs for three independent experiments are illustrated. Within the same type of cells, the significance levels were * $p < 0.05$, ** $p < 0.01$, and *** $p < 0.001$ related to PLA (*) and PLA/Ch (+).

Regarding the effectiveness of PLA-coated films against *P. putida* biofilm growth (Figure 8b), it was also evident that they were effective in reducing the number of viable, VBNC, and culturable cells by, on average, 73%, 52%, and 87%, respectively. These percentages exclude the cell numbers of the PLA/ChoC surface (i.e., the PLA coated by the β-chitooligosaccharide of higher Mw). Despite having a smaller number of culturable cells than PLA (67%, $p < 0.001$), this coating showed equal or higher numbers of the remaining types of cells.

Looking at the results of the two bacterial strains together (Figure 8a,b), they suggest that the surfaces with the greatest antimicrobial activity were those coated with the native β-chitosan (Mn = 206 kDa/Mw = 294 kDa) and the depolymerized β-chitosan of the highest molecular weight (ChoA, chitosan of Mn = 138 kDa/Mw = 186 kDa). On the other hand, no linear relationship was found between the molecular weight of the tested chitosans obtained from the *Loligo opalescens* pen and their antimicrobial performance under the conditions tested in this study.

The effect of immobilized chitosan and its derivatives against *E. coli* and *P. putida* biofilm formation was also analyzed by CLSM. Both bacteria formed dense and thick biofilms, regardless of the tested surface (Figure 9). Nevertheless, microscopic images revealed that, in general, *E. coli* and *P. putida* biofilms grown on uncoated PLA surfaces were thicker than those developed on PLA films coated with chitosan, which may be related to its antimicrobial activity (Figure 8). These differences in biofilm thickness were particularly evident for PLA/Ch and PLA/ChoA surfaces in the case of *E. coli* (Figure 9b,c), and for PLA/Ch, PLA/ChoA, and PLA/ChoB films with *P. putida* (shadow projection on the right of Figure 9g–i). Furthermore, quantitative data showed a decrease of up to 26% in the average thickness of *E. coli* biofilms formed on PLA/Ch and PLA/ChoA surfaces (shadow projection on the right of Figure 9b), whereas *P. putida* biofilms developed on the same surfaces had approximately 44% and 36% less thickness and biovolume, respectively, than those grown on PLA (shadow projection on the right of Figure 9c,d). Thus, besides bactericidal activity, the native chitosan and its higher Mw derivative also prevented biofilm growth.

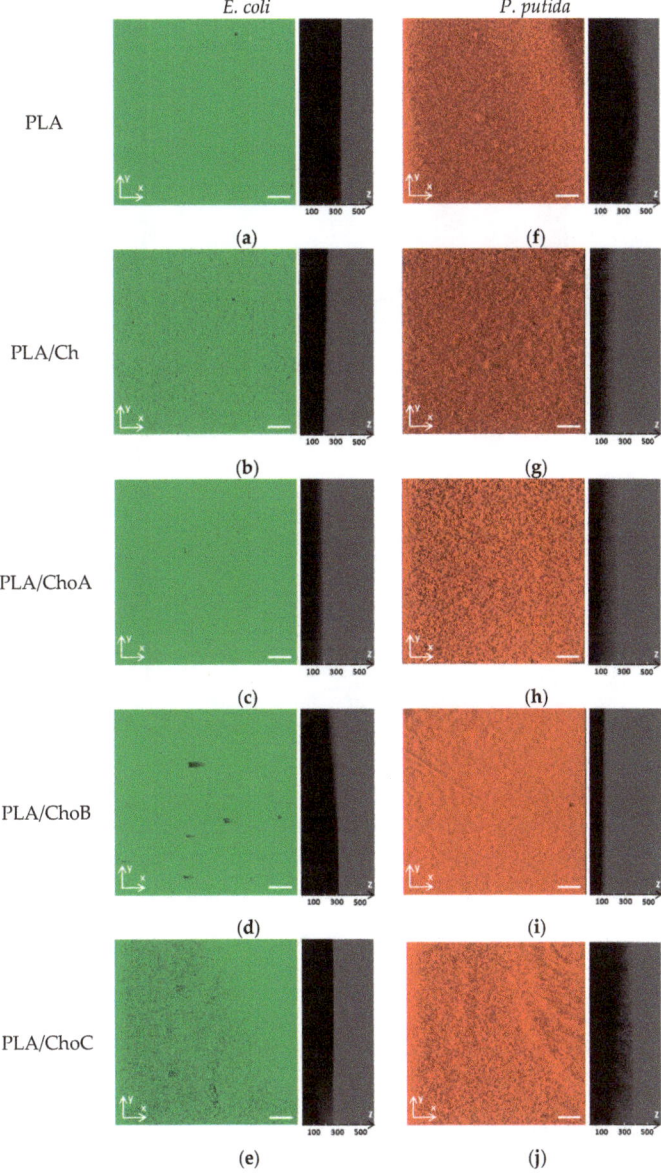

Figure 9. Representative biofilm structures of (**a**–**e**) *E. coli* and (**f**–**j**) *P. putida* on PLA and Ch-based surfaces. These images were obtained from confocal z-stacks using IMARIS software and present an aerial, three-dimensional (3D) view of the biofilms (images on the left). The shadow on the right represents the vertical projection of the biofilm. The white scale bar is 200 μm and the numerical scale indicated in each panel is in μm.

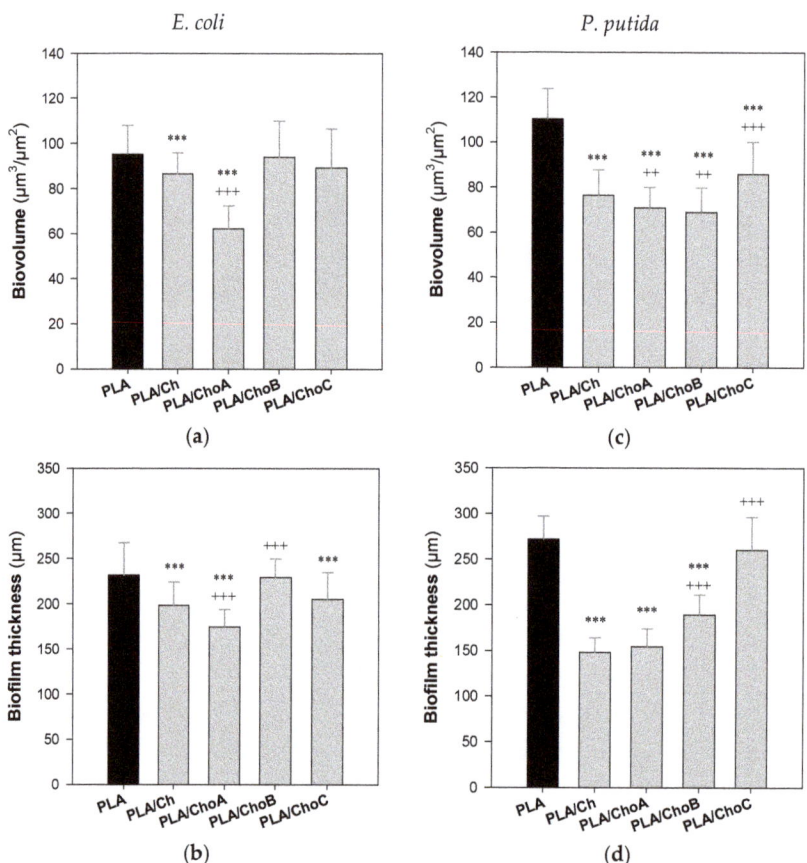

Figure 10. Biovolume and thickness of (**a**,**b**) *E. coli* and (**c**,**d**) *P. putida* biofilms formed on PLA and Ch-based surfaces. The values were obtained from the confocal z-stacks using the COMSTAT2 tool associated with the ImageJ software. Statistical analysis was performed using one-way analysis of variance (ANOVA) and the significance levels were * $p < 0.05$, ** $p < 0.01$, and *** $p < 0.001$ related to PLA (*) and PLA/Ch (+).

3. Discussion

The demand for bio-based and safer materials is increasing due to the growth of the human population, industrial development, and environmental concerns. Among known biopolymers, chitosan was selected to confer antibacterial properties to poly(lactic acid) surfaces as it presents remarkable characteristics such as non-toxicity, biocompatibility, and biodegradability [10–12]. From the particular perspective of food packaging, easy film formation and antimicrobial activity are considered the most important properties of chitosan, which have been extensively studied [5,7,12,14,47].

Poly(lactic acid) is a polyester formed from 100% renewable raw materials and is highly transparent, hence its intensive use in many disposable packaging solutions. One of the strategies to modify PLA is to apply a surface treatment using a plasma process in order to improve the wettability, adhesion, and biocompatibility of this biopolymer. As expected, the wettability of PLA films used in the present study increased after treatment with oxygen plasma. Identical behavior was reported by Jordá-Vilaplana et al. [40], who used atmospheric plasma treatment to improve the adhesion capacity of PLA films.

In this work, chitosan and its depolymerized derivatives were successfully obtained from a *Loligo opalescens* squid pen by-products via a combination of enzymatic and alkaline treatments [39] and immobilized onto PLA films through plasma oxygen treatment followed by dip-coating. In the last few years, a considerable number of studies have been published on the production of new polymeric systems incorporating chitosan. Some studies have focused on the synthesis of PLA/Ch composites by solution mixing and film casting [19,48,49], but others prepared PLA films by extrusion, coated them with a Ch solution, and used crosslinking agents [20].

Most of the commercial chitosan solutions reported in the literature revealed a viscoelastic behavior, i.e., a high dependence of viscosity with shear rate, except for the low-concentration solutions (lower than 0.25–0.5% (w/v)) [50,51]. On the contrary, the results here obtained at 1% (w/v) of Ch and derivatives showed a Newtonian behavior, i.e. null dependence of viscosity with shear rate. Other authors observed the same flow behavior, with a Newtonian plateau at a low chitosan concentration of 1.7%, but no Newtonian behavior could be observed at higher chitosan concentrations [52], which suggests that the viscosity of chitosan solutions may be affected by other factors, such as the degree of deacetylation, molecular weight, temperature, and pH [53–55]. Additionally, the decrease in viscosity with the decrease in molecular weight among β-Ch and β-Cho was in agreement with the data collected by Chattopadhyay and Inamdar [54]. These authors demonstrated that the viscosity of chitosan is influenced by its Mw and that the intrinsic viscosity of different grades of chitosan decreased approximately ten-fold when the viscosity average molecular weight dropped from 285 to 21 [54]. Furthermore, the decrease in viscosity of β-Cho compared to native chitosan can facilitate the formulation of coatings for application in food technology [56,57].

After the synthesis of the PLA/Ch surfaces, they were tested against two bacterial strains (*E. coli* and *P. putida*) in conditions that simulated the short-term food packaging environment (refrigeration without agitation and 1 day of contact with the cell suspensions). To the best of our knowledge, this is one of the very few studies that evaluates the antibiofilm effect of PLA surfaces coated with native chitosan and derivatives without adding any other compounds, such as essential oils or metallic nanoparticles, to reinforce the antimicrobial properties of coatings and extend the shelf-life of packaged food products [58]. In general, the native chitosan surfaces demonstrated bactericidal activity against the Gram-negative bacteria tested. They decreased the number of biofilm viable, viable but nonculturable, and culturable cells by up to 73%, 74%, and 87%, respectively, compared to PLA. Although the exact mechanism of antibacterial activity of chitosan is still unclear, several mechanisms have been proposed. First, the antimicrobial activity of Ch films is dependent on the degree of deacetylation since the presence of charged amino groups on chitosan molecules can disturb the negatively charged phosphoryl groups on the bacterial cell membrane, leading to its degradation followed by cell death [47]. Chitosan may also form an impermeable layer around the bacterial cell and block the exchange of essential solutes between the intra- and extracellular environment, affecting the physiological state of bacteria and, ultimately, causing cell death [59]. This biopolymer can also diffuse through the cell wall, disrupt the cytoplasmic membrane of bacteria and affect its integrity, as well as suppress the synthesis of RNA and proteins by binding to DNA molecules [58,59].

The antimicrobial activity of chitosan and its derivatives relies on numerous intrinsic and extrinsic factors, including pH, microorganism species, degree of deacetylation of Ch, Mw, concentration, hydrophilic/hydrophobic characteristics, etc. [33,34]. In this work, the surfaces with immobilized chitosan showed different bactericidal performance and inhibited biofilm growth differently. Since the water contact angles and SEM images were identical for all Ch-based surfaces, it is believed that the physicochemical properties and morphology of the films did not affect their antibacterial behavior. Therefore, the main parameter influencing this behavior seems to be the molecular weight of chitosan. Several studies have discussed the relation between bactericidal activity and chitosan Mw, although with contradictory results. Some authors indicated that increasing chitosan Mw leads to decreasing chitosan activity against *Escherichia coli*, while others suggested that high Mw chitosan displays greater activity than low Mw chitosan [34,60]. Hirano et al. [61] showed that chitosans with a Mw of 1.5–4.5 kDa exhibited better inhibitory activities than those with a higher Mw (6.5–12.0 kDa). On the other hand, Tokura et al. [60] disclosed that a 9.3 kDa chitosan inhibited the growth of *E. coli*, whereas a 2.2 kDa chitosan increased bacterial growth. Moreover, some authors have shown that intermediate molecular weights are more effective [34,62]. For instance, Li et al. [62] demonstrated that chitosan suppressed *E. coli* growth, but its inhibitory activity differed with Mw (from 3 to 1000 kDa), with the Ch of 50 kDa Mw having the strongest effect. Similar to Li et al. [62], no linear relationship was found between the Mw of the tested chitosans obtained from the *Loligo opalescens* pen and their antimicrobial performance under the tested conditions. Moreover, the results indicate that the surfaces with the greatest antibiofilm activity were those coated with the native β-chitosan and the depolymerized β-chitosan of the highest molecular weight (ChoA). It is possible that the chitosan of higher Mw interacted with the bacterial cells adhered to the substrate and altered cell permeability, resulting in cell lysis [34]. At the same time, the positive charge of Ch given by the functional amino groups (NH_3^+) of N-acetylglucosamine units is expected to react electrostatically with the negatively charged biofilm components such as EPS, proteins, and DNA [57,63], which may explain the lower biovolume and thickness of biofilms exposed to surfaces coated with higher Mw chitosan. It is also reported that high Mw water-soluble chitosan and solid chitosan may form an impermeable layer around the cell surface, thus blocking the transport of nutrients into the cell and causing cell lysis [64,65].

Another interesting result of this work is the capacity that the chitosan-based films showed to reduce the number of viable but nonculturable cells in the biofilms formed by both microorganisms when compared to uncoated PLA (up to 74%). The VBNC state is a unique survival strategy of many bacteria in the environment in response to adverse conditions. The foodborne pathogens may enter the VBNC state during food processing operations, such as disinfection, preservation, and low-temperature storage, and represent a threat to food safety and public health as cells in this state are not detectable through conventional food and water testing methods [66,67]. Indeed, VBNC bacteria cannot be cultured on routine microbiological media, but they remain viable and retain virulence. Therefore, this study suggests that replacing PLA films with PLA coated with chitosan may be an interesting solution to eliminate most VBNC cells in the food packaging environment, preventing foodborne infections and increasing food safety. These Ch-based surfaces may also be beneficial in improving the shelf-life of food products, which is dependent on microbial contamination since certain microorganisms can modify the odor, flavor, color, and textural properties of food products [68].

4. Materials and Methods

4.1. Production and Chemical Characterization of Chitosan and Chitooligosaccharides

Chitosan previously isolated from the pen of *Loligo opalescens* squid [69] was depolymerized by reaction with sodium nitrite [70]. High molecular weight chitosan of 206 kDa (Mn, number average molecular weight) was initially purified by overnight dissolution in 5% (*v/v*) acetic acid at 9 g/L, followed by filtration (FILTER-LAB®ref. 1250, 10–13 µm; Filtros Anoia, S.A., Barcelona, Spain) and precipitation with methanol:25% ammonia in a proportion 1:3 (*v/v*) chitosan solution:methanolic ammonia. The mixture was left at 4 °C for 1 h, then centrifuged in 1 L bottles at 13,261× *g* on a Beckman Coulter Avanti J-25I centrifuge (Beckman Coulter, Inc, Indianapolis, IN, USA). The precipitates were washed three times with water followed by a final acetone wash, dried overnight at 50 °C on a stove, and freeze-dried. Purified chitosan was milled to a fine powder and dissolved overnight in triplicate in 0.05 M HCl at 8 g/L. Depolymerization reactions were carried out under stirring at room temperature by adding the appropriate amounts of a 1.6 g/L sodium nitrite solution to each chitosan solution, according to the following equation [39]:

$$\frac{1}{M_f} - \frac{1}{M_o} = \frac{n}{m} \tag{1}$$

where M_f is the molecular weight of chitosan after depolymerization, M_0 the initial molecular weight of chitosan, n the moles of sodium nitrite, and m the initial mass of chitosan. After 4 h of reaction, chitosan was precipitated with 5 M NaOH, the solids separated by centrifugation as described above for the purification process, and washed with water until neutrality. Finally, depolymerized samples were freeze-dried and milled to a fine powder.

The degree of acetylation of chitosan was estimated from nuclear magnetic resonance (NMR) experiments. Chitosan samples (7 g/L) were dissolved in 0.056 M deuterated trifluoroacetic acid (TFA-d in D_2O), and the corresponding 1H NMR spectra were recorded at 400 MHz (Bruker Avance II; Brucker, USA). The degree of acetylation was calculated from the relative integrals of acetyl (N-acetyl and AcOH) and combined H2–H6 protons (GlcN and GlcNAc) [71,72]. Chemical shifts were expressed in ppm with the HOD solvent signal acting as a reference. Mestrenova 10.0 software (Mestrelab Research, S.L., Santiago de Compostela, Spain) was used for spectral processing.

The molecular weight of chitosan samples was determined by gel permeation chromatography (GPC) on an Agilent 1260 system equipped with a quaternary pump, injector, column oven, and refractive index and static dual-angle light scattering detectors. Chitosan was separated with a set of four columns: Novema Precolumn (10 mm, 8 × 50 mm), Novema 30 Å (10 mm, 8 × 300 mm), Novema 1000 Å (10 mm, 8 × 300 mm), and Novema 1000 Å (10 mm, 8 × 300 mm) from Polymer Standards Service, Mainz, Germany. Column oven and light scattering detector were kept at 30 °C and the refractive index detector was maintained at 40 °C. Samples were eluted with 0.15 M ammonium acetate–0.2 M acetic acid (pH 4.5) as mobile phase at 1 mL/min. Chitosan samples were dissolved in the GPC buffer at a concentration of 1 g/L. Detectors were calibrated with a polyethylene oxide standard of 106 kDa and polydispersity index (PDI) of 1.06 (PSS Polymer Standards Service GmbH, Mainz, Germany). Molecular weight of chitosan was estimated using a refractive index increment (dn/dC) value of 0.18 [73]. From this, two types of chitosan size determination were considered: (1) the average molecular weight of the biopolymer (Mw) and (2) the number average molecular weight of the biopolymer (Mn).

4.2. Immobilization of Chitosan and Chitooligosaccharides onto Poly(lactic acid) (PLA) Films

Solutions of chitosan (Ch) and three chitooligosaccharides (ChoA, ChoB, and ChoC) at 1% (w/v) were immobilized onto poly(lactic acid) (PLA) films (Goodfellow, UK). For the immobilization of chitosan and derivatives onto the surfaces of PLA films, a plasma oxygen treatment (Harrick Plasma, PJS-14-0240) was applied using a moderate intensity for 15 min. After this, PLA films with dimensions of 1 cm × 1 cm were dipped in the different solutions (Ch, ChoA, ChoB, and ChoC) for 15 min and dried with nitrogen for 5 min.

4.3. Rheological Measurements of Chitosan Solutions

Flow curves were obtained using a Discovery Hybrid Rheometer (DHR1) from TA Instruments (New Castle, DE, USA) with Peltier temperature set to 25 °C. TRIOS Software (New Castle, DE, USA) was used to control the equipment and to acquire rheological parameters. A stainless-steel cone-plate geometry of 60 mm, with an angle of 2.006° and truncation of 64 µm, was used due to its capability of generating a uniform shear rate across the samples. Steady-state flow curves were obtained working in a controlled-stress mode, over the shear rate range of 1–300 s^{-1}. All the samples (Ch, ChoA, ChoB, and ChoC at 1% (w/v)) were measured in triplicate.

4.4. Surface Characterization
4.4.1. Water Contact Angle

Films' surface hydrophobicity was evaluated through the measurement of contact angle by sessile drop technique using a DSA 100E drop shape analysis system (Kruss Gmbh, Hamburg, Germany). A water droplet (2 µL) was deposited at different points on the film surface, and afterwards, a digital camera connected to DSA 3 drop shape image analysis software recorded drop images. The image produced was used to calculate the contact angle via circle fitting method [74]. At least 10 measurements were taken per tested film.

4.4.2. Fourier-Transform Infrared Spectroscopy (FTIR)

FTIR spectra of the films were recorded with VERTEX 80v FTIR spectrometer (Bruker, Germany) in the wavelength range 4000–400 cm^{-1} at a resolution of 4 cm^{-1}, using Platinum Attenuated Total Reflection mode (ATR) (Bruker, Germany). The absorbance of each FTIR spectrum was normalized between 0 and 1 [75].

4.4.3. X-ray Diffraction (XRD)

XRD was used to investigate the presence and influence of chitosan on the crystalline structure of the polymer matrix. The XRD patterns of PLA films with and without chitosan were determined using a diffractometer (PanAnalytical X Pert PRO MRD system, Malvern, UK). The scanning range varied from $2\theta = 10°$ to $50°$ [76].

4.4.4. Scanning Electron Microscopy (SEM)

The morphology of the film's surface was observed using a scanning electron microscope (Quanta 650 FEG, FEI Europe B.V., Eindhoven, The Netherlands) with an accelerating voltage of +5 kV at different magnifications [75]. The samples were cut with a blade and mounted on sample holders with double-sided adhesive and sputtered with a 10 nm layer of gold.

4.5. Antimicrobial Activity of Functionalized PLA Films

4.5.1. Bacterial Strains and Culture Conditions

A model food pathogen—*Escherichia coli* SS2 expressing the green fluorescent protein (GFP) (*E. coli* SS2 GFP)—and an industrial isolate from a salad processing plant—*Pseudomonas putida*—were the bacteria chosen for this study [35,36,77]. Stock cultures were maintained at −80 °C in Tryptone Soy Broth (TSB; BioMérieux, Marcy-l'Étoile, France) containing 20% (*v/v*) glycerol. Before each experiment, frozen cells were subcultured twice in TSB at 30 °C with a constant orbital agitation of 120 rpm [36].

4.5.2. Biofilm Formation

Biofilm assays were performed on 12-well plates (VWR International, Carnaxide, Portugal) for 1 day at 5 °C under static conditions in order to mimic the conditions typically found in short-term food packaging. Before each experiment, the PLA film and the PLA-coated surfaces produced as described in Section 4.2 were sterilized by ultraviolet (UV) radiation for 30 min. Then, the sterilized surfaces were placed on the wells and inoculated with 3 mL of an overnight culture of *E. coli* SS2 GFP or *P. putida* in TSB adjusted to an optical density (OD) of 0.01 at 610 nm (1:10 dilution from an initial cell suspension at OD$_{610}$ nm = 0.1). The microplates were then kept at 5 °C for 1 h to promote bacterial attachment to the surface materials [36,77]. After this adhesion step, the wells were emptied and refilled with 3 mL of sterile TSB, and the microplates were incubated to allow biofilm development. Furthermore, 3 mL of TSB was added to the wells containing sterilized surfaces to monitor their sterility throughout the experiments.

Biofilm formation experiments were performed in three independent assays, each one with three technical replicates.

4.5.3. Biofilm Cell Quantification

Biofilm cell suspensions were obtained by dipping each surface in 2 mL 0.85% (*v/v*) NaCl and vortexing for 3 min. Biofilm cell culturability was assessed after serial dilutions in Tryptone Soy Agar plates (TSA; BioMérieux, Marcy-l'Étoile, France) in the case of *P. putida*, and TSA plates supplemented with 0.1 g/L of ampicillin for *E. coli* SS2 GFP. In turn, biofilm viability was evaluated by staining the biofilm suspension with the Live/Dead® BacLight™ Bacterial Viability kit (Invitrogen Life Technologies, Alfagene, Portugal) as previously described [78] and observing it in an epifluorescence microscope (Leica DM LB2; Leica Microsystems, Wetzlar, Germany). A minimum of twenty fields of view was analyzed for each stained sample using the ImageJ software (version 1.52p, U.S. National Institutes of Health, Bethesda, MD, USA) and the number of viable cells was counted. Finally, the number of VBNC cells was determined by subtracting the number of culturable cells from that of viable cells [79]. The number of culturable cells was presented as CFU/cm^2, whereas the numbers of viable and VBNC cells were expressed as $cells/cm^2$.

4.5.4. Confocal Scanning Electron Microscopy (CLSM)

Single-species biofilms of *E. coli* and *P. putida* that developed after 1 day on all tested surfaces were observed using a 10× dry objective (Leica HC PLAN APO CS) in an inverted microscope Leica DMI6000-CS (Leica Microsystems, Wetzlar, Germany). *E. coli* cells were pinpointed from the GFP expression, while *P. putida* biofilms were stained in red with 5 µM SYTO® 61 (Invitrogen Life Technologies, Alfagene, Portugal), a cell-permeant fluorescent nucleic acid marker. For this reason, *E. coli* biofilms were observed with a 488 nm argon laser, whereas *P. putida* biofilm samples were scanned at an excitation wavelength of 633 nm (helium-neon laser) [36]. A minimum of six stacks of horizontal plane images (512 × 512 pixels, corresponding to 1550 × 1550 µm) with a z-step of 1 µm were acquired for each sample.

Three-dimensional (3D) projections of biofilm structures were reconstructed using the "Easy 3D" tool of IMARIS 9.1 software (Bitplane, Zurich, Switzerland) directly from the CLSM acquisitions. The plug-in COMSTAT2 associated with the ImageJ software was used to determine the biovolume ($µm^3/µm^2$) and biofilm thickness (µm) [80].

4.6. Statistical Analysis

Descriptive statistics were used to calculate the mean and standard deviations (SDs) for the number of viable, VBNC, and culturable cells (Figure 8), and biovolume and biofilm thickness (Figure 10). Differences in the number of cells in relation to PLA and PLA/Ch (Figure 8) were evaluated using unpaired *t*-tests or Mann–Whitney tests according to the normality of the variables' distributions. Quantitative parameters obtained from confocal microscopy (Figure 10) were compared using a one-way analysis of variance (ANOVA). All tests were performed with a confidence level of 95% (p-values < 0.05). Data analysis was performed using IBM SPSS Statistics version 24.0 for Windows (IBM SPSS, Inc., Chicago, IL, USA).

5. Conclusions

The recent increase in sensitivity towards environmental issues arising from plastic packaging has fostered an interest in alternative sustainable packaging materials. Chitosan and its derivatives were efficiently prepared from fishery waste and immobilized onto PLA films. Their antimicrobial effects were demonstrated in the composite films, with a strong reduction in viable, VBNC, and culturable cell counts in *E. coli* and *P. putida* biofilms. Furthermore, the surfaces with the highest antibiofilm activity were those coated with the native Ch and the Cho with the highest Mw. This is the first time that PLA/Ch surfaces have been shown to be able to eliminate most VBNC cells in the food environment, which is a very interesting result given that such cells retain a public health risk. Further research is needed to bring this biopolymer to industrial levels for food packaging applications.

Author Contributions: Conceptualization, F.J.M., J.A.V. and L.P.; methodology, L.C.G., S.I.F., J.A.V., J.V., A.I.B. and M.A.C.; formal analysis, L.C.G. and S.I.F.; investigation, L.C.G., S.I.F., J.A.V., J.V., A.I.B. and M.A.C.; resources, F.J.M. and L.P.; data curation, L.C.G. and S.I.F.; writing—original draft preparation, L.C.G.; writing—review and editing, F.J.M., J.A.V., J.V., A.I.B. and M.A.C.; supervision, F.J.M. All authors have read and agreed to the published version of the manuscript.

Funding: This research was funded by Base Funding—UIDB/00511/2020 of the Laboratory for Process Engineering, Environment, Biotechnology and Energy (LEPABE) funded by national funds through the FCT/MCTES (PIDDAC), and "CVMAR+I—Industrial Innovation and Marine Biotechnology Valorization" project, funded by INTERREG V Espanha Portugal (POCTEP) (0302_CVMAR_I_1_P). The research was also supported by the SurfSAFE project funded by the European Union's Horizon 2020 research and innovation programme under grant agreement no. 952471. L.C.G. thanks the Portuguese Foundation for Science and Technology (FCT) for the financial support of her work contract through the Scientific Employment Stimulus—Individual Call—(CEECIND/01700/2017). J.A.V. and J.V. also offer their thanks to Xunta de Galicia by Xunta de Galicia (Grupos de Potencial Crecimiento, IN607B 2018/2019) for the financial support.

Institutional Review Board Statement: Not applicable.

Informed Consent Statement: Not applicable.

Data Availability Statement: The data presented in this study are available on request from the corresponding author. The data are not publicly available yet as some data sets are being used for additional publications.

Conflicts of Interest: The authors declare no conflict of interest.

References

1. Díez-Pascual, A.M. Antimicrobial Polymer-Based Materials for Food Packaging Applications. *Polymers* **2020**, *12*, 731. [CrossRef] [PubMed]
2. Andrade, G.C.; Gombi-Vaca, M.F.; da Costa Louzada, M.L.; Azeredo, C.M.; Levy, R.B. The consumption of ultra-processed foods according to eating out occasions. *Public Health Nutr.* **2020**, *23*, 1041–1048. [CrossRef] [PubMed]
3. Ketelsen, M.; Janssen, M.; Hamm, U. Consumers' response to environmentally-friendly food packaging-a systematic review. *J. Clean. Prod.* **2020**, *254*, 120123. [CrossRef]
4. Jamróz, E.; Kulawik, P.; Kopel, P. The effect of nanofillers on the functional properties of biopolymer-based films: A review. *Polymers* **2019**, *11*, 675. [CrossRef] [PubMed]
5. Riaz, A.; Lagnika, C.; Abdin, M.; Hashim, M.M.; Ahmed, W. Preparation and Characterization of Chitosan/Gelatin-Based Active Food Packaging Films Containing Apple Peel Nanoparticles. *J. Polym. Environ.* **2020**, *28*, 411–420. [CrossRef]
6. Sullivan, D.J.; Azlin-Hasim, S.; Cruz-Romero, M.; Cummins, E.; Kerry, J.P.; Morris, M.A. Antimicrobial effect of benzoic and sorbic acid salts and nano-solubilisates against *Staphylococcus aureus*, *Pseudomonas fluorescens* and chicken microbiota biofilms. *Food Control* **2020**, *107*, 106786. [CrossRef]
7. Bi, F.; Zhang, X.; Bai, R.; Liu, Y.; Liu, J.; Liu, J. Preparation and characterization of antioxidant and antimicrobial packaging films based on chitosan and proanthocyanidins. *Int. J. Biol. Macromol.* **2019**, *134*, 11–19. [CrossRef] [PubMed]
8. Olszewska, M.A.; Gędas, A.; Simões, M. Antimicrobial polyphenol-rich extracts: Applications and limitations in the food industry. *Int. Food Res. J.* **2020**, *134*, 109214. [CrossRef]
9. Arcan, I.; Yemenicioğlu, A. Incorporating phenolic compounds opens a new perspective to use zein films as flexible bioactive packaging materials. *Food Res. Int.* **2011**, *44*, 550–556. [CrossRef]
10. Dutta, J.; Tripathi, S.; Dutta, P.K. Progress in antimicrobial activities of chitin, chitosan and its oligosaccharides: A systematic study needs for food applications. *Food Sci. Technol. Int.* **2012**, *18*, 3–34. [CrossRef]
11. Mujtaba, M.; Morsi, R.E.; Kerch, G.; Elsabee, M.Z.; Kaya, M.; Labidi, J.; Khawar, K.M. Current advancements in chitosan-based film production for food technology; A review. *Int. J. Biol. Macromol.* **2019**, *121*, 889–904. [CrossRef]
12. Lago, M.A.; Sendón, R.; de Quirós, A.R.-B.; Sanches-Silva, A.; Costa, H.S.; Sánchez-Machado, D.I.; Valdez, H.S.; Angulo, I.; Aurrekoetxea, G.P.; Torrieri, E.; et al. Preparation and Characterization of Antimicrobial Films Based on Chitosan for Active Food Packaging Applications. *Food Bioprocess. Tech.* **2014**, *7*, 2932–2941. [CrossRef]
13. Aider, M. Chitosan application for active bio-based films production and potential in the food industry: Review. *LWT Food Sci. Technol.* **2010**, *43*, 837–842. [CrossRef]
14. Sagoo, S.; Board, R.; Roller, S. Chitosan inhibits growth of spoilage micro-organisms in chilled pork products. *Food Microbiol.* **2002**, *19*, 175–182. [CrossRef]
15. Elsabee, M.Z.; Abdou, E.S. Chitosan based edible films and coatings: A review. *Mater. Sci. Eng. C* **2013**, *33*, 1819–1841. [CrossRef]
16. Haghighi, H.; Licciardello, F.; Fava, P.; Siesler, H.W.; Pulvirenti, A. Recent advances on chitosan-based films for sustainable food packaging applications. *Food Packag. Shelf Life* **2020**, *26*, 100551. [CrossRef]
17. Siracusa, V.; Blanco, I.; Romani, S.; Tylewicz, U.; Rocculi, P.; Rosa, M.D. Poly(lactic acid)-modified films for food packaging application: Physical, mechanical, and barrier behavior. *J. Appl. Polym. Sci.* **2012**, *125*, E390–E401. [CrossRef]
18. Sébastien, F.; Stéphane, G.; Copinet, A.; Coma, V. Novel biodegradable films made from chitosan and poly(lactic acid) with antifungal properties against mycotoxinogen strains. *Carbohydr. Polym.* **2006**, *65*, 185–193. [CrossRef]
19. Grande, R.; Carvalho, A.J. Compatible ternary blends of chitosan/poly(vinyl alcohol)/poly(lactic acid) produced by oil-in-water emulsion processing. *Biomacromolecules* **2011**, *12*, 907–914. [CrossRef] [PubMed]
20. Soares, F.C.; Yamashita, F.; Müller, C.M.O.; Pires, A.T.N. Thermoplastic starch/poly(lactic acid) sheets coated with cross-linked chitosan. *Polym. Test.* **2013**, *32*, 94–98. [CrossRef]

21. Bonilla, J.; Fortunati, E.; Vargas, M.; Chiralt, A.; Kenny, J.M. Effects of chitosan on the physicochemical and antimicrobial properties of PLA films. *J. Food Eng.* **2013**, *119*, 236–243. [CrossRef]
22. Chang, S.-H.; Chen, Y.-J.; Tseng, H.-J.; Hsiao, H.-I.; Chai, H.-J.; Shang, K.-C.; Pan, C.-L.; Tsai, G.-J. Antibacterial Activity of Chitosan–Polylactate Fabricated Plastic Film and Its Application on the Preservation of Fish Fillet. *Polymers* **2021**, *13*, 696. [CrossRef] [PubMed]
23. Vázquez, J.A.; Ramos, P.; Mirón, J.; Valcarcel, J.; Sotelo, C.G.; Pérez-Martín, R.I. Production of Chitin from *Penaeus vannamei* By-Products to Pilot Plant Scale Using a Combination of Enzymatic and Chemical Processes and Subsequent Optimization of the Chemical Production of Chitosan by Response Surface Methodology. *Mar. Drugs* **2017**, *15*, 180. [CrossRef] [PubMed]
24. Caligiani, A.; Marseglia, A.; Leni, G.; Baldassarre, S.; Maistrello, L.; Dossena, A.; Sforza, S. Composition of black soldier fly prepupae and systematic approaches for extraction and fractionation of proteins, lipids and chitin. *Food Res. Int.* **2018**, *105*, 812–820. [CrossRef]
25. Wu, T.; Zivanovic, S.; Draughon, F.A.; Conway, W.S.; Sams, C.E. Physicochemical Properties and Bioactivity of Fungal Chitin and Chitosan. *J. Agric. Food. Chem.* **2005**, *53*, 3888–3894. [CrossRef] [PubMed]
26. Vázquez, J.A.; Rodríguez-Amado, I.; Montemayor, M.; Fraguas, J.; González, M.; Murado, M.Á. Chondroitin sulfate, hyaluronic acid and chitin/chitosan production using marine waste sources: Characteristics, applications and eco-friendly processes: A review. *Mar. Drugs* **2013**, *11*, 747. [CrossRef]
27. Domard, A. A perspective on 30 years research on chitin and chitosan. *Carbohydr. Polym.* **2011**, *84*, 696–703. [CrossRef]
28. FAO. *Fishery and Aquaculture Statistics 2017/FAO Annuaire*; FAO: Rome, Italy, 2017.
29. Zeidberg, L.D. Doryteuthis opalescens, Opalescent Inshore Squid. In *Advances in Squid Biology, Ecology and Fisheries. Part I—Myopsid Squids*; Rosa, R., O'Dor, R., Pierce, G., Eds.; Nova Science Publishers, Inc.: New York, NY, USA, 2013; pp. 159–204.
30. Yan, N.; Chen, X. Sustainability: Don't waste seafood waste. *Nature* **2015**, *524*, 155–157. [CrossRef]
31. Dai, J.; Li, F.; Fu, X. Towards Shell Biorefinery: Advances in Chemical-Catalytic Conversion of Chitin Biomass to Organonitrogen Chemicals. *ChemSusChem* **2020**, *13*, 6498–6508. [CrossRef]
32. Hülsey, M.J. Shell biorefinery: A comprehensive introduction. *Green Energy Environ.* **2018**, *3*, 318–327. [CrossRef]
33. Hosseinnejad, M.; Jafari, S.M. Evaluation of different factors affecting antimicrobial properties of chitosan. *Int. J. Biol. Macromol.* **2016**, *85*, 467–475. [CrossRef] [PubMed]
34. Kong, M.; Chen, X.G.; Xing, K.; Park, H.J. Antimicrobial properties of chitosan and mode of action: A state of the art review. *Int. J. Food Microbiol.* **2010**, *144*, 51–63. [CrossRef] [PubMed]
35. Meireles, A.; Fulgêncio, R.; Machado, I.; Mergulhão, F.J.M.; Melo, L.F.; Simões, M.V. Characterization of the heterotrophic bacteria from a minimally processed vegetables plant. *LWT Food Sci. Technol.* **2017**, *85*, 293–300. [CrossRef]
36. Gomes, L.C.; Piard, J.-C.; Briandet, R.; Mergulhão, F.J.M. *Pseudomonas grimontii* biofilm protects food contact surfaces from *Escherichia coli* colonization. *LWT Food Sci. Technol.* **2017**, *85*, 309–315. [CrossRef]
37. Hadawey, A.; Tassou, S.A.; Chaer, I.; Sundararajan, R. Unwrapped food product display shelf life assessment. *Energy Procedia* **2017**, *123*, 62–69. [CrossRef]
38. Franzetti, L.; Scarpellini, M. Characterisation of *Pseudomonas* spp. isolated from foods. *Ann. Microbiol.* **2007**, *57*, 39–47. [CrossRef]
39. Allan, G.G.; Peyron, M. Molecular weight manipulation of chitosan II: Prediction and control of extent of depolymerization by nitrous acid. *Carbohydr. Res.* **1995**, *277*, 273–282. [CrossRef]
40. Jordá-Vilaplana, A.; Fombuena, V.; García-García, D.; Samper, M.D.; Sánchez-Nácher, L. Surface modification of polylactic acid (PLA) by air atmospheric plasma treatment. *Eur. Polym. J.* **2014**, *58*, 23–33. [CrossRef]
41. Wang, J.; Wu, Y.; Cao, Y.; Li, G.; Liao, Y. Influence of surface roughness on contact angle hysteresis and spreading work. *Colloid Polym. Sci.* **2020**, *298*, 1107–1112. [CrossRef]
42. Kaya, M.; Khadem, S.; Cakmak, Y.S.; Mujtaba, M.; Ilk, S.; Akyuz, L.; Salaberria Asier, M.; Labidi, J.; Abdulqadir, A.H.; Deligöz, E. Antioxidative and antimicrobial edible chitosan films blended with stem, leaf and seed extracts of *Pistacia terebinthus* for active food packaging. *RSC Adv.* **2018**, *8*, 3941–3950. [CrossRef]
43. Stoleru, E.; Dumitriu, R.P.; Munteanu, B.S.; Zaharescu, T.; Tănase, E.E.; Mitelut, A.; Ailiesei, G.-L.; Vasile, C. Novel procedure to enhance PLA surface properties by chitosan irreversible immobilization. *Appl. Surf. Sci.* **2016**, *367*, 407–417. [CrossRef]
44. Srithep, Y.; Pholharn, D. Plasticizer effect on melt blending of polylactide stereocomplex. *e-Polymers* **2017**, *17*, 409–416. [CrossRef]
45. Cardoso, E.; Parra, D.F.; Scagliusi, S.R.; Sales, R.M.; Caviquioli, F.; Lugao, A.B. Study of Bio-Based Foams Prepared from PBAT/PLA Reinforced with Bio-Calcium Carbonate and Compatibilized with Gamma Radiation. In *Use of Gamma Radiation Techniques in Peaceful Applications*; Almayah, B.A., Ed.; IntechOpen: London, UK, 2019.
46. Julkapli, N.M.; Ahmad, Z.; Akil, H.M. X-ray Diffraction Studies of Cross Linked Chitosan With Different cross Linking Agents for Waste Water Treatment Application. *AIP Conf. Proc.* **2010**, *1202*, 106–111.
47. Latou, E.; Mexis, S.F.; Badeka, A.V.; Kontakos, S.; Kontominas, M.G. Combined effect of chitosan and modified atmosphere packaging for shelf life extension of chicken breast fillets. *LWT Food Sci. Technol.* **2014**, *55*, 263–268. [CrossRef]
48. Chen, C.; Dong, L.; Cheung, M.K. Preparation and characterization of biodegradable poly(l-lactide)/chitosan blends. *Eur. Polym. J.* **2005**, *41*, 958–966. [CrossRef]
49. Li, L.; Ding, S.; Zhou, C. Preparation and degradation of PLA/chitosan composite materials. *J. Appl. Polym. Sci.* **2004**, *91*, 274–277. [CrossRef]

50. Calero, N.; Muñoz, J.; Ramírez, P.; Guerrero, A. Flow behaviour, linear viscoelasticity and surface properties of chitosan aqueous solutions. *Food Hydrocoll.* **2010**, *24*, 659–666. [CrossRef]
51. Hwang, J.; Shin, H.-H. Rheological properties of chitosan solutions. *Korea Aust. Rheol. J.* **2000**, *12*, 175–179.
52. Doench, I.; Torres-Ramos, M.E.W.; Montembault, A.; Nunes de Oliveira, P.; Halimi, C.; Viguier, E.; Heux, L.; Siadous, R.; Thiré, R.M.S.M.; Osorio-Madrazo, A. Injectable and Gellable Chitosan Formulations Filled with Cellulose Nanofibers for Intervertebral Disc Tissue Engineering. *Polymers* **2018**, *10*, 1202. [CrossRef]
53. Wang, W.; Xu, D. Viscosity and flow properties of concentrated solutions of chitosan with different degrees of deacetylation. *Int. J. Biol. Macromol.* **1994**, *16*, 149–152. [CrossRef]
54. Chattopadhyay, D.P.; Inamdar, M.S. Aqueous Behaviour of Chitosan. *Int. J. Polym. Sci.* **2010**, *2010*, 939536. [CrossRef]
55. Elhefian, E.A.; Yahaya, A. Rheological Study of Chitosan and Its Blends: An Overview. *Maejo Int. J. Sci. Technol.* **2010**, *4*, 210–220.
56. Liaqat, F.; Eltem, R. Chitooligosaccharides and their biological activities: A comprehensive review. *Carbohydr. Polym.* **2018**, *184*, 243–259. [CrossRef] [PubMed]
57. Rivera Aguayo, P.; Bruna Larenas, T.; Alarcón Godoy, C.; Cayupe Rivas, B.; González-Casanova, J.; Rojas-Gómez, D.; Caro Fuentes, N. Antimicrobial and Antibiofilm Capacity of Chitosan Nanoparticles against Wild Type Strain of *Pseudomonas* sp. Isolated from Milk of Cows Diagnosed with Bovine Mastitis. *Antibiotics* **2020**, *9*, 551. [CrossRef] [PubMed]
58. Wang, H.; Qian, J.; Ding, F. Emerging Chitosan-Based Films for Food Packaging Applications. *J. Agric. Food Chem.* **2018**, *66*, 395–413. [CrossRef] [PubMed]
59. Youssef, A.M.; El-Sayed, S.M.; El-Sayed, H.S.; Salama, H.H.; Dufresne, A. Enhancement of Egyptian soft white cheese shelf life using a novel chitosan/carboxymethyl cellulose/zinc oxide bionanocomposite film. *Carbohydr. Polym.* **2016**, *151*, 9–19. [CrossRef]
60. Tokura, S.; Ueno, K.; Miyazaki, S.; Nishi, N. Molecular weight dependent antimicrobial activity by Chitosan. *Macromol. Symp* **1997**, *120*, 199–207. [CrossRef]
61. Hirano, S.; Tsuchida, H.; Nagao, N. N-acetylation in chitosan and the rate of its enzymic hydrolysis. *Biomaterials* **1989**, *10*, 574–576. [CrossRef]
62. Li, X.-F.; Feng, X.-Q.; Yang, S.; Fu, G.-Q.; Wang, T.-P.; Su, Z.-X. Chitosan kills *Escherichia coli* through damage to be of cell membrane mechanism. *Carbohydr. Polym.* **2010**, *79*, 493–499. [CrossRef]
63. Khan, F.; Pham, D.T.N.; Oloketuyi, S.F.; Manivasagan, P.; Oh, J.; Kim, Y.-M. Chitosan and their derivatives: Antibiofilm drugs against pathogenic bacteria. *Colloids Surf. B* **2020**, *185*, 110627. [CrossRef] [PubMed]
64. Choi, B.K.; Kim, K.Y.; Yoo, Y.J.; Oh, S.J.; Choi, J.H.; Kim, C.Y. In vitro antimicrobial activity of a chitooligosaccharide mixture against *Actinobacillus actinomycetemcomitans* and *Streptococcus mutans*. *Int. J. Antimicrob. Agents* **2001**, *18*, 553–557. [CrossRef]
65. Eaton, P.; Fernandes, J.C.; Pereira, E.; Pintado, M.E.; Malcata, X.F. Atomic force microscopy study of the antibacterial effects of chitosans on *Escherichia coli* and *Staphylococcus aureus*. *Ultramicroscopy* **2008**, *108*, 1128–1134. [CrossRef]
66. Ayrapetyan, M.; Oliver, J.D. The viable but non-culturable state and its relevance in food safety. *Curr. Opin. Food Sci.* **2016**, *8*, 127–133. [CrossRef]
67. Zhao, X.; Zhong, J.; Wei, C.; Lin, C.-W.; Ding, T. Current Perspectives on Viable but Non-culturable State in Foodborne Pathogens. *Front. Microbiol.* **2017**, *8*, 580. [CrossRef]
68. Valdés, A.; Ramos, M.; Beltrán, A.; Jiménez, A.; Garrigós, M.C. State of the Art of Antimicrobial Edible Coatings for Food Packaging Applications. *Coatings* **2017**, *7*, 56. [CrossRef]
69. Vázquez, J.A.; Ramos, P.; Valcarcel, J.; Antelo, L.T.; Novoa-Carballal, R.; Reis, R.L.; Pérez-Martín, R.I. An integral and sustainable valorisation strategy of squid pen by-products. *J. Clean. Prod.* **2018**, *201*, 207–218. [CrossRef]
70. Allan, G.G.; Peyron, M. Molecular weight manipulation of chitosan. I: Kinetics of depolymerization by nitrous acid. *Carbohydr. Res.* **1995**, *277*, 257–272. [CrossRef]
71. Fernandez-Megia, E.; Novoa-Carballal, R.; Quiñoá, E.; Riguera, R. Optimal routine conditions for the determination of the degree of acetylation of chitosan by 1H-NMR. *Carbohydr. Polym.* **2005**, *61*, 155–161. [CrossRef]
72. Novoa-Carballal, R.; Fernandez-Megia, E.; Riguera, R. Dynamics of Chitosan by 1H NMR Relaxation. *Biomacromolecules* **2010**, *11*, 2079–2086. [CrossRef] [PubMed]
73. Sorlier, P.; Rochas, C.; Morfin, I.; Viton, C.; Domard, A. Light scattering studies of the solution properties of chitosans of varying degrees of acetylation. *Biomacromolecules* **2003**, *4*, 1034–1040. [CrossRef]
74. Martins, V.D.F.; Cerqueira, M.A.; Fuciños, P.; Garrido-Maestu, A.; Curto, J.M.R.; Pastrana, L.M. Active bi-layer cellulose-based films: Development and characterization. *Cellulose* **2018**, *25*, 6361–6375. [CrossRef]
75. Costa, M.J.; Pastrana, L.M.; Teixeira, J.A.; Sillankorva, S.M.; Cerqueira, M.A. Characterization of PHBV films loaded with FO1 bacteriophage using polyvinyl alcohol-based nanofibers and coatings: A comparative study. *Innov. Food Sci Emerg. Technol.* **2021**, *69*, 102646. [CrossRef]
76. Martins, A.J.; Silva, P.; Maciel, F.; Pastrana, L.M.; Cunha, R.L.; Cerqueira, M.A.; Vicente, A.A. Hybrid gels: Influence of oleogel/hydrogel ratio on rheological and textural properties. *Food Res. Int.* **2019**, *116*, 1298–1305. [CrossRef] [PubMed]
77. Gomes, L.C.; Deschamps, J.; Briandet, R.; Mergulhão, F.J. Impact of modified diamond-like carbon coatings on the spatial organization and disinfection of mixed-biofilms composed of *Escherichia coli* and *Pantoea agglomerans* industrial isolates. *Int. J. Food Microbiol.* **2018**, *277*, 74–82. [CrossRef] [PubMed]
78. Gomes, L.C.; Silva, L.N.; Simões, M.; Melo, L.F.; Mergulhão, F.J. *Escherichia coli* adhesion, biofilm development and antibiotic susceptibility on biomedical materials. *J. Biomed. Mater. Res.* **2015**, *103*, 1414–1423. [CrossRef]

79. Alves, P.; Gomes, L.C.; Vorobii, M.; Rodriguez-Emmenegger, C.; Mergulhão, F.J. The potential advantages of using a poly(HPMA) brush in urinary catheters: Effects on biofilm cells and architecture. *Colloids Surf. B* **2020**, *191*, 110976. [CrossRef]
80. Heydorn, A.; Nielsen, A.T.; Hentzer, M.; Sternberg, C.; Givskov, M.; Ersbøll, B.K.; Molin, S. Quantification of biofilm structures by the novel computer program COMSTAT. *Microbiology* **2000**, *146*, 2395–2407. [CrossRef] [PubMed]

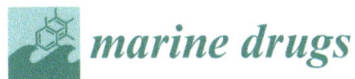

Article

Insights into the Synthesis, Secretion and Curing of Barnacle Cyprid Adhesive via Transcriptomic and Proteomic Analyses of the Cement Gland

Guoyong Yan [1,2], Jin Sun [3], Zishuai Wang [4], Pei-Yuan Qian [3] and Lisheng He [1,*]

1. Institute of Deep-sea Science and Engineering, Chinese Academy of Sciences, Sanya 572000, China; yanguoyong@idsse.ac.cn
2. Center for Human Tissues and Organs Degeneration, Institute of Biomedicine and Biotechnology, Shenzhen Institutes of Advanced Technology, Chinese Academy of Sciences, Shenzhen 518055, China
3. Department of Ocean Science, Division of Life Science and Hong Kong Branch of The Southern Marine Science and Engineering Guangdong Laboratory (Guangzhou), The Hong Kong University of Science and Technology, Hong Kong 999077, China; sunjinsd@gmail.com (J.S.); boqianpy@ust.hk (P.-Y.Q.)
4. Department of Computer Science, City University of Hong Kong, Hong Kong 999077, China; zishuwang2-c@my.cityu.edu.hk
* Correspondence: he-lisheng@idsse.ac.cn; Tel.: +86-898-8838-0060

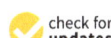

Received: 4 March 2020; Accepted: 29 March 2020; Published: 31 March 2020

Abstract: Barnacles represent one of the model organisms used for antifouling research, however, knowledge regarding the molecular mechanisms underlying barnacle cyprid cementation is relatively scarce. Here, RNA-seq was used to obtain the transcriptomes of the cement glands where adhesive is generated and the remaining carcasses of *Megabalanus volcano* cyprids. Comparative transcriptomic analysis identified 9060 differentially expressed genes, with 4383 upregulated in the cement glands. Four cement proteins, named Mvcp113k, Mvcp130k, Mvcp52k and Mvlcp1-122k, were detected in the cement glands. The salivary secretion pathway was significantly enriched in the Kyoto Encyclopedia of Genes and Genomes (KEGG) enrichment analysis of the differentially expressed genes, implying that the secretion of cyprid adhesive might be analogous to that of saliva. Lysyl oxidase had a higher expression level in the cement glands and was speculated to function in the curing of cyprid adhesive. Furthermore, the KEGG enrichment analysis of the 352 proteins identified in the cement gland proteome partially confirmed the comparative transcriptomic results. These results present insights into the molecular mechanisms underlying the synthesis, secretion and curing of barnacle cyprid adhesive and provide potential molecular targets for the development of environmentally friendly antifouling compounds.

Keywords: barnacle; cement gland; cyprid adhesive; transcriptome; cement protein

1. Introduction

Barnacles are major marine fouling organisms that can secrete adhesives to attach themselves permanently to underwater substrates on which they live [1]. The adhesive generated by barnacles has been termed barnacle adhesive or barnacle cement [2], usually, the adhesive is a thin layer only a few microns thick, but it is nevertheless capable of adhering barnacles tightly to different foreign materials throughout their entire lifespan without failure, even under conditions of strong wave action [3]. Due to its robust strength and durability underwater, barnacle adhesive has attracted the attention of scientists from different fields. Some scientists have attempted to develop biomimetic underwater glues [4], and others have engaged in developing antifouling compounds to prevent the adhesive attraction [5]; however, both lines of research require a good understanding of the molecular mechanisms underlying the regulation of barnacle cyprid cementation.

The life cycle of barnacles includes the nauplius I-VI, cyprid, juvenile and adult stages. The cyprid stage is the last planktonic stage during which barnacle cyprids search for suitable substrates on which to attach and metamorphose. The adhesive that cyprid larvae secrete from the attachment discs on their antennules is named cyprid adhesive, which is synthesized in a pair of cement glands. The cement glands are composed of two cell types, α cells and β cells, both of which are secretory; these cells synthesize proteins and lipids, respectively [6,7]. After settlement, the cement glands disappear gradually, and only cement cells spread over the connective tissue on the base plates of adult barnacles [8,9]. An adult adhesive is generated in the cement cells and is secreted into the adhesive interface through a well-developed duct system [8,10], and a recent study showed that acorn barnacles secrete phase-separating fluid, which is rich in lipids and reactive oxygen species to clean the surface before cement deposition [11].

Although both cyprid and adult barnacles can generate adhesive, it is almost impossible to collect enough cyprid adhesive for common research use; thus, almost all related research has been based on adult barnacle adhesive. Previous research has found that barnacle adhesive consists of proteins (90%), lipids (1%), carbohydrates (1%) and inorganic ash (4%) [2], indicating that the majority of the secretion is proteinaceous. Detailed analysis of the components of barnacle adhesive was hindered by its inherent insolubility [12] until Kamino and his colleagues developed a nonhydrolytic method of dissolving most of the barnacle adhesive from adult *Megabalanus rosa*, leading to the identification of the barnacle cement proteins Mrcp100k, Mrcp68k, Mrcp52k, Mrcp20k and Mrcp19k [12–15] and their homologues in different species [16–19]. In the past few years, high-throughput transcriptomic and proteomic approaches have facilitated the discovery of novel cement proteins, such as cp114k and cp43k; and many other genes and proteins that might be related to cementation, such as peroxidases and lysyl oxidases, have also been identified [20–22].

In contrast to the well-studied proteins in mussel and tube worm adhesives, barnacle cement proteins have no 3,4-dihydroxyphenylalanine (DOPA) [3,23]. There are no phosphorylation modifications in any characterized cement protein, although phosphoproteins have been reported in the cement gland and adhesive interface [3,7,24]. Quinone-type cross-linking has been thought to be responsible for the adhesion of barnacle adhesive [25,26], but sufficient evidence is lacking [23]. Dickinson and colleagues hypothesized that the barnacle cement polymerization process was similar to blood clotting caused by transglutaminase cross-linking [27], but this hypothesis was repudiated by Kamino [28]. Recently, growing evidence has demonstrated that hydrophobic interactions among cement proteins and amyloid-like conformations might play important roles in the self-assembly and curing of barnacle adhesive [13,29]. It is highly possible that barnacle adhesive functions through multiple mechanisms.

Here, to the best of our knowledge, for the first time, we obtained the transcriptome of cement glands dissected from *Megabalanus volcano* cyprids through RNA-seq. Comparative analysis with the carcass transcriptome was performed to screen for Differentially Expressed Genes (DEGs). Cement proteins produced in the cyprid cement gland were identified and characterized. Further analysis of the DEGs was performed to identify genes and pathways that might be involved in the synthesis, secretion and curing of barnacle cyprid adhesive. The proteome of the cement gland was also obtained by LC–MS/MS analysis, and Kyoto Encyclopedia of Genes and Genomes (KEGG) enrichment analysis was performed to verify and complement the comparative transcriptomic analysis results.

2. Results

2.1. Transcriptome Sequencing, Assembly and Annotation

The pair of cement glands was isolated from the whole body of *M. volcano* cyprids (Figure 1), and the remaining parts were collected together and defined as the carcass. The cement glands and carcasses were separately subjected to RNA extraction, cDNA library construction and Illumina high-throughput sequencing. In total, 65.60 M raw reads each were obtained for the cement glands and carcasses, and 65.36 M (99.63%) and 65.44 M (99.76%) clean reads remained, respectively, after poor-quality reads were filtered out. All clean reads for the cement glands and carcasses were subjected to *de novo* assembly, and a total of 38,538 and 55,537 unigenes were obtained, with mean lengths of 679 bp and 565 bp and N50 values of 1092 bp and 779 bp, respectively. Redundancy was further removed for the unigenes from the cement glands and carcasses to obtain a global dataset (all-unigenes). Finally, 67,299 unigenes remained, with a mean length of 613 bp and an N50 value of 928 bp (Table 1). Benchmarking Universal Single-Copy Orthologs (BUSCO) was used to assess the completeness of the transcriptome assembly, and the results showed that 76.8% of the BUSCOs were complete, 12.5% were fragmented and 10.7% were missing.

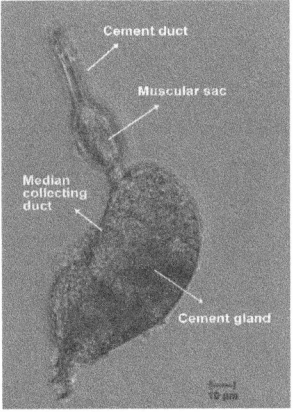

Figure 1. Dissected cement gland of a *Megabalanus volcano* cyprid.

Table 1. Summary of sequencing, assembly and annotation results.

Result	Cement Gland	Carcass	All
Output result			
Raw reads (M)	65.60	65.60	
Clean reads (M)	65.36 (99.76%)	65.44 (99.63%)	
Clean read Q20	97.43%	96.80%	
Clean read Q30	94.11%	93.34%	
Assembly result			
Number of unigenes	38,538	55,573	67,299
Unigene mean length (nt)	679	565	613
Unigene N50 (nt)	1092	779	928
GC (%)	55.97	55.04	55.15
Annotation result			
Nr	19,234	21,389	27,793
Nt	11,216	12,307	15,978
Swiss-Prot	15,963	16,802	21,906
KEGG	15,416	16,610	21,600
COG	9078	8828	12,584
GO	9258	9546	6830
Coding sequence prediction			
CDS predicted from BLAST result	19,624	21,842	28,522
CDS predicted by ESTScan	3401	4208	5360
Total CDSs predicted	23,025	26,050	33,882

To determine the gene functions of the assembled unigenes, six public databases were searched for annotations. In total, 22,139 (57.45%), 25,099 (45.16%) and 32,505 (48.30%) unigenes were annotated for the cement gland, carcass and global datasets, respectively. The detailed annotation results are summarized in Table 1. The coding regions of unannotated unigenes were predicted with ESTScan, and 5360 were predicted to have coding regions. Ultimately, 33,882 protein-coding unigenes were obtained from the transcriptome. To gain an overview of the functions of all the unigenes, the Gene Ontology (GO), Cluster of Orthologous Groups (COG) and KEGG databases were used for unigene classification. The GO classification results showed that 6830 nr-annotated unigenes were assigned to the three major functional categories. In detail, the unigenes were annotated in 19, 25 and 19 subcategories in the GO Cellular Component (GOCC), GO Biological Process (GOBP) and GO Molecular Function (GOMF) categories, respectively (Figure S1A). With regards to the COG database, 12,584 unigenes were annotated and further classified into 25 categories (Figure S1B). Moreover, the KEGG analysis showed that 21,600 unigenes were mapped to 235 pathways.

2.2. Comparative Transcriptomic Analysis and Characterization of DEGs

Genes that have different expression levels in different organs or tissues are thought to have specific functions consistent with the roles that the organs or tissues play in the whole body. Hence, comparative transcriptomic analysis was performed to screen for DEGs between cement glands and carcasses based on Fragments Per Kilobase of Transcript Per Million Mapped Reads (FPKM) values. As a result, a total of 9060 DEGs were identified, among which 4383 DEGs were upregulated and 4677 were downregulated in the cement glands compared with carcasses (Figure 2A). The numerous DEGs between cement glands and carcasses reflect the great differences between these samples at the transcriptional level, which are caused by tissue/organ-specific gene expression.

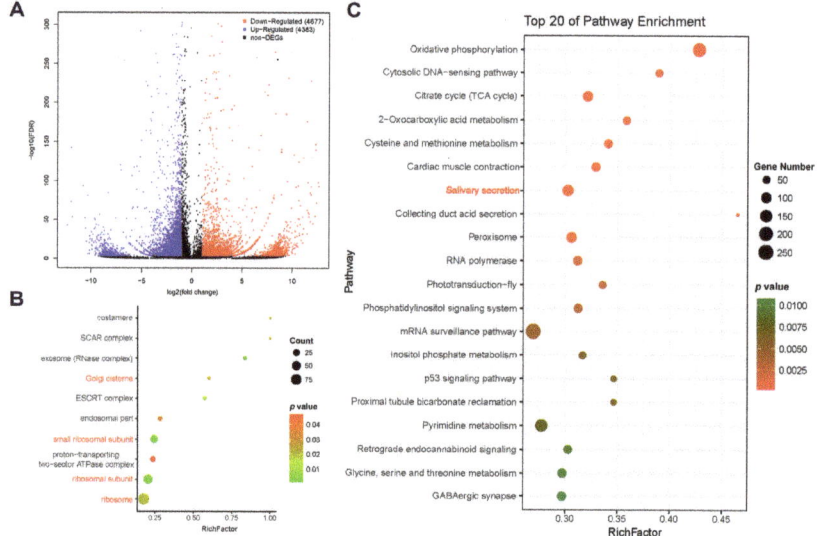

Figure 2. Comparative analysis of unigene expression levels between cement glands and carcasses. **A.** Volcano plot of the Differentially Expressed Genes (DEGs) between cement glands and carcasses. The blue spots indicate unigenes that were upregulated in cement glands, the red spots indicate downregulated unigenes, and the black spots indicate unigenes that were not differentially expressed. **B.** Gene Ontology (GO) enrichment analysis of the upregulated DEGs in cement glands, terms related to protein synthesis and protein modification are in red. **C.** KEGG enrichment analysis of all the DEGs between cement glands and carcasses, salivary secretion pathway (ko04970) is in red.

DEGs that were upregulated in cement glands were subjected to GO enrichment analysis to determine the functions of the overrepresented gene set. In the GOCC category, 10 terms were significantly enriched ($p < 0.05$; Figure 2B). Among them, four terms (GO: 0005840, ribosome; GO: 0044391, ribosomal subunit; GO: 0015935, small ribosomal subunit and GO: 0031985, Golgi cisterna) were related to protein synthesis and further protein modification, which is consistent with the role of the cement gland in generating cement proteins [6,7]. In total, 508 of the 4383 DEGs upregulated in cement glands were predicted to be transcription factors based on AnimalTFDB 2.0 (Table S1). In addition, 622 of the 4383 had no hits in any public databases, but 148 of them were predicted to have coding regions by ESTScan. The SignalP and TMHMM servers were used to analyze the sequence characteristics of the 148 DEGs [30]. Seven of the DEGs with predicted signal peptides but without transmembrane domains were suggested to be putative cement gland-secreted proteins (Table S2). These putative secreted proteins that are highly expressed in cement glands also have the potential to be novel cement proteins.

Further KEGG enrichment analysis was performed on all the DEGs to identify the predominant pathways that might be involved in the specific function of the cement gland. The results showed that eight pathways were significantly enriched ($p < 0.001$; Figure 2C). These pathways included oxidative phosphorylation (ko00190), the citrate cycle (TCA cycle; ko00020), 2-oxocarboxylic acid metabolism (ko01210) and cysteine and methionine metabolism (ko00270), which are involved in fundamental material and energy metabolism; the cytosolic DNA-sensing pathway (ko04623), which plays important roles in the innate immune response; and salivary secretion (ko04970), collecting duct acid secretion (ko04966) and cardiac muscle contraction (ko04260), which function in the secretion and release of secretory substances. These pathways are closely related to the role of the cement gland as a synthetic and secretory organ.

2.3. Characterization of Cement Proteins in the Cement Gland

According to the BLASTx results, four barnacle cement proteins were identified in the cement gland transcriptome, and they were named Mvcp113k, Mvcp130k, Mvcp52k and Mvlcp1-122k. Mvcp113k had the highest similarity (81%) with Mrcp100k from *M. rosa*, and Mvcp130k had the highest similarity (65%) with Aacp100k from *Amphibalanus amphitrite*. The sequence similarity between Mvcp113k and Mvcp130k was 51.7% (Figure 3A). Sequence alignment of the six cp100k homologues from four species of acorn barnacle revealed that they were conserved in different species, especially at the *N*-terminus (Figure S2). Comparative analysis of the amino acid composition of the six cp100k homologues revealed that they also had similar amino acid composition and theoretical pI values, which ranged from 9.63 to 9.99 (Table S3). Mvcp52k had the highest similarity (83%) with Mrcp52k from *M. rosa*. Sequence analysis showed that Mvcp52k also contained four repeat sequences with lengths of 129, 124, 120 and 113 amino acids, respectively, and that each repeat sequence contained a Cys residue located in nearly the same region (Figure 4A,B). Mvlcp1-122k had the highest similarity (89.6%) with the newly reported Mr-lcp1-122k, a cement gland-specific protein from *M. rosa* [31]. Sequence analysis found that Mvlcp1-122k and Mr-lcp1-122k were predicted to have one *N*-glycosylation site and seven mucin type GalNAc O-glycosylation sites (Figure 5A). The transcriptome quantitative results showed that Mvcp113k, Mvcp130k and Mvcp52k were almost exclusively expressed in the cement glands (Figures 3B and 4C), and Mvlcp1-122k was expressed in both cement glands and carcasses and had especially high expression level in the cement glands, which ranked the 91st of all the unigenes (Figure 5B).

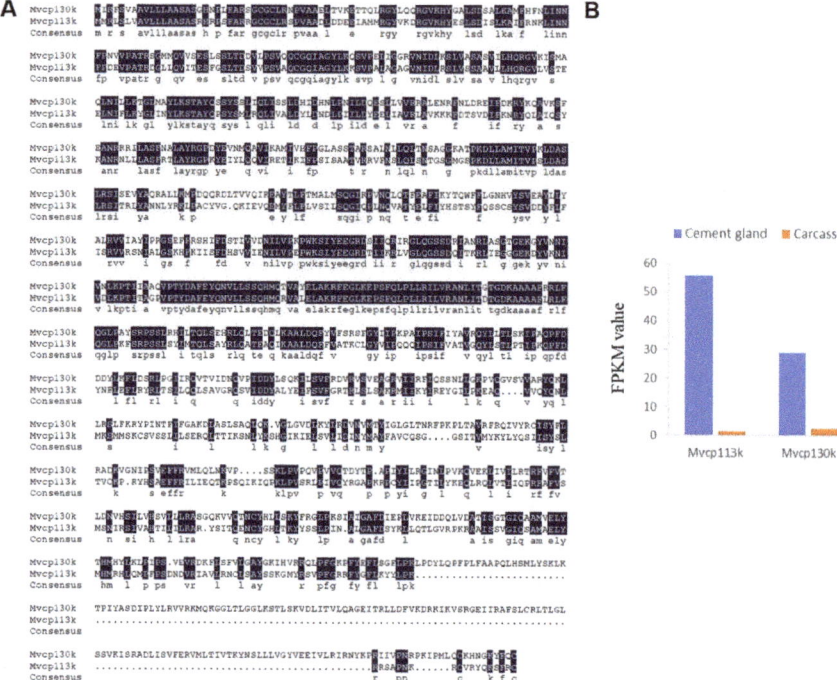

Figure 3. Cement protein-100 kDa homologues expressed in cement glands. **A**. Sequence alignment of Mvcp113k (MK336236) and Mvcp130k (MK336237) of *M. volcano*, the homology level of the sequences = 100% are shaded in black. **B**. Expression levels (Fragments Per Kilobase of Transcript Per Million Mapped Reads (FPKM) values) of Mvcp113k and Mvcp130k in cement glands and carcasses.

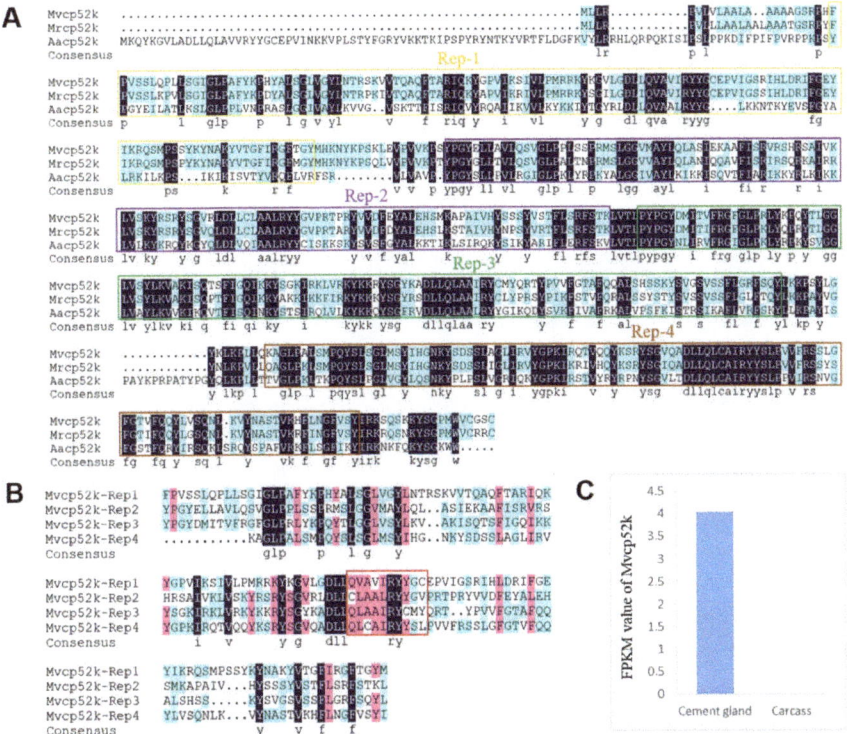

Figure 4. Cement protein-52 kDa homologue expressed in cement glands. **A**. Sequence alignment of Mvcp52k (MK336235), Mrcp52k (BAL22342.1) from *M. rosa* and Aacp52k (AKZ20820.1) from *A. amphitrite*, the homology level of the sequences = 100% and ≥ 50% are shaded in black and blue; 4 repeat sequences are labeled as Rep-1, -2, -3 and -4, and boxed in yellow, purple, green and orange rectangles respectively. **B**. Sequence alignment of the four repeat sequences of Mvcp52k, the homology level of the sequences = 100%, ≥ 75% and ≥ 50% are shaded in black, pink and blue, locations of a Cys residues are boxed in red rectangle. **C**. Expression levels (FPKM values) of Mvcp52k in cement glands and carcasses.

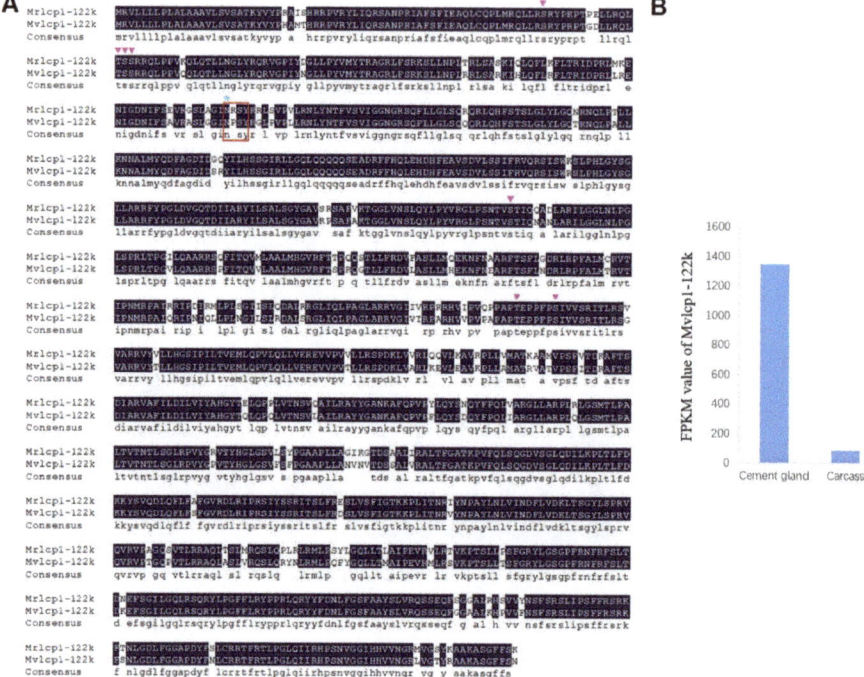

Figure 5. Cement gland-specific protein 122 kDa homologues expressed in cement glands. **A.** Sequence alignment of Mvlcp1-122k (MT024661) and Mrlcp1-122k (MK490677) of *M. rosa*, the homology level of the sequences = 100% are shaded in black. Asn-Xaa-Ser/Thr sequon is boxed in red rectangle, and the Asparagine predicted to be *N*-glycosylation site is marked with blue asterisk, predicted mucin type GalNAc O-glycosylation sites are marked with inverted purple triangle. **B.** Expression levels (FPKM values) of Mvlcp1-122k in cement glands and carcasses.

2.4. Characterization of Enzymes in the Cement Gland

All the enzyme-coding unigenes in the cement gland transcriptome were summarized according to their KEGG annotation results, and a total of 5913 enzyme-coding unigenes were ultimately identified. These unigenes were classified into six groups according to the enzyme commission scheme, with 946 classified as oxidoreductases, 2204 classified as transferases, 2091 classified as hydrolases, 207 classified as lyases, 214 classified as isomerases and 251 classified as ligases; furthermore, 1026 of the 5913 enzyme-coding unigenes were upregulated in the cement glands (Table S4). Lysyl oxidase (MvLOX), a homologue of AaLOX-1 in *A. amphitrite*, which has been detected in the adult barnacle adhesive interface [20,21], was also identified in the cement gland transcriptome of *M. volcano*. The putative protein sequence of MvLOX contained 510 amino acids and had the highest similarity (75%) to AaLOX-1, it had a conserved lysyl oxidase domain located at the C-terminus, and a predicted signal peptide indicating that it could be secreted out of cells (Figure 6A). MvLOX had higher expression level in the cement gland than the carcass (Figure 6B), suggesting that it might be involved in cyprid cementation. In addition, enzymes that involve in chitin synthesis (chitin synthase) and degradation (chitinase) were expressed in the cement gland as well as in the carcass (Table S5).

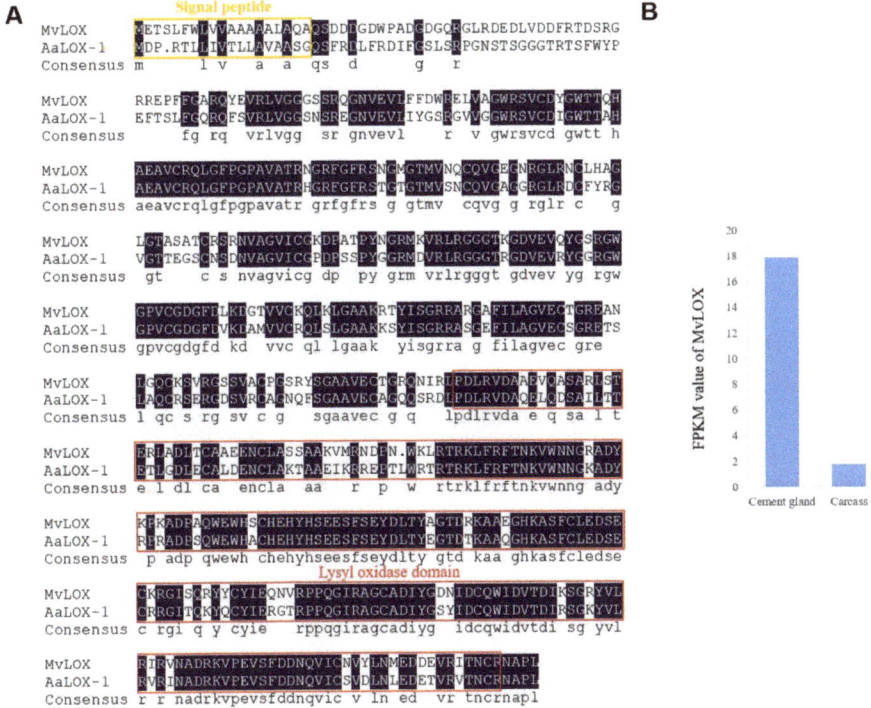

Figure 6. Characterization of *M. volcano* lysyl oxidase. **A**. Sequence alignment of MvLOX and AaLOX-1 (AQY78507.1) from *A. amphitrite*, the homology level of the sequences = 100% are shaded in black, predicted signal peptide is boxed in yellow rectangle and conserved lysyl oxidase domain is boxed in red rectangle. **B**. Expression levels (FPKM values) of MvLOX in the cement glands and carcasses.

2.5. Proteomic Analysis of the Cement Gland

LC–MS/MS analysis was performed to obtain the proteome of the cement glands, and a total of 352 proteins were identified based on 1504 peptides. All of the identified proteins were mapped to 77 pathways. KEGG enrichment analysis showed that pathways related to protein synthesis (ribosome (ko03010)) and energy metabolism (oxidative phosphorylation (ko00190), fructose and mannose metabolism (ko00051) and sulfur metabolism (ko00920)) were highly enriched, confirming that the production and secretion of the adhesive requires adequate energy supply. The salivary secretion pathway (ko04970) was also significantly enriched (Figure 7), which is consistent with the transcriptomic analysis results. The proteomic analysis partially validated the results from the comparative transcriptomic analysis.

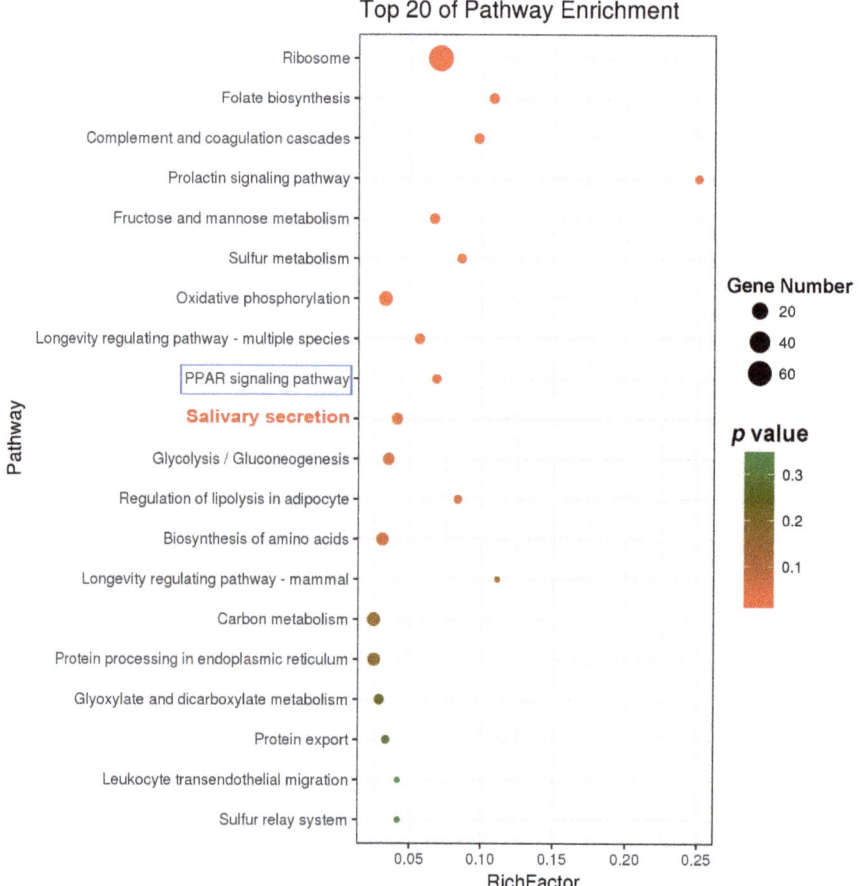

Figure 7. KEGG enrichment analysis of all the proteins identified in the cement gland proteome. The salivary secretion pathway (ko04970) is in red, and the PPAR signaling pathway (ko03320) is boxed in blue rectangle.

Furthermore, the PPAR signaling pathway (ko03320), which is mainly involved in lipid metabolism, was also significantly enriched (Figure 7). Lipid-binding proteins are important components of the PPAR signaling pathway (ko03320), and two lipid-binding proteins were identified in the cement gland proteome (Table S6). Conserved domain database (CDD) analysis showed that these two proteins had hits in the lipocalin (pfam00061) and lipocalin_7 (pfam14651) domain families, respectively (Figure S3), which belong to the lipocalin superfamily (cl21528). These findings indicate the basic function of these lipid-binding proteins as lipocalins that transport small hydrophobic molecules such as lipids. Mv-FABP1 (Unigene13631_All) was found to be upregulated in the cement glands according to the comparative transcriptomic results, suggesting that it is likely involved in the regulation of lipid accumulation and metabolism in the cement glands. Lipids have been found to be integral components in mussel adhesion [32], and lipid-binding proteins have also been identified in the adhesive glands of marine tube-building polychaetes [33], implying their universal importance for marine adhesives.

3. Discussion

The cement gland is the primary organ responsible for the synthesis and secretion of barnacle cyprid adhesive, and it plays an indispensable role in the larval settlement of barnacles. However, because cyprids are very small and have a pair of carapaces [34], it is very difficult to harvest the pair of cement glands (Figure 1). Therefore, research on barnacle cyprid adhesive system is relatively rare, especially research at the molecular level. In this study, three-day-old *M. volcano* cyprids were chosen for cement glands dissection, when temporary settlement behavior began to appear, suggesting that most of the cyprids were in the preparation for settlement. Sufficient cement glands for RNA-seq were isolated successfully, and the transcriptomes of cement glands and carcasses were obtained for the first time. The high occupation of clean reads, complete BUSCO and high N50 value indicated that the quality of the transcriptome was sufficient for further analyses [18,35]. Comparative transcriptomic analysis is an efficient and reliable method for screening DEGs involved in specific regulatory functions. Here, a false discovery rate (FDR) ≤ 0.001 rather than the common FDR ≤ 0.01 was used to improve the confidence level of the differential analysis results because of no biological replicates. In total, 9060 DEGs were identified, 4383 of which were upregulated in the cement glands. Unigenes that might function in cyprid cementation were further characterized with the aim to decipher the underlying molecular mechanisms.

Transcription is the first step in gene expression, while transcription factors control whether genes are transcribed and the rate of transcription [36]. Those transcription factors that had a higher expression level in the cement glands might play transcriptional regulatory roles during the initial expression of cement proteins and other related proteins in the cement glands [37]. However, due to the lack of whole genome information of barnacles, we are currently incapable of obtaining the promoter sequences of the cement protein-coding genes; otherwise, we could identify the upstream transcription factors that regulate the transcription of these genes based on predicted transcription factor binding sites in their promoter sequences [38].

Barnacle larval settlement is a highly energy-consuming process [39,40]. Here, several energy metabolism pathways were enriched in both transcriptomic and proteomic analyses (Figures 2C and 6), suggesting that a portion of energy might be used for adhesive synthesis and secretion. This finding is consistent with the findings of studies on organs that are analogous or homologous to cement glands, such as silkworm silk glands [41], planthopper salivary glands [42] and scorpion venom glands [43], in which abundant protein synthesis and high energy metabolism are demanded. In addition, in the marine environment, biofilms are crucial mediators of barnacle larval settlement [44], which means that larvae are exposed to active and dense microbial environments that include potential pathogens. Cement glands are attractive targets for pathogens because they connect to the external environment directly via the cement ducts in the antennules; however, it is possible that cyprids protect themselves from invading pathogens through the cytosolic DNA-sensing pathway, which can detect foreign DNA and induce further immune responses [45]; acid secretion regulated by the collecting duct acid secretion pathway might also be involved in maintaining a sterile interior and surface cleaning.

Until now, studies on adhesive secretion have focused only on morphological and physiological characteristics, and exocytosis was found to be the major mode of adhesive secretion, but detailed molecular mechanisms underlying this process are poorly understood [46,47]. The significant enrichment of the salivary secretion pathway found in this study implies that the molecular mechanisms underlying cyprid adhesive secretion by cement glands might be analogous to that of saliva secretion by salivary glands [48,49]. In secretory cells, suitable environment cues for settlement are transformed into neural signals. On the one hand, these signals cause adenylyl cyclase activation and intracellular cAMP accumulation, and elevated cAMP induces the secretion of proteins such as cement protein. On the other hand, these signals also activate phospholipase C, causing increases in intracellular Ca^{2+} that lead to ion and water secretion. In cyprids, the secretion of adhesive from the secretory cells and the release of these adhesive from the cement gland are two separate processes. It is presumed that secreted adhesive is accumulated by the median collecting duct and is temporarily stored in the cement duct and/or muscular sac; once a suitable substrate for permanent attachment has been found, the adhesive is released explosively through the adhesive disc with the pumping action of the muscular sac [46,47,50]. The muscular sac is composed of a layer of circular muscle (Figure 1) [50]. As the cardiac muscle contraction pathway was also found to be enriched in the current study, we speculated that the contraction of the muscular sac might be the same as that of cardiac muscle, which is initiated by electrical excitation of myocytes and is mediated by calcium cycling and signaling [51].

Protein is the dominant component of both cyprid and adult adhesive [6,7,12], but whether the two types of adhesive possess the same kinds of cement protein remains unclear. Cyprid and adult adhesive have been thought to be different but share a portion of cement proteins [3]. According to the transcriptome of adult *M. volcano* [34], Mvcp130k, Mvcp113k and Mvcp52k that identified in the cement glands of cyprids are also expressed at the adult stage. The place where larval adhesive generated is quite different from adults and they have different ways to be released to the surface [9,10], suggesting that there might be potential larval-specific cement proteins compared to well-studied adult cement proteins [21]. Recently, Aldred et al. (2020) reported the existence of a cement gland-specific protein (lcp1-122k) in barnacle *A. amphitrite* and *M. rosa*, and speculated that it functioned through glycosylation with chitin [31]. The homologue of lcp1-122k was also identified in the cyprid of *M. volcano* in this study, while it was not found in the transcriptome of adult *M. volcano* [34]. Chitin metabolism related enzymes express in the cement gland, implying that chitin could be generated in the cement gland. Further identification of potential glycosylation sites in the lcp1-122k homologues provide increased evidence that cement gland-specific protein lcp1-122k might be a glycoprotein (Figure 5A). Cheung and Nigrelli observed that the cement gland at the nauplius VI stage presented considerable biosynthetic activity while the activity in the cement gland at the cyprid stage was relatively low [8], no direct evidence has shown that cement proteins are produced at the nauplius VI stage up to now. Here, a high level of cement protein-coding gene mRNAs (Mvcp130k, Mvcp113k, Mvcp52k and Mvlcp1-122k) was detected in the cyprid cement gland transcriptome, indicating that the cement proteins used for settlement are *de novo* synthesized in the cement gland at the cyprid stage. In the present study, we reported the existence of two cp100k homologues in *Megabalanus* barnacles and detected the expression of cp52k in barnacle cyprids for the first time. Two cp100k homologues of the barnacle species *M. volcano* were identified in this study, and three cp20k homologues and two cp100k homologues were also found in previous studies [52], but the different roles that these homologous cement proteins might play have not been clarified based on their sequence characteristics and predicted physical and chemical properties. We speculated that the diversity of cement protein homologues might be a mechanism for guaranteeing the successful settlement of barnacles under different circumstances. Notably, gene duplication has played vital roles in spider silk gland evolution [53]; however, whether similar gene duplication has occurred in the evolution of the barnacle cement gland will be difficult to determine until the whole barnacle genome is available.

Enzymes have been reported to play important roles in secretory glands, such as snail salivary glands [30] and tube worm adhesive glands [33]. What is more, many enzymes have been proposed as specific targets for antifouling compounds [5]. In adult barnacle adhesive, lysyl oxidase has been predicted to oxidize the lysine in cement proteins to reactive allysine and further form durable lysine protein cross-links that involve three proximate allysines and a lysine side chain [20]. The elevated expression level of MvLOX in the cement gland suggests that MvLOX has the potential to play the same role in cyprid adhesive, indicating that allysine-mediated cross-links might be at least one of the factors involved in cyprid adhesive curing. Inexplicably, neither phenoloxidase nor catecholoxidase was identified in the cement gland transcriptome, although phenoloxidase and catecholoxidase activity have been reported in barnacle cyprid cement glands [2,6]. In well-studied marine tube worm cement proteins and mussel foot proteins, post-translational modification of tyrosine residues into DOPA is of great importance for adhesion [54,55]. Seven types of enzymes have been reported to contribute to the L-DOPA metabolic pathway, including phenylalanine dehydrogenase, phenylalanine hydroxylase, tyrosine aminotransferase, aspartate aminotransferase, histidinol-phosphate aminotransferase, L-amino-acid oxidase, tyrosinase and peroxidase [33]; however, most of these enzymes were absent in the cement gland transcriptome except aspartate aminotransferase and peroxidase, suggesting that the functional mechanism of barnacle cyprid adhesive differs from that of marine adhesives that rely on DOPA.

In total, 352 proteins were identified in the cement glands by LC–MS/MS. Notably, no cement proteins were identified, which is probably due to the technical limitations of mass spectrometry, because some abundant proteins might increase the difficulty of identifying cement proteins expressed at relatively low levels [22]. Protein database based on a whole genome might be more helpful for protein identification, considering the spatial and temporal expression difference of transcriptomes. The significant enrichment of lipid metabolism-related pathways implies that lipids play important roles in cementation, which is consistent with the discovery that cyprid adhesive is a biphasic system consisting of phosphoproteins and lipids and that lipids are secreted first to create a conducive environment for phosphoproteins and modulate the protein phase simultaneously [7]. Moreover, lipids have been reported to augment amyloid-beta (Aβ) peptide generation, and various lipids and their assemblies can interact with amphiphilic Aβ peptide to change Aβ aggregation [56]. Considering previous findings that amyloid-like nanofibrils are the main components of adhesive plaques from the barnacle *Balanus amphitrite* [57] and that certain peptides from a bulk 52 kDa cement protein [29] and a full-length 19 kDa cement protein [58,59] can self-assemble into amyloid fibrils, we hypothesize that lipids might also participate in the curing of barnacle adhesive by affecting cement protein amyloid fibril aggregation.

In the present study, comparative transcriptomic analysis and proteomic analysis were used to screen for genes, proteins and pathways that were involved in barnacle cyprid cementation, which is of great importance to decipher the molecular mechanisms underlying the synthesis, secretion and curing of barnacle cyprid adhesive. As adhesive production/release has been reported to be the most common targets for antifouling compounds development, and antifouling compounds that have specific molecular targets are considered more likely to be non-toxic rather than function through toxic killing [5]; thus, these genes, proteins and pathways have the potential to be molecular targets for novel non-toxic antifouling compounds. In recent years, many antifouling biocides with potential environmental risk, such as tributyltin (TBT), were restricted to use, and non-toxic antifouling compounds with specific targets are urgently need; we hope that our findings in this research to be helpful for the development of environmentally friendly antifoulants.

4. Materials and Methods

4.1. Larval Culture

Larval culture was performed as described in our previous study [34]. Briefly, adult *M. volcano* barnacles were collected from the rocky shore, cleaned thoroughly in the laboratory. After drying in the air for 24 h, they were transferred into 0.22 μm-filtered sea water (FSW) to release embryos. The released embryos were collected and hatched in FSW at 28 °C to obtain swimming nauplii; then, all the nauplii were transferred into another tank and cultured at a density of 1 larva mL^{-1} in autoclaved FSW at 25 °C with the light:dark cycle of 12 h:12 h, and were fed with *Chaetoceros gracilis* at about 1×10^6 cells/mL every day until they transformed into cyprids.

4.2. Cement Gland Dissection

Dissection of the cement gland from *M. volcano* cyprids was performed following a protocol described for *M. rosa* [46]. Three-day-old cyprids were placed into modified barnacle saline [60] containing 462 mM NaCl, 8 mM KCl, 32 mM MgCl$_2$ and 10 mM HEPES (pH = 7.5) for relaxation. Relaxed cyprids were dissected under a stereoscope with a pair of finely etched tungsten needles. The swimming appendages were removed first, and then the bivalved carapaces were separated to expose the internal cavity; the pair of cement glands was carefully pulled away from adjacent tissues with the needles without touching them directly to avoid being damaged. The isolated cement glands were sucked out with a pipette, and the remaining parts were all collected as the carcass. The cement glands and carcasses were separately transferred to RNAlater (Invitrogen, Carlsbad, CA, USA) and stored at −80 °C until use.

4.3. RNA Extraction, cDNA Library Construction and Sequencing

Thirty cement glands and 10 carcasses of *M. volcano* cyprids were pooled together, respectively. Total RNA from the cement gland and carcass samples was extracted with TRIzol Reagent (Invitrogen) following the manufacturer's instructions. The quality and quantity of the RNA samples were measured with an Agilent Bioanalyzer 2100 system (Agilent Technologies, Santa Clara, CA, USA). RNA-seq for the cement glands and carcasses was performed by BGI China using equal amount of RNA. Briefly, sequencing libraries were constructed using a Nextera XT DNA Library Preparation Kit (Illumina Inc., San Diego, CA, USA) according to the manufacturer's instructions, and high-throughput sequencing was performed on an Illumina HiSeq 4000 platform (Illumina Inc.) with the model of paired-end (PE) 101 bp.

4.4. De Novo Assembly and Annotation

The raw sequence reads were filtered to obtain high-quality clean reads by removing reads with adaptor sequences, more than 5% unknown nucleotides, or more than 20% low-quality bases with SOAPnuke version 1.5.2 [61]. The read data have been submitted to the SRA of NCBI under the accession numbers SRR6516776 and SRR6516777. Clean reads were used for all the following analyses. The clean reads for the cement glands and carcasses were separately subjected to de novo assembly with the Trinity algorithm version 2.0.6 [62]; they were further assembled and redundancy was removed with TGICL version 2.1 [63], using the parameters of "repeat_stringency = 0.95, minmatch = 35, minscore = 35". The completeness of transcriptome assembly was assessed by BUSCO version 3.0 with the arthropoda_odb9 database [64]. The assembled unigenes were annotated by searching against public databases including the NCBI nonredundant (nr) database, the nucleotide (Nt) database, Swiss-Prot, the COG database and the KEGG database (e-value < 0.00001) using BLASTx version 2.2.23 [65]; GO classification was performed with Blast2GO [66]. ESTScan version 3.0.2 was used to predict the coding regions of the unigenes that had no hits in any databases [67].

4.5. Comparative Transcriptomic Analysis

The clean reads for the cement glands and carcasses were mapped to the assembled whole transcriptome (all-unigenes) with software Bowtie 2 version 2.2.5 [68]. The number of reads mapped to every unigene was counted with SAMtools [69]. The expression levels of the unigenes were quantified as FPKM [70]. DEGs were analyzed with the in-house software PossionDis [71,72] based on the Poisson distribution according to Audic and Claverie (1997), which can provide a quantitative assessment of differential expression without replicates [73]. p-values were then corrected by the FDR [74] in multiple testing. The threshold of FDR ≤ 0.001 and |$\log_2$ Fold Change| ≥ 1 was used to determine the DEGs. GO and KEGG enrichment analyses were performed based on the cumulative hypergeometric distribution method using the online OmicShare tools (version 1.0, http://www.omicshare.com/tools).

4.6. Protein Extraction and in-Solution Digestion

The same cement gland sample that was used for RNA extraction with TRIzol Reagent (Invitrogen) was also subjected to protein extraction according to the manufacturer's protocol. Briefly, after phase separation, the interphase and organic phenol-chloroform phase was subjected to a protein isolation procedure; in the last protein resuspension step, 100 μL of 10 M urea with 50 mM DTT (Sigma, St. Louis, MO, USA) was added to the protein pellet. The mixture was vortexed thoroughly and centrifuged at 16,000× g for 10 min, and the supernatant was transferred into a new tube. The protein concentration was quantified with an RC-DC kit (Bio-Rad, Hercules, CA, USA) following the manufacturer's instructions. For in-solution digestion, protein was alkylated by incubation in 40 mM iodoacetamide (Sigma) for 20 min at room temperature in the dark and then diluted 10-fold with 25 mM tetraethylammonium bromide (TEAB; Sigma). Trypsin (Promega, Madison, WI, USA) was added at an enzyme-to-substrate ratio of 1:50 (*w/w*), and the mixture was incubated for 16 h at 37 °C. After tryptic digestion, the peptide solution was desalted with Sep-Pak C18 cartridges (Waters, Milford, MA, USA) and dried using a SpeedVac (Thermo Electron, Waltham, MA, USA).

4.7. LC–MS/MS Analysis

Dried peptide fractions were reconstituted with 0.1% formic acid and analyzed two times using an LTQ-Orbitrap Elite coupled to an Easy-nLC system (Thermo Fisher, Bremen, Germany) as described previously [75]. Raw data obtained from LC–MS/MS analysis were converted into MGF format files with the software Proteome Discovery version 1.3.0.339 (Thermo Finnigan, San Jose, CA, USA) and then searched against the protein database deduced from the *M. volcano* cyprid transcriptome with 67,764 sequences including both 'target' and 'decoy' sequences with Mascot version 2.3.02 (Matrix Sciences, London, UK). The search parameters used were identical to those described by Mu and colleagues [75], except that the ion score cut-off was set to 25 to achieve 95% confidence in identification. Proteins with at least one matched unique peptide were retained, and the threshold of 1% FDR was used for the final protein identification. Proteomic data are available via ProteomeXchange with identifier PXD012779.

4.8. Sequence Analysis

Transcription factor identification was performed with the software DIAMOND version 0.8.23 [76] based on AnimalTFDB version 2.0 [77]. The SignalP 4.1 server was used to predict the presence and location of signal peptide cleavage sites [78], and the TMHMM Server 2.0 was used to predict transmembrane helices in proteins [79]. The NetNGlyc 1.0 Server and NetOGlyc 4.0 Server were used to predict *N*-Glycosylation sites and mucin type GalNAc O-glycosylation sites in proteins [80]. Sequence alignment was performed with ClustalX 2.1 (EMBL, Heidelberg, Germany) with the deduced protein sequences as input. Sequence alignment results were shaded with DNAMAN 8.0 (Lynnon Biosoft, San Ramon, CA, USA).

Supplementary Materials: The following are available online at http://www.mdpi.com/1660-3397/18/4/186/s1, Figure S1: All-unigenes classification, Figure S2: Sequence alignment of cp100k homologues from different species, Figure S3: CDD analysis of the lipid-binding proteins, Table S1: List of predicted transcription factor-coding unigenes that were upregulated in the cement gland transcriptome, Table S2: List of potential novel cement proteins, Table S3: Amino acid composition of cp100k homologues from different species, Table S4: Classification of all the enzyme-coding unigenes in the cement gland transcriptome, Table S5: List of enzymes involve in chitin synthesis and degradation, Table S6: List of lipid-binding proteins identified in the cement gland proteome.

Author Contributions: L.H., P.-Y.Q. and G.Y. conceived and designed the project. G.Y. prepared the samples, performed the wet experiments and drafted the manuscript. G.Y. and Z.W. performed the bioinformatics analysis. J.S. performed the protein search with Mascot. All authors reviewed the manuscript. L.H. supervised the work. All authors have read and agreed to the published version of the manuscript.

Funding: This work was supported by grants from the National Key Research and Development Program of China (2016YFC0302504), the National Natural Science Foundation of China (31460092), the National Key Research and Development Program of China (2016YFC0304905) and the Hong Kong Branch of Southern Marine Science and Engineering Guangdong Laboratory (SMSEGL20Sc01).

Acknowledgments: Special thanks to Ling Fang from the Instrumental Analysis and Research Center of Sun Yat-Sen University for performing the LC–MS/MS analysis.

Conflicts of Interest: The authors declare no conflict of interest.

References

1. Holm, E.R. Barnacles and biofouling. *Integr. Comp. Biol.* **2012**, *52*, 348–355. [CrossRef] [PubMed]
2. Walker, G. The Biochemical Composition of the Cement of two Barnacle Species, Balanus Hameri and Balanus Crenatus. *J. Mar. Biol. Assoc. U. K.* **1972**, *52*, 429–435. [CrossRef]

3. Kamino, K. Barnacle Underwater Attachment. In *Biological Adhesives*; Smith, A.M., Ed.; Springer International Publishing: Cham, Switzerland, 2016; pp. 153–176. [CrossRef]
4. Kamino, K. Mini-review: Barnacle adhesives and adhesion. *Biofouling* **2013**, *29*, 735–749. [CrossRef] [PubMed]
5. Qian, P.-Y.; Chen, L.; Xu, Y. Mini-review: Molecular mechanisms of antifouling compounds. *Biofouling* **2013**, *29*, 381–400. [CrossRef] [PubMed]
6. Walker, G. A study of the cement apparatus of the cypris larva of the barnacle Balanus balanoides. *Mar. Biol.* **1971**, *9*, 205–212. [CrossRef]
7. Gohad, N.V.; Aldred, N.; Hartshorn, C.M.; Lee, Y.J.; Cicerone, M.T.; Orihuela, B.; Clare, A.S.; Rittschof, D.; Mount, A.S. Synergistic roles for lipids and proteins in the permanent adhesive of barnacle larvae. *Nat. Commun.* **2014**, *5*. [CrossRef]
8. Cheung, P.J.; Nigrelli, R.F. Secretory activity of the cement gland in different developmental stages of the barnacle Balanus eburneus. *Mar. Biol.* **1975**, *32*, 99–103. [CrossRef]
9. Walker, G. The histology, histochemistry and ultrastructure of the cement apparatus of three adult sessile barnacles, Elminius modestus, Balanus balanoides and Balanus hameri. *Mar. Biol.* **1970**, *7*, 239–248. [CrossRef]
10. Walker, G. The early development of the cement apparatus in the barnacle, Balanus balanoides (L.) (Crustacea: Cirripedia). *J. Exp. Mar. Biol. Ecol.* **1973**, *12*, 305–314. [CrossRef]
11. Fears, K.P.; Orihuela, B.; Rittschof, D.; Wahl, K.J. Acorn Barnacles Secrete Phase-Separating Fluid to Clear Surfaces Ahead of Cement Deposition. *Adv. Sci.* **2018**, *5*. [CrossRef]
12. Kamino, K.; Inoue, K.; Maruyama, T.; Takamatsu, N.; Harayama, S.; Shizuri, Y. Barnacle cement proteins - Importance of disulfide bonds in their insolubility. *J. Biol. Chem.* **2000**, *275*, 27360–27365. [CrossRef] [PubMed]
13. Kamino, K.; Nakano, M.; Kanai, S. Significance of the conformation of building blocks in curing of barnacle underwater adhesive. *Febs J.* **2012**, *279*, 1750–1760. [CrossRef] [PubMed]
14. Mori, Y.; Urushida, Y.; Nakano, M.; Uchiyama, S.; Kamino, K. Calcite-specific coupling protein in barnacle underwater cement. *Febs J.* **2007**, *274*, 6436–6446. [CrossRef]
15. Urushida, Y.; Nakano, M.; Matsuda, S.; Inoue, N.; Kanai, S.; Kitamura, N.; Nishino, T.; Kamino, K. Identification and functional characterization of a novel barnacle cement protein. *Febs J.* **2007**, *274*, 4336–4346. [CrossRef] [PubMed]
16. He, L.S.; Zhang, G.; Wang, Y.; Yan, G.Y.; Qian, P.Y. Toward understanding barnacle cementing by characterization of one cement protein-100kDa in Amphibalanus amphitrite. *Biochem. Biophys. Res. Commun.* **2018**, *495*, 969–975. [CrossRef] [PubMed]
17. Liang, C.; Li, Y.Q.; Liu, Z.M.; Wu, W.J.; Hu, B.R. Protein Aggregation Formed by Recombinant cp19k Homologue of Balanus albicostatus Combined with an 18 kDa N-Terminus Encoded by pET-32a(+) Plasmid Having Adhesion Strength Comparable to Several Commercial Glues. *PLoS ONE* **2015**, *10*. [CrossRef]
18. Lin, H.-C.; Wong, Y.H.; Tsang, L.M.; Chu, K.H.; Qian, P.-Y.; Chan, B.K.K. First study on gene expression of cement proteins and potential adhesion-related genes of a membranous-based barnacle as revealed from Next-Generation Sequencing technology. *Biofouling* **2014**, *30*, 169–181. [CrossRef]
19. He, L.-S.; Zhang, G.; Qian, P.-Y. Characterization of Two 20kDa-Cement Protein (cp20k) Homologues in Amphibalanus amphitrite. *PLoS ONE* **2013**, *8*. [CrossRef]
20. So, C.R.; Scancella, J.M.; Fears, K.P.; Essock-Burns, T.; Haynes, S.E.; Leary, D.H.; Diana, Z.; Wang, C.Y.; North, S.; Oh, C.S.; et al. Oxidase Activity of the Barnacle Adhesive Interface Involves Peroxide-Dependent Catechol Oxidase and Lysyl Oxidase Enzymes. *Acs Appl. Mater. Interfaces* **2017**, *9*, 11493–11505. [CrossRef]
21. So, C.R.; Fears, K.P.; Leary, D.H.; Scancella, J.M.; Wang, Z.; Liu, J.L.; Orihuela, B.; Rittschof, D.; Spillmann, C.M.; Wahl, K.J. Sequence basis of Barnacle Cement Nanostructure is Defined by Proteins with Silk Homology. *Sci. Rep.* **2016**, *6*. [CrossRef]
22. Wang, Z.; Leary, D.H.; Liu, J.; Settlage, R.E.; Fears, K.P.; North, S.H.; Mostaghim, A.; Essock-Burns, T.; Haynes, S.E.; Wahl, K.J.; et al. Molt-dependent transcriptomic analysis of cement proteins in the barnacle Amphibalanus amphitrite. *BMC Genomics* **2015**, *16*. [CrossRef] [PubMed]
23. Power, A.M.; Klepal, W.; Zheden, V.; Jonker, J.; McEvilly, P.; von Byern, J. Mechanisms of Adhesion in Adult Barnacles. In *Biological Adhesive Systems: From Nature to Technical and Medical Application*; von Byern, J., Grunwald, I., Eds.; Springer: Vienna, Austria, 2010; pp. 153–168. [CrossRef]

24. Dickinson, G.H.; Yang, X.; Wu, F.H.; Orihuela, B.; Rittschof, D.; Beniash, E. Localization of Phosphoproteins within the Barnacle Adhesive Interface. *Biol. Bull.* **2016**, *230*, 233–242. [CrossRef] [PubMed]
25. Crisp, D.J. Mechanisms of adhesion of fouling organisms. In Proceedings of the 3rd International Congress on Marine Corrosion and Fouling, Gaithersburg, MD, USA, 2–6 October 1972; pp. 691–709.
26. Lindner, E.; Dooley, C.A. Chemical bonding in cirriped adhesive. In Proceedings of the 3rd International Congress on Marine Corrosion and Fouling, Gaithersburg, MD, USA, 2–6 October 1972; pp. 653–673.
27. Dickinson, G.H.; Vega, I.E.; Wahl, K.J.; Orihuela, B.; Beyley, V.; Rodriguez, E.N.; Everett, R.K.; Bonaventura, J.; Rittschof, D. Barnacle cement: A polymerization model based on evolutionary concepts. *J. Exp. Biol.* **2009**, *212*, 3499–3510. [CrossRef] [PubMed]
28. Kamino, K. Absence of cross-linking via trans-glutaminase in barnacle cement and redefinition of the cement. *Biofouling* **2010**, *26*, 755–760. [CrossRef] [PubMed]
29. Nakano, M.; Kamino, K. Amyloid-like conformation and interaction for the self-assembly in barnacle underwater cement. *Biochemistry* **2015**, *54*, 826–835. [CrossRef]
30. Bose, U.; Wang, T.; Zhao, M.; Motti, C.A.; Hall, M.R.; Cummins, S.F. Multiomics analysis of the giant triton snail salivary gland, a crown-of-thorns starfish predator. *Sci. Rep.* **2017**, *7*. [CrossRef]
31. Aldred, N.; Chan, V.B.S.; Emami, K.; Okano, K.; Clare, A.S.; Mount, A.S. Chitin is a functional component of the larval adhesive of barnacles. *Commun. Biol.* **2020**, *3*, 31. [CrossRef]
32. He, Y.H.; Sun, C.J.; Jiang, F.H.; Yang, B.; Li, J.X.; Zhong, C.; Zheng, L.; Ding, H.B. Lipids as integral components in mussel adhesion. *Soft Matter* **2018**, *14*, 7145–7154. [CrossRef]
33. Buffet, J.P.; Corre, E.; Duvernois-Berthet, E.; Fournier, J.; Lopez, P.J. Adhesive gland transcriptomics uncovers a diversity of genes involved in glue formation in marine tube-building polychaetes. *Acta Biomater.* **2018**, *72*, 316–328. [CrossRef]
34. Yan, G.Y.; Zhang, G.; Huang, J.M.; Lan, Y.; Sun, J.; Zeng, C.; Wang, Y.; Qian, P.Y.; He, L.S. Comparative Transcriptomic Analysis Reveals Candidate Genes and Pathways Involved in Larval Settlement of the Barnacle Megabalanus volcano. *Int. J. Mol. Sci.* **2017**, *18*, 2253. [CrossRef]
35. Chandramouli, K.H.; Al-Aqeel, S.; Ryu, T.; Zhang, H.; Seridi, L.; Ghosheh, Y.; Qian, P.Y.; Ravasi, T. Transcriptome and proteome dynamics in larvae of the barnacle Balanus Amphitrite from the Red Sea. *BMC Genomics* **2015**, *16*, 1063. [CrossRef] [PubMed]
36. Qin, J.; Hu, Y.H.; Ma, K.Y.; Jiang, X.S.; Ho, C.H.; Tsang, L.M.; Yi, L.F.; Leung, R.W.T.; Chu, K.H. CrusTF: A comprehensive resource of transcriptomes for evolutionary and functional studies of crustacean transcription factors. *BMC Genomics* **2017**, *18*. [CrossRef] [PubMed]
37. Hennebert, E.; Maldonado, B.; Ladurner, P.; Flammang, P.; Santos, R. Experimental strategies for the identification and characterization of adhesive proteins in animals: A review. *Interface Focus* **2015**, *5*. [CrossRef] [PubMed]
38. Cartharius, K.; Frech, K.; Grote, K.; Klocke, B.; Haltmeier, M.; Klingenhoff, A.; Frisch, M.; Bayerlein, M.; Werner, T. MatInspector and beyond: Promoter analysis based on transcription factor binding sites. *Bioinformatics* **2005**, *21*, 2933–2942. [CrossRef] [PubMed]
39. Lucas, M.; Walker, G.; Holland, D.; Crisp, D. An energy budget for the free-swimming and metamorphosing larvae of Balanus balanoides (Crustacea: Cirripedia). *Mar. Biol.* **1979**, *55*, 221–229. [CrossRef]
40. Thiyagarajan, V.; Harder, T.; Qian, P.Y. Relationship between cyprid energy reserves and metamorphosis in the barnacle Balanus amphitrite Darwin (Cirripedia; Thoracica). *J. Exp. Mar. Biol. Ecol.* **2002**, *280*, 79–93. [CrossRef]
41. Wang, S.; You, Z.; Feng, M.; Che, J.; Zhang, Y.; Qian, Q.; Komatsu, S.; Zhong, B. Analyses of the Molecular Mechanisms Associated with Silk Production in Silkworm by iTRAQ-Based Proteomics and RNA-Sequencing-Based Transcriptomics. *J. Proteome Res.* **2016**, *15*, 15–28. [CrossRef]
42. Huang, H.J.; Lu, J.B.; Li, Q.; Bao, Y.Y.; Zhang, C.X. Combined transcriptomic/proteomic analysis of salivary gland and secreted saliva in three planthopper species. *J. Proteomics* **2018**, *172*, 25–35. [CrossRef]
43. Alvarenga, É.R.; Mendes, T.M.; Magalhães, B.F.; Siqueira, F.F.; Dantas, A.E.; Barroca, T.M.; Horta, C.C.; Kalapothakis, E. Transcriptome analysis of the Tityus serrulatus scorpion venom gland. *Open J. Genet.* **2012**, *2*, 210. [CrossRef]
44. Qian, P.Y.; Lau, S.C.K.; Dahms, H.U.; Dobretsov, S.; Harder, T. Marine biofilms as mediators of colonization by marine macroorganisms: Implications for antifouling and aquaculture. *Mar. Biotechnol.* **2007**, *9*, 399–410. [CrossRef]

45. Yanai, H.; Savitsky, D.; Tamura, T.; Taniguchi, T. Regulation of the cytosolic DNA-sensing system in innate immunity: A current view. *Curr. Opin. Immunol.* **2009**, *21*, 17–22. [CrossRef]
46. Okano, K.; Shimizu, K.; Satuito, C.; Fusetani, N. Visualization of cement exocytosis in the cypris cement gland of the barnacle Megabalanus rosa. *J. Exp. Biol.* **1996**, *199*, 2131–2137. [PubMed]
47. Odling, K.; Albertsson, C.; Russell, J.T.; Martensson, L.G.E. An in vivo study of exocytosis of cement proteins from barnacle Balanus improvisus (D.) cyprid larva. *J. Exp. Biol.* **2006**, *209*, 956–964. [CrossRef] [PubMed]
48. Turner, R.J.; Sugiya, H. Understanding salivary fluid and protein secretion. *Oral Dis.* **2002**, *8*, 3–11. [CrossRef] [PubMed]
49. Catalan, M.A.; Nakamoto, T.; Melvin, J.E. The salivary gland fluid secretion mechanism. *J. Med. Investig. JMI* **2009**, *56*, 192–196. [CrossRef]
50. Walley, L.J.; Rees, E.I.S. Studies on the Larval Structure and Metamorphosis of Balanus balanoides (L.). *Philos. Trans. R. Soc. Lond. B Biol. Sci.* **1969**, *256*, 237–280.
51. Bers, D.M. Calcium cycling and signaling in cardiac myocytes. *Annu. Rev. Physiol.* **2008**, *70*, 23–49. [CrossRef]
52. Rocha, M.; Antas, P.; Castro, L.F.C.; Campos, A.; Vasconcelos, V.; Pereira, F.; Cunha, I. Comparative Analysis of the Adhesive Proteins of the Adult Stalked Goose Barnacle Pollicipes pollicipes (Cirripedia: Pedunculata). *Mar. Biotechnol. (N. Y.)* **2018**. [CrossRef]
53. Clarke, T.H.; Garb, J.E.; Hayashi, C.Y.; Arensburger, P.; Ayoub, N.A. Spider Transcriptomes Identify Ancient Large-Scale Gene Duplication Event Potentially Important in Silk Gland Evolution. *Genome Biol. Evol.* **2015**, *7*, 1856–1870. [CrossRef]
54. Waite, J.H.; Jensen, R.A.; Morse, D.E. Cement precursor proteins of the reef-building polychaete Phragmatopoma californica (Fewkes). *Biochemistry* **1992**, *31*, 5733–5738. [CrossRef]
55. Lee, H.; Scherer, N.F.; Messersmith, P.B. Single-molecule mechanics of mussel adhesion. *Proc. Natl. Acad. Sci. USA* **2006**, *103*, 12999–13003. [CrossRef] [PubMed]
56. Morgado, I.; Garvey, M. Lipids in Amyloid-beta Processing, Aggregation, and Toxicity. *Adv. Exp. Med. Biol.* **2015**, *855*, 67–94. [CrossRef] [PubMed]
57. Barlow, D.E.; Dickinson, G.H.; Orihuela, B.; Kulp, J.L., 3rd; Rittschof, D.; Wahl, K.J. Characterization of the adhesive plaque of the barnacle Balanus amphitrite: Amyloid-like nanofibrils are a major component. *Langmuir* **2010**, *26*, 6549–6556. [CrossRef] [PubMed]
58. Liu, X.P.; Liang, C.; Zhang, X.K.; Li, J.Y.; Huang, J.Y.; Zeng, L.; Ye, Z.H.; Hu, B.R.; Wu, W.J. Amyloid fibril aggregation: An insight into the underwater adhesion of barnacle cement. *Biochem. Biophys. Res. Commun.* **2017**, *493*, 654–659. [CrossRef] [PubMed]
59. Liang, C.; Ye, Z.; Xue, B.; Zeng, L.; Wu, W.; Zhong, C.; Cao, Y.; Hu, B.; Messersmith, P.B. Self-Assembled Nanofibers for Strong Underwater Adhesion: The Trick of Barnacles. *ACS Appl. Mater. Interfaces* **2018**, *10*, 25017–25025. [CrossRef] [PubMed]
60. Hayashi, J.H.; Stuart, A.E. Currents in the presynaptic terminal arbors of barnacle photoreceptors. *Visual Neurosci.* **1993**, *10*, 261–270. [CrossRef] [PubMed]
61. Chen, Y.X.; Chen, Y.S.; Shi, C.M.; Huang, Z.B.; Zhang, Y.; Li, S.K.; Li, Y.; Ye, J.; Yu, C.; Li, Z.; et al. SOAPnuke: A MapReduce acceleration-supported software for integrated quality control and preprocessing of high-throughput sequencing data. *Gigascience* **2017**, *7*. [CrossRef]
62. Grabherr, M.G.; Haas, B.J.; Yassour, M.; Levin, J.Z.; Thompson, D.A.; Amit, I.; Adiconis, X.; Fan, L.; Raychowdhury, R.; Zeng, Q.; et al. Full-length transcriptome assembly from RNA-Seq data without a reference genome. *Nat. Biotechnol.* **2011**, *29*, 644–652. [CrossRef]
63. Pertea, G.; Huang, X.; Liang, F.; Antonescu, V.; Sultana, R.; Karamycheva, S.; Lee, Y.; White, J.; Cheung, F.; Parvizi, B.; et al. TIGR Gene Indices clustering tools (TGICL): A software system for fast clustering of large EST datasets. *Bioinformatics* **2003**, *19*, 651–652. [CrossRef]
64. Simao, F.A.; Waterhouse, R.M.; Ioannidis, P.; Kriventseva, E.V.; Zdobnov, E.M. BUSCO: Assessing genome assembly and annotation completeness with single-copy orthologs. *Bioinformatics* **2015**, *31*, 3210–3212. [CrossRef]
65. Altschul, S.F.; Gish, W.; Miller, W.; Myers, E.W.; Lipman, D.J. Basic local alignment search tool. *J. Mol. Biol.* **1990**, *215*, 403–410. [CrossRef]
66. Conesa, A.; Gotz, S.; Garcia-Gomez, J.M.; Terol, J.; Talon, M.; Robles, M. Blast2GO: A universal tool for annotation, visualization and analysis in functional genomics research. *Bioinformatics* **2005**, *21*, 3674–3676. [CrossRef] [PubMed]

67. Iseli, C.; Jongeneel, C.V.; Bucher, P. ESTScan: A program for detecting, evaluating, and reconstructing potential coding regions in EST sequences. In Proceedings of the International Conference on Intelligent Systems for Molecular Biology, Heidelberg, Germany, 6–10 August 1999; pp. 138–148.
68. Langmead, B.; Salzberg, S.L. Fast gapped-read alignment with Bowtie 2. *Nat. Methods* **2012**, *9*, 357–359. [CrossRef]
69. Li, H.; Handsaker, B.; Wysoker, A.; Fennell, T.; Ruan, J.; Homer, N.; Marth, G.; Abecasis, G.; Durbin, R.; Genome Project Data Processing Subgroup. The Sequence Alignment/Map format and SAMtools. *Bioinformatics* **2009**, *25*, 2078–2079. [CrossRef]
70. Mortazavi, A.; Williams, B.A.; McCue, K.; Schaeffer, L.; Wold, B. Mapping and quantifying mammalian transcriptomes by RNA-Seq. *Nat. Methods* **2008**, *5*, 621–628. [CrossRef]
71. Liu, H.; Chen, C.H.; Gao, Z.X.; Min, J.M.; Gu, Y.M.; Jian, J.B.; Jiang, X.W.; Cai, H.M.; Ebersberger, I.; Xu, M.; et al. The draft genome of blunt snout bream (Megalobrama amblycephala) reveals the development of intermuscular bone and adaptation to herbivorous diet. *Gigascience* **2017**, *6*. [CrossRef]
72. Zhao, L.; Zhang, X.M.; Qiu, Z.Y.; Huang, Y. De Novo Assembly and Characterization of the Xenocatantops brachycerus Transcriptome. *Int. J. Mol. Sci.* **2018**, *19*, 520. [CrossRef]
73. Audic, S.; Claverie, J.M. The significance of digital gene expression profiles. *Genome Res.* **1997**, *7*, 986–995. [CrossRef]
74. Benjamini, Y.; Drai, D.; Elmer, G.; Kafkafi, N.; Golani, I. Controlling the false discovery rate in behavior genetics research. *Behav. Brain Res.* **2001**, *125*, 279–284. [CrossRef]
75. Mu, H.; Sun, J.; Heras, H.; Chu, K.H.; Qiu, J.W. An integrated proteomic and transcriptomic analysis of perivitelline fluid proteins in a freshwater gastropod laying aerial eggs. *J. Proteomics* **2017**, *155*, 22–30. [CrossRef] [PubMed]
76. Buchfink, B.; Xie, C.; Huson, D.H. Fast and sensitive protein alignment using DIAMOND. *Nat. Methods* **2015**, *12*, 59–60. [CrossRef] [PubMed]
77. Zhang, H.M.; Liu, T.; Liu, C.J.; Song, S.; Zhang, X.; Liu, W.; Jia, H.; Xue, Y.; Guo, A.Y. AnimalTFDB 2.0: A resource for expression, prediction and functional study of animal transcription factors. *Nucleic Acids Res.* **2015**, *43*, D76–D81. [CrossRef] [PubMed]
78. Nielsen, H. Predicting Secretory Proteins with SignalP. *Methods Mol. Biol.* **2017**, *1611*, 59–73. [CrossRef] [PubMed]
79. Krogh, A.; Larsson, B.; von Heijne, G.; Sonnhammer, E.L. Predicting transmembrane protein topology with a hidden Markov model: Application to complete genomes. *J. Mol. Biol.* **2001**, *305*, 567–580. [CrossRef] [PubMed]
80. Steentoft, C.; Vakhrushev, S.Y.; Joshi, H.J.; Kong, Y.; Vester-Christensen, M.B.; Schjoldager, K.T.; Lavrsen, K.; Dabelsteen, S.; Pedersen, N.B.; Marcos-Silva, L.; et al. Precision mapping of the human O-GalNAc glycoproteome through SimpleCell technology. *EMBO J.* **2013**, *32*, 1478–1488. [CrossRef]

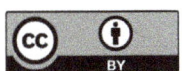

© 2020 by the authors. Licensee MDPI, Basel, Switzerland. This article is an open access article distributed under the terms and conditions of the Creative Commons Attribution (CC BY) license (http://creativecommons.org/licenses/by/4.0/).

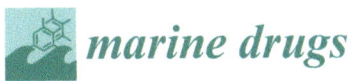

Review

Marine Microbial-Derived Antibiotics and Biosurfactants as Potential New Agents against Catheter-Associated Urinary Tract Infections

Shuai Zhang [1], Xinjin Liang [2,3], Geoffrey Michael Gadd [3] and Qi Zhao [4,*]

[1] School of Mechanical and Aerospace Engineering, Queen's University Belfast, Belfast BT9 5AH, UK; shuai.zhang@qub.ac.uk
[2] The Bryden Center, School of Chemical and Chemistry Engineering, Queen's University Belfast, Belfast BT7 1NN, UK; x.liang@qub.ac.uk
[3] School of Life Sciences, University of Dundee, Dundee DD1 5EH, UK; g.m.gadd@dundee.ac.uk
[4] School of Science and Engineering, University of Dundee, Dundee DD1 4HN, UK
* Correspondence: q.zhao@dundee.ac.uk

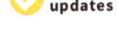

Citation: Zhang, S.; Liang, X.; Gadd, G.M.; Zhao, Q. Marine Microbial-Derived Antibiotics and Biosurfactants as Potential New Agents against Catheter-Associated Urinary Tract Infections. *Mar. Drugs* 2021, 19, 255. https://doi.org/10.3390/md19050255

Academic Editor: Tom Turk

Received: 1 April 2021
Accepted: 27 April 2021
Published: 29 April 2021

Publisher's Note: MDPI stays neutral with regard to jurisdictional claims in published maps and institutional affiliations.

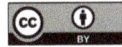

Copyright: © 2021 by the authors. Licensee MDPI, Basel, Switzerland. This article is an open access article distributed under the terms and conditions of the Creative Commons Attribution (CC BY) license (https://creativecommons.org/licenses/by/4.0/).

Abstract: Catheter-associated urinary tract infections (CAUTIs) are among the leading nosocomial infections in the world and have led to the extensive study of various strategies to prevent infection. However, despite an abundance of anti-infection materials having been studied over the last forty-five years, only a few types have come into clinical use, providing an insignificant reduction in CAUTIs. In recent decades, marine resources have emerged as an unexplored area of opportunity offering huge potential in discovering novel bioactive materials to combat human diseases. Some of these materials, such as antimicrobial compounds and biosurfactants synthesized by marine microorganisms, exhibit potent antimicrobial, antiadhesive and antibiofilm activity against a broad spectrum of uropathogens (including multidrug-resistant pathogens) that could be potentially used in urinary catheters to eradicate CAUTIs. This paper summarizes information on the most relevant materials that have been obtained from marine-derived microorganisms over the last decade and discusses their potential as new agents against CAUTIs, providing a prospective proposal for researchers.

Keywords: marine microorganisms; urinary catheter; antibiofilm; antifouling; coating

1. Introduction

Urinary catheters are hollow, partially flexible tubes that are designed to drain urine from the bladder. The earliest use of urinary catheters can be traced back to the third century B.C., but the modern indwelling catheter, called the 'Foley' catheter, was designed by Frederick B. Foley in the mid-1930s [1]. To date, over 100 million urinary catheters are used worldwide per year since catheterization rates remain high at 20% in non-intensive care units and 61% in intensive care units (ICUs) [2]. Despite the care taken to avoid contamination, catheters are still susceptible to infections as they provide direct access for uropathogens from the outside environment into the urinary tract, impairing local host defence mechanisms of the bladder [3,4]. Opportunistic uropathogens (Table 1) are mainly faecal or skin microbiota from the patients that can enter the bladder through the catheter lumen (34%) or along the catheter–urethral interface (66%) causing infections and complications, such as encrustation, bladder stones, bacteriuria, pyelonephritis, septicaemia and endotoxic shock (Figure 1) [3,5–7]. According to the European Centre for Disease Prevention and Control (ECDC), catheter-associated urinary tract infections (CAUTIs) account for 27% of all hospital-acquired infections in developed countries, and over 1 million cases occur in the USA and Europe [1,8]. In the UK, CAUTIs cost the NHS GBP 1–2.5 billion and account for approximately 2100 deaths annually [9].

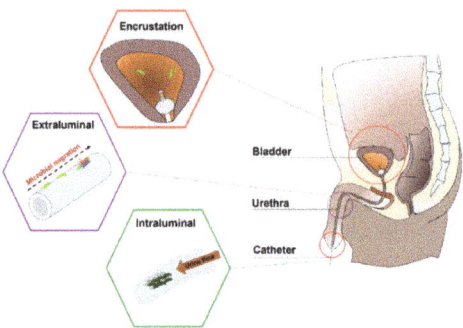

Figure 1. Anatomical cross-section of the renal system in a male showing CAUTIs.

Depending on clinical indications, the duration of catheterization may be short- (<7 days) or long-term (>28 days). Early work showed that 10–50% of patients undergoing short-term catheterization developed bacteriuria, and all patients undergoing long-term catheterization became infected, regardless of whether the catheter system was open or closed [10]. As a basic survival strategy, bacteria that encounter a catheter surface submerged in urine become attached within minutes [11]. These attached bacteria begin to phenotypically change, producing extracellular polymeric substances (EPS) (mainly exopolysaccharides and proteins) that allow the emerging biofilm community to develop a complex, three-dimensional structure within hours. Once established, the biofilms are very difficult to eradicate and exhibit a high tolerance to antibiotics and other biocidal treatments, making them a continuous focus for infections that can only be eliminated by the constant removal of the catheters [3,7,12–15]. Furthermore, in the presence of urease-positive bacteria (e.g., *Proteus mirabilis*), urease catalyses the hydrolysis of urea into carbon dioxide and ammonia, which increases the urine pH, leading to the precipitation of calcium and magnesium phosphate crystals (encrustation) and the formation of crystalline biofilms on the catheter, which eventually results in the complete blockage of the catheter [7,16,17]. Previous attempts to prevent CAUTIs include improving sterile techniques to inhibit the access of microbes into the urinary tract and limiting microbial accumulation on the catheter surface by intermittent catheterization. However, clinical evidence shows that these efforts do not lead to a noticeable reduction in CAUTIs [15]. Therefore, developing novel urinary catheters with antibiofilm and antiencrustation properties remains the most direct and promising strategy for this significant clinical problem.

Table 1. Common pathogens causing CAUTI.

Short-Term Catheterization	Type	References
Escherichia coli	GN bacterium	[18]
Serratia spp.	GN bacterium	[19]
Staphylococcus epidermidis	GP bacterium	[20]
Enterococcus spp.	GP bacterium	[21]
Bacillus subtilis	GP bacterium	[3]
Long-Term Catheterization	**Type**	**References**
Providencia aeruginosa	GN bacterium	[1]
Proteus mirabilis	GN bacterium	[7]
Providencia stuartii	GN bacterium	[22]
Morganella morganii	GN bacterium	[6]
Klebsiella pneumoniae	GN bacterium	[23]
Staphylococcus aureus	GP bacterium	[24]
Candida spp.	Fungus	[25]

GN: Gram-negative; GP: Gram-positive.

2. Current Anti-Infection Strategies against CAUTIs and Challenges

Current commercial urinary catheters can be generally classified as standard and antimicrobial catheters (Figure 2). Owing to their superior malleability, several materials used for making standard catheters include polyvinyl chloride (PVC), polyurethane (PU), silicone and latex [20]. Of these, silicone has emerged as the material of choice for urinary catheters due to distinct advantages, including excellent biocompatibility, no allergic reactions, superior chemical and thermal stability and good mechanical strength [2,26]. Morris et al. [27] compared the antiencrustation performance of 18 types of catheter and found that all-silicone urinary catheters took the longest time to encrust and block. The main reason for this lies in that the all-silicone catheter has a wider lumen, allowing a faster urine flow, which prevents the accumulation of crystalline deposits. However, recent studies demonstrated that there was no significant difference between the development of infections or bacterial adherence on silicone catheters as compared to other types of catheters [20,26,28,29].

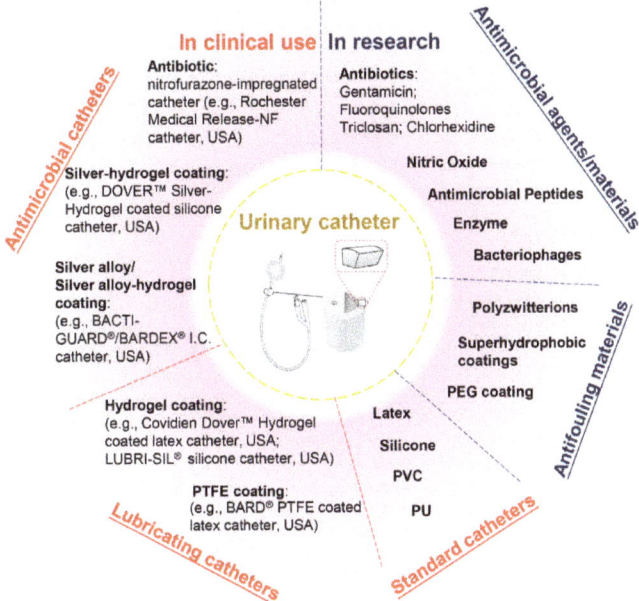

Figure 2. Classification of urinary catheters in clinical use and recently reported antimicrobial and antifouling materials for the prevention of CAUTIs.

Given that bacterial adhesion is the critical step in the progression of biofilm formation, numerous attempts have been made to endow the catheters with antiadhesive or antimicrobial properties, or both. Antiadhesive coatings are designed to prevent microbial adhesion through mechanisms of steric repulsion, electrostatic repulsion or low surface energy instead of killing the microbes [15]. To date, hydrogel- and polytetrafluoroethylene (PTFE)-coated catheters are commercially available, but clinical studies demonstrate that their efficacies against CAUTI are insignificant when compared with standard catheters [2,4,26,30]. Despite their lubricating features that may help improve patient comfort, hydrogel- or PTFE-coated catheters are only suitable for short- or medium-term catheterization (<28 days). Antimicrobial coatings are characterized by bactericidal or bacteriostatic activities that protect the catheters from microbial adhesion and migration. Recent reviews of commercial antimicrobial catheters identified two main strategies used: silver-based coatings and antibiotic impregnation [1,7,31]. However, all these catheters have only been reported to yield positive results for short-term application [7,20,32].

Silver is among the few FDA-approved antimicrobial materials for urinary catheter coatings, and its antimicrobial activity is associated with the release of silver ions. To date, silver has been applied in catheter coatings in the forms of bulk silver, silver alloy (silver/gold or palladium) and silver-hydrogels. Silver is very prone to oxidation in aqueous conditions, and the release of silver ions from these coatings often undergoes an initial burst-release phase followed by a slow-release phase. In clinical trials, the long-term antimicrobial efficacy of these silver-based coatings has proven limited [1,28,33]. In this scenario, attempts have been made to introduce silver nanoparticles into catheter coatings to attain enhanced antimicrobial efficacy. However, concerns have also been raised about the potential toxicity towards patients due to the fast and excessive release of silver ions [33,34]. In comparison, despite studies suggesting that the overuse of antibiotics may result in the development of antibiotic resistance, certain types of antibiotic-impregnated catheters have been proven to be more effective than silver-based antimicrobial catheters in preventing CAUTIs [3,20,35–37]. For example, nitrofurazone-impregnated catheters are commercially available, and studies comparing silver-alloy coated catheters, silver-hydrogel coated catheters, and nitrofurazone-impregnated catheters have found that nitrofurazone could effectively reduce the risk of symptomatic CAUTI and bacteriuria in short-term catheterization by impairing bacterial adherence and planktonic growth, while silver-based catheters have only demonstrated minimal effects [28,38]. Pickard et al. [33] compared the ability of silver-alloy-coated catheters and nitrofural-impregnated catheters for the reduction in incidence of symptomatic CAUTIs in adults requiring short-term catheterization via a clinical model, and the results demonstrated that nitrofural-impregnated catheters were more effective than the silver-alloy-coated catheters. In addition, impregnating antibiotics into catheters provides a cost-effective strategy to manufacture antimicrobial catheters, as this can be achieved by simply submerging swollen catheters in antibiotic-containing solutions for antibiotic encapsulation [31]. However, there are still certain concerns about using nitrofurazone in urinary catheters, such as patient discomfort [38] and the potential risks of developing tumours [39] and resistance in bacteria. This has hindered research in this field, and there is a growing demand for developing new antibiotics instead.

Apart from silver and antibiotics, recent research has also focused on a variety of antifouling materials (e.g., poly(ethylene glycol) (PEG) and polyzwitterions) [2,40] and biocidal materials (e.g., nitric oxide, antimicrobial peptides, enzymes and bacteriophages) [41–44] for urinary catheter coatings and has reported with varying levels of success, which offers potential for complete protection against CAUTIs. However, the promising performance of anti-infection coatings under laboratory conditions has not been translated into clinical success to date. Therefore, exploring novel anti-infection materials for urinary catheters will remain a current and broad interest in the upcoming decade.

3. Marine Microbiota as a Source of Novel Anti-Infection Materials

For short-term urinary catheters, the use of antibiotics has proven to be a cost-efficient strategy to prevent CAUTIs in clinical trials, but a major concern is the development of antibiotic resistance, particularly the increasing emergence of new forms of multidrug resistance among uropathogens that can render these antibiotics useless after repeated applications. Therefore, the identification of new resources for novel antibiotics with new modes of action has become the research focus over the past two decades. Currently, over 75% of the antibiotics currently available on the market are derived from terrestrial organisms, and the discovery of new antibiotics has declined considerably (only two new classes of antibiotics have been commercialized since 1962) due to difficulties in identifying novel and effective compounds [45–47].

Oceans cover 71% of the Earth's surface, but less than 5% have been explored to date, presenting an unexplored area of opportunity [48,49]. In recent decades, significant progress in the clinical development of marine-derived drugs has been achieved, and the discovery of novel antimicrobial substances from marine organisms has indicated their potential to combat existing medical device-related infections [50–54]. However, there are concerns that the overexploration of marine organisms may affect the balance between ecological constraints and economic activity. In this scenario, marine microbiota are emerging as a viable source of bioactive materials [55]. Diverse marine habitats provide unique conditions for marine microorganisms to develop into complex and diverse assemblages, and the isolation and extraction of bioactive secondary metabolites from such organisms are relevant to the discovery of novel anti-infection agents [56–59]. Therefore, microbes isolated from previously unexplored marine habitats may lead to the discovery of novel structures with potent antibiotic activity, and marine microbial-derived antibiotics are believed to be a promising alternative to overcome existing problems [60–62].

For long-term catheters, microbes are more prone to colonize and build biofilms on the surfaces with the attenuation of antimicrobial efficacy. Catheters with only biocidal activity are considered insufficient to eradicate CATUIs, as recent studies demonstrated that a 'foundation layer' composed of both dead and live bacteria can form on the catheter surface in long-term catheterization, which protects bacteria from contact with underlying biocidal substances [4,63]. To solve this problem, more research has focused on endowing catheter surfaces with both biocidal and antiadhesion properties [4,9,15,64]. Biosurfactants (BSs) are amphipathic secondary metabolites produced by microorganisms and have become a promising anti-infection material for medical applications [65–67]. Recent studies of the anti-infection functions of biosurfactants have identified three main routes, including killing microbes or inhibiting microbial growth, resisting microbial adhesion and disrupting biofilm formation [68–70]. For example, several BSs isolated from terrestrial-derived microbes, such as surfactin [71] and iturin [72], display potent antimicrobial activities, which make them relevant molecules in combating infections. Van Hoogmoed et al. [73] reported that biosurfactants released by *Streptococcus thermophilus* significantly inhibited *Candida* spp. adhesion to silicone rubber, which indicates their potential for use as a defence against colonizing strains on urinary catheters. These biosurfactants are mostly obtained from terrestrial-derived microorganisms, while biosurfactants produced by marine microorganisms have been less explored. Over the last decade, marine microbial-derived biosurfactants have attracted increasing interest, as marine microbes may exhibit unique metabolic and physiological capabilities producing novel metabolites with potent biological activities. To date, a considerable number of marine microbial-derived biosurfactants with antimicrobial, antiadhesive and antibiofilm activities have been obtained, and several have been proven to be effective against a broad spectrum of uropathogens, including Gram-positive and Gram-negative bacteria, as well as the yeast *Candida albicans*, which could potentially offer a new solution to the problems associated with long-term catheterization.

In this review, we summarize the diversity of marine microbial-derived antibiotics and biosurfactants discovered over the past 10 years and discuss their potential for use in combatting CAUTIs in short-term and long-term urinary catheters.

4. Marine Microbial-Derived Antibiotics with Broad-Spectrum Antimicrobial Activity

Antibiotics are low-molecular-weight compounds produced by microorganisms that kill or inhibit the growth of other microorganisms at low concentrations [74]. The current understanding of the biological activity of antibiotics is mainly centered on their primary cellular targets. The mechanisms of antibiotic action can be classified into 5 categories: (1) inhibition of cell wall synthesis (the most common mechanism), (2) inhibition of protein synthesis, (3) alteration of cell membranes, (4) inhibition of nucleic acid synthesis and (5) antimetabolite activity [75,76]. However, not all antibiotics have broad-spectrum antimicrobial activity, and their efficiency decays along with catheterization due to a limited shelf-life. Some microbes may be inherently resistant to certain antibiotics, while they may also mutate and/or exchange genetic material with other microbes, leading to the development of multidrug resistance [77,78]. Furthermore, some antibiotics may exhibit toxicity at or close to their therapeutic dose [47]. Considering the diversity of uropathogen species, the ideal antibiotic for urinary catheters should exhibit broad-spectrum antimicrobial activity and avoid developing resistance without inducing cytotoxicity in patients.

Generally, antibiotic compounds based on their structures and/or biosynthetic origins can be classified as alkaloids [79], quinones [80], phenols [81], polyketides [82], terpenes [83], polyketides [84,85] and peptides [86]. Table 2 lists the recent discoveries of marine microbial-derived compounds with broad-spectrum antimicrobial activity. Although very few of them have been developed into clinical trial phases, several have demonstrated to be effective against a broad spectrum of uropathogens, including Gram-positive and Gram-negative bacteria, fungi, as well as methicillin-resistant *Staphylococcus aureus* (MRSA). Therefore, they could be an alternative to conventional antibiotics for short-term catheters against CAUTIs caused by those pathogens.

Over the last two decades, the most studied group of microbes producing antimicrobial substances is the Firmicutes phylum (particularly the genus *Bacillus*) [87]. Tareq et al. [88–91] reported the discovery of four types of bioactive molecules with broad-spectrum antimicrobial activity against both Gram-positive and Gram-negative bacteria and fungi. Gageostatins A–C (Figure 3a) and gageopeptides A–D (Figure 3b) are two types of non-cytotoxic linear lipopeptides isolated from a marine *Bacillus subtilis* 109GGC020. The authors proposed a biosynthetic pathway based on nonribosomal peptide synthetases (NRPS) for the production of gageotetrins. Comparative studies showed that gageostatins A–C were more active against fungi than bacteria with minimum inhibitory concentration (MIC) values of 0.02–0.04 µM. Gageopeptides A–D exhibited potent antifungal and moderately broad antibacterial activity, while not showing cytotoxicity to human myeloid leukaemia K-562 and mouse leukemic macrophage RAW 264.7 cell lines. Gageomacrolactins A–C (Figure 3c) are three macrolactin derivatives obtained from the secondary metabolites of marine *Bacillus subtilis* 109GGC020 and displayed strong broad-spectrum activity against Gram-negative and Gram-positive bacteria and fungi. By comparing the structure-function of the gageomacrolactins A–C with that of known macrolactins 4–7, the authors demonstrated that antibacterial activity was not affected by the position of the epoxide group but highly dependent on the hydroxyl group at C-15 of the macrolactone ring. Ieodoglucomides 1 and 2 (Figure 3d) are two unique glycolipopeptides produced by a marine *Bacillus licheniformis* 09IDYM23 which act as moderate antimicrobial molecules. Podilapu et al. [92] reported the successful synthesis of ieodoglucomides A and B through a high-yielding route using per-O-TMS glucosyl iodide, making them promising candidates for industrial application.

Apart from *Bacillus* spp., Uzair et al. [93] reported the isolation of 4-[(Z)-2 phenyl ethenyl] benzoic acid (kocumarin) from the marine *Kocuria marina* CMG S2, which exhibited pronounced and rapid growth inhibition against fungi and pathogenic bacteria, including methicillin-resistant *Staphylococcus aureus* (MRSA). Although its antimicrobial mechanism has not been clearly elucidated, research on the functional groups involved in the molecular mechanism would reveal further insights into this atypical class of antibiotics. Schumacher et al. [84] described the first antimicrobial polyketide (bonactin) isolated from the liquid culture of a *Streptomyces* sp. BD21-2, a compound displaying antifungal and broad-spectrum antibacterial activity against microbes, including *Bacillus megaterium*, *Micrococcus luteus*, *Klebsiella pneumoniae*, *Staphylococcus aureus*, *Alcaligenes faecalis*, *Escherichia coli* and *Saccharomyces cerevisiae*. However, such marine microbial-derived compounds with activity against both bacteria and fungi are still very rare to date.

Over the past 10 years, numerous molecules possessing broad-spectrum antibacterial or antifungal activities have been isolated from marine microorganisms. Glycosylated macrolactins A1 and B1 (Figure 3e) were isolated from a marine *Streptomyces* sp. KJ371985, which inhibited *Bacillus subtilis*, *Escherichia coli*, *Pseudomonas aeruginosa* and *Staphylococcus aureus* with MICs of 0.03–0.22 µM. These compounds inhibit the peptidyl transferase activity and binding of the acceptor substrate to bacterial ribosomes. The higher solubility in the polar solvents of sugar-containing macrolactins could be an advantage in clinical applications [94]. Bacteriocins are natural peptides synthesized by bacteria for the purpose of killing/inhibiting other bacterial strains whilst not harming the producing bacteria through specific immunity proteins [95]. Elayaraja et al. [96] purified a bacteriocin from marine *Lactobacillus murinus* AU06, which exhibited a broad inhibitory spectrum against both Gram-positive and -negative bacteria. Marinocine is a broad-spectrum antibacterial protein synthesized by the melanogenic marine bacterium *Marinomonas mediterranea*, which generates hydrogen peroxide that kills bacteria [97]. However, recent studies demonstrated that the molecular basis of the antibacterial activity was L-lysine dependent, and activity was inhibited under anaerobic conditions. Mollemycin A (Figure 3f) is an antibacterial glyco-hexadepsipeptide-polyketide isolated from an Australian marine-derived *Streptomyces* sp. (CMB-M0244), which exhibited exceptionally potent and selective growth inhibitory activity against Gram-positive and Gram-negative bacteria (IC50 10–50 nM) but did not show any antifungal activity against *Candida albicans*. The cytotoxicity test also showed that mollemycin A was proportionately less cytotoxic toward human neonatal foreskin fibroblast cells [98]. Thiomarinols A–G (Figure 3g) were discovered as a class of polyketide antibiotics from marine *Alteromonas rava* SANK 73390, which displayed broad-spectrum activity against Gram-positive and Gram-negative bacterial species [99]. These thiomarinols act through inhibiting bacterial isoleucyl-transfer RNA synthetase and have pronounced activity against MRSA, with MICs $\leq$ 0.01 µg/mL [60]. Similar antibacterial compounds were also obtained from actinobacteria, such as *Pseudonocardia carboxydivorans* M-227 [100] and *Streptomyces* sp. JRG-04 [101]. Fungi (primarily *Candida species*) account for 20–30% of CAUTI cases, and *Candida albicans* is the most prevalent pathogen found in CAUTI biofilms [1,37]. Antifungal (particularly anti-*Candida*) compounds derived from marine microbes have been reported for metabolites produced by *Streptomyces* sp. ZZ338 [102], *Streptomyces* sp. SNM55 [103], *Bacillus subtilis* KC433737 [104], *Janthinobacterium* spp. ZZ145 and ZZ148 [105], *Trichoderma* sp. MF106 [106] and *Stagonosporopsis cucurbitacearum*-strain G019 [107]. These microbial strains, respectively produced actinomycins D, V and $X_{0\beta}$ (Figure 4a) (MIC, 9.83–9.96 µM); mohangamides A and B (Figure 4b) (IC50, 4.4 and 20.5 µM); 5-hydroxymethyl-2-furaldehyde (5HM2F) (Figure 4c) (MBIC, 400 µg/mL); janthinopolyenemycin A and B (Figure 4d) (MIC, 15.6 µg/mL, MBC, 31.25 µg/mL); trichodin A (Figure 4e) (IC50, 25.38 ± 0.41 µM); and didymellamide A (Figure 4f) (MIC, 3.1 µg/mL).

Table 2. Marine microbial-derived compounds with broad-spectrum antimicrobial activity.

Compound	Molecular Class	Source	Target	Reference
Gageotetrins A–C	Peptide	*Bacillus subtillis* 109GGC020	B/F	[90]
Gageopeptides A–D	Peptide	*Bacillus subtillis* 109GGC020	B/F	[91]
Ieodoglucomide 1, 2	Peptide	*Bacillus licheniformis* 09IDYM23	B/F	[88]
Bacteriocin	Peptide	*Lactobacillus murinus* AU06	B	[96]
Actinomycins D, V, $X_{0\beta}$	Peptide	*Streptomyces* sp. ZZ338	F	[102]
Mohangamides A, B	Peptide	*Streptomyces* sp. SNM55	F	[103]
Gageomacrolactins A–C	Macrolide	*Bacillus subtillis* 109GGC020	B/F	[89]
Glycosylated macrolactins A1, B1	Macrolide	*Streptomyces* sp. (KJ371985)	B	[94]
Bonactin	Acyclic ester	*Streptomyces* sp. BD21-2	B/F	[86]
Butenolide	Lactone	*Streptomyces* sp.	B	[108]
Mollemycin A	Peptide-polyketide	*Streptomyces* sp. CMB-M0244	B	[98]
Thiomarinols A-G	Polyketide	*Alteromonas rava* SANK 73390	B	[99]
Branimycin B, C	Polyketide	*Pseudonocardia carboxydivorans* M-227	B	[100]
UN	Polyketide	*Streptomyces* sp. JRG-04	B	[101]
Janthinopolyenemycin A, B	Polyketide	*Janthinobacterium* spp. ZZ145 and ZZ148	F	[105]
Kocumarin	Benzoic acid	*Kocuria marina* CMG S2	B/F	[93]
Marinocine	Protein	*Marinomonas mediterranea* MMB-1	B	[109]
5HM2F	Furan	*Bacillus subtilis* KC433737	F	[104]
Trichodin A	Pyridone	*Trichoderma* sp. MF106	F	[106]

B: Gram-positive and Gram-negative bacteria; F: fungi; UN: unnamed material.

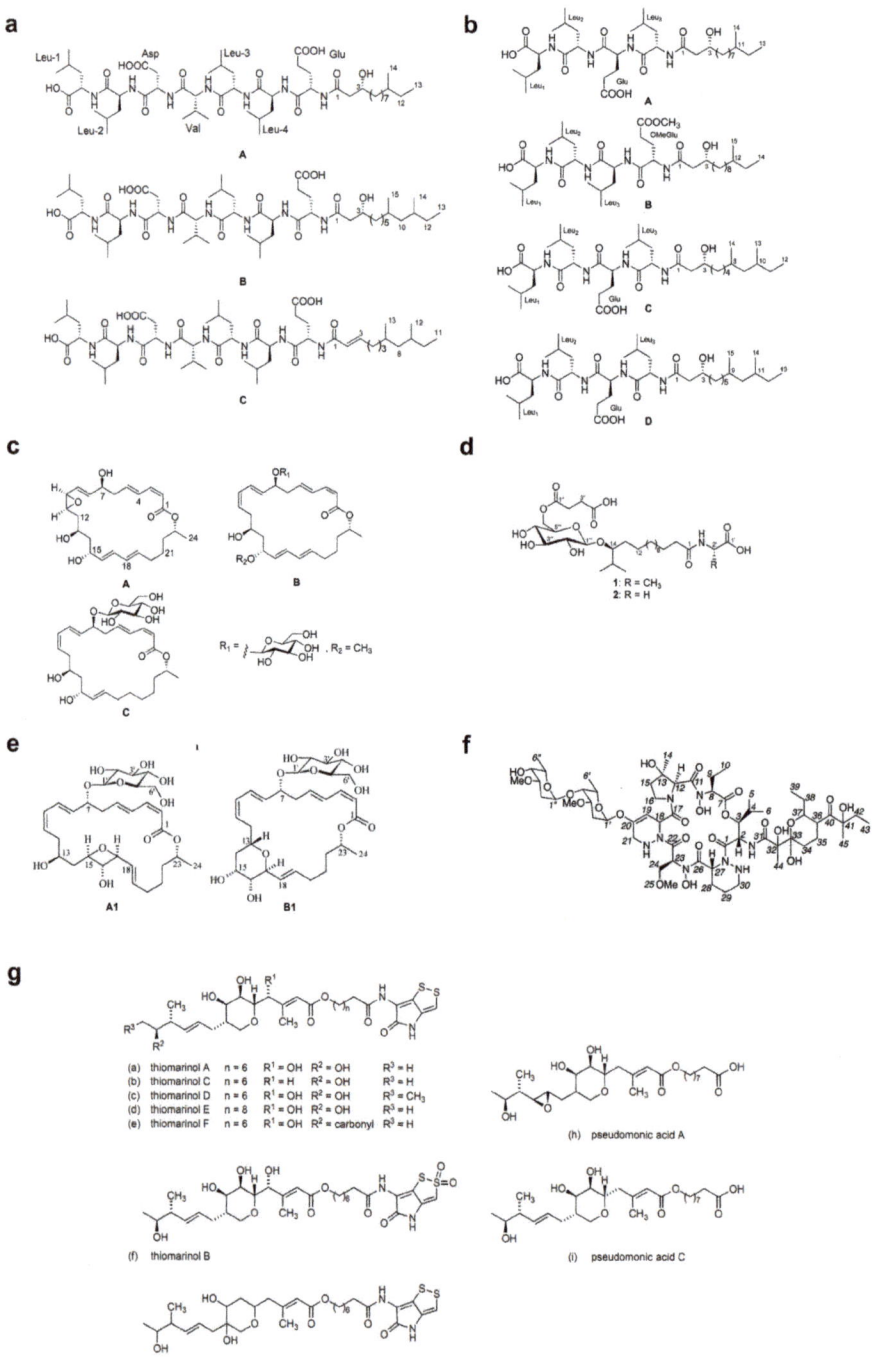

Figure 3. Structures of (**a**) gageosatins A–C [90], (**b**) gageopeptides A–D [91], (**c**) gageomacrolactins A–C [89], (**d**) ieodoglucomides 1 and 2 [88], (**e**) glycosylated macrolactins A1 and B1 [94], (**f**) mollemycin A [98], and (**g**) thiomarinols A–G [99].

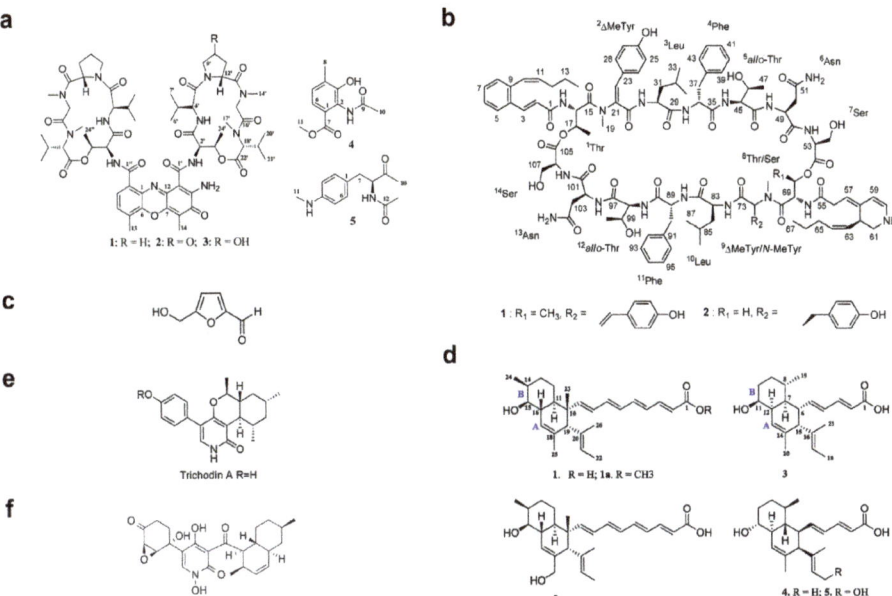

Figure 4. Structures of (**a**) actinomycins D, V and X$_{0\beta}$ [102], (**b**) mohangamides A and B [103], (**c**) 5-hydroxymethyl-2-furaldehyde (5HM2F) [104], (**d**) janthinopolyenemycin A and B [105], (**e**) trichodin A [106], and (**f**) didymellamide A [107].

5. Marine Microbial-Derived Biosurfactants: New Agents against CAUTIs

Biosurfactants (BSs) are amphipathic secondary metabolites produced by microorganisms that consist of both hydrophilic and hydrophobic moieties [45]. Compared to conventional chemical surfactants, these biomolecules have many advantages, such as low toxicity; high biodegradability; biocompatibility; low critical micelle concentrations (CMC); an ability to function over wide ranges of pH, temperature and salinity; as well as greater selectivity, and can be produced from renewable, cheaper substrates [110,111]. Such characteristics allow BSs to play a key role in multidisciplinary applications in industrial and environmental fields and make them a green alternative to their chemical counterparts. Furthermore, some BSs have been reported for their specific bioactivities, which play an essential role in the survival of microbial producers against other competing microbes [69,112]. In nature, BSs can be secreted extracellularly or remain attached to cell surfaces, reducing surface tension at the interface, thereby reducing surface contamination and aiding microbial motility in potentially hostile environments [113]. BSs may also have a range of therapeutic and biomedical benefits and could be used instead of conventional antibiotics to combat infections [114]. Current research regarding BSs has mostly focused on microbes from terrestrial sources (particularly soil-isolated microbes such as species of *Bacillus*, *Pseudomonas* and yeasts) [45,112], while practical applications of BSs in healthcare are still limited [115]. For this reason, marine habitats have again emerged as a potential source for isolating new BSs, and the discovery of new BS-producing microorganisms is attracting increasing interest.

BSs according to their molecular weight can be grouped into two categories: (a) high-molecular-mass (HMW) molecules (also called bioemulsifiers), such as polysaccharides, proteins, lipopolysaccharides, lipoproteins and lipoheteropolysaccharides, and (b) low-molecular-mass (LWM) molecules (generally 500 to 1500 Da), which can be further subdivided into glycolipids, lipopeptides, phospholipids, polymeric compounds and neutral lipids based on their chemical composition and microbial origin [45,65,116]. Recent research has mainly focused on the LWM BSs, and several have been reported to display antimicrobial, antiadhesive and antibiofilm activities against a broad spectrum of uropathogens (including multidrug-resistant pathogens), indicating their use as promising anti-infection materials for urinary catheters (Table 3).

5.1. Antimicrobial Activity

Biosurfactants have been reported to exhibit antimicrobial activity via different mechanisms of action, which primarily destroy the cell wall or plasma membrane by disrupting their integrity and permeability [65,68,117,118]. More specifically, their amphiphilic characteristics and affinity for lipid bilayers allow BSs to interact with cell membranes, leading to cell lysis and metabolite leakage, which ultimately results in cell death [116]. To date, various marine microbes have been reported to produce antimicrobial BSs, of which glycolipids and lipopeptides are the two primary isolated families that display broad-spectrum antimicrobial activity.

Glycolipids are a class of carbohydrate molecules made of mono-, di-, tri- and tetrasaccharides in combination with long-chain aliphatic acids or hydroxyaliphatic acids [119], of which trehalolipids, rhamnolipids and sophorolipids are of the most interest [120]. Reported marine microbial-derived glycolipid BSs with broad-spectrum antimicrobial activity against both bacteria and fungi are listed in Table 3. A glycolipid BS isolated from a marine *Staphylococcus saprophyticus* SBPS 15 exhibited dual functions: (1) excellent antibacterial and antifungal activities against a broad spectrum of clinical human pathogens, including Gram-positive bacteria (*Bacillus subtilis* and *Staphylococcus aureus*), Gram-negative bacteria (*Escherichia coli*, *Pseudomonas aeruginosa*, *Klebsiella pneumoniae* and *Salmonella paratyphi*) and fungi (*Aspergillus niger*, *Candida albicans* and *Cryptococcus neoformans*), and (2) potent surface tension-reducing activity (32 mN/m). This BS also showed superior stability over a broad range of pH (3–9) and temperature (up to 80 °C) [121]. Another glycolipid BS purified from extracts of a tropical marine strain of *Serratia marcescens* demonstrated similar dual functions, inhibiting the growth of *Candida albicans* and *Pseudomonas aeruginosa* with MIC values of >25.0 μg/mL and preventing adhesion by up to 99% [122]. The glycolipid BS also displayed biofilm disrupting activities against the test strains, which were believed to result from synergistic antimicrobial and surfactant activity. Glycolipid BSs were also isolated from the marine actinobacteria *Brevibacterium casei* MSA19, *Streptomyces* sp. MAB36 and *Brachybacterium paraconglomeratum* MSA21. The MSA19 glycolipid was bacteriostatic and could inhibit microbial attachment and disrupt both fungal and bacterial biofilms in both individual strains and mixed cultures at 30 μg/mL [123]. The MAB36 glycolipid also possessed strong antimicrobial activity against pathogenic bacteria and fungi and demonstrated excellent stability over a wide range of pH, temperature and ion concentrations [124]. The BS produced by the sponge-associated *Brachybacterium paraconglomeratum* MSA21 displayed broad antibiotic activity and it was suggested that the discovery of polyketide synthase (pks II) genes might pave the way for making new BSs by exploiting the microbial genes and enzymes, making the green production of BSs possible in the future [125]. Another glycolipid BS was isolated from a marine halotolerant bacterium (*Buttiauxella* sp. M44) that exhibited significant stability over a broad range of pH (7–8), temperature (20–60 °C) and salinity (0–3%) and potent antimicrobial activity against both bacteria and fungi [126]. Moreover, the combination of a cheap energy and carbon source (e.g., molasses) as well as a response surface method (RSM) could favor production and expand possible uses in the future.

Lipopeptides (LPs) are composed of peptide chains (short linear or cyclic structures) with lipid moieties and are the most widely reported class of biosurfactants with antimicrobial activity. *Bacillus* species are the most studied LP-producing strains that have been reported to produce several antimicrobial lipopeptide biosurfactants (LPBs), such as surfactin, iturin and fengycin, although most of these strains are from terrestrial ecosystems [70,72]. Liu et al. [71] reported the first surfactin (mainly composed of the nC14- and anteiso-C15-surfactin) isolated from marine *Bacillus velezensis* H3, which exhibited antimicrobial activity against a broad range of pathogens, including *Staphyloccocus aureus*, *Klebsiella peneumoniae*, *Pseudomonas aeruginosa* and *Candida albicans*. The surfactin demonstrated a lower inhibitory effect than the antibiotic polymixin B but greater antifungal activity against *Candida albicans* than the antibiotic vancomycin. Similar antibacterial and antifungal activities were also found for the BSs produced by *Halobacterium salinarum* [127]. Another surfactin produced by the marine actinobacterium *Nocardiopsis alba* MSA10 was shown to effectively inhibit the growth of *Enterococcus faecalis*, *Klebsiella pneumoniae*, *Micrococcus luteus*, *Proteus mirabilis*, *Staphylococcus aureus*, *Staphylococcus epidermidis* and *Candida albicans*, however, without effects on *Escherichia coli* and *Pseudomonas aeruginosa* [128]. Apart from surfactin, Balan et al. [129] first reported the discovery of aneurinifactin from the marine *Aneurinibacillus aneurinilyticus* SBP-11, which showed broad-spectrum antibacterial activity against *Klebsiella pneumoniae*, *Escherichia coli*, *Staphylococcus aureus*, *Pseudomonas aeruginosa*, *Bacillus subtilis* and *Vibrio cholerae*. The antibacterial mechanism was proposed to be derived from the anchoring of the BS on the bacterial cell membrane that disrupted its integrity, resulting in the production of hydroxyl radicals, which in turn caused lipid peroxidation and pore formation in the membrane [129]. However, antifungal activity was not investigated. It was also reported that a LPB (pontifactin) produced by marine *Pontibacter korlensis* SBK-47 displayed high antibacterial activity against *Streptococcus mutans*, *Micrococcus luteus*, *Salmonella typhi* and *Klebsiella oxytoca* and moderate activity against *Klebsiella pneumonia* and *Vibrio cholerae*. The molecule also showed antiadhesion potential against *Bacillus subtilis*, *Staphylococcus aureus*, *Salmonella typhi* and *Vibrio cholerae* [130]. Lawrance et al. [131] discovered an antibacterial LPB from the marine sponge-associated bacterium *Bacillus licheniformis* NIOT-AMKV06, which displayed significant bacteriostatic activity against a range of human pathogens, including *Enterococcus faecalis*, *Klebsiella pneumoniae*, *Micrococcus luteus*, *Proteus mirabilis*, *Salmonella typhi*, *Shigella flexneri*, *Staphylococcus aureus* and *Vibrio cholerae*. The production of these biosurfactants in heterologous host strains was achieved by cloning three gene clusters (sfp, sfpO and srfA) in *Escherichia coli*, with production being increased three-fold over the original strain. In addition, a lipopeptide BS produced by the marine *Bacillus circulans* is the only one found to be effective against multidrug-resistant (MDR) clinical strains while not having any haemolytic activity, indicating its potential to combat infections caused by such pathogens [132].

5.2. Antiadhesive and Antibiofilm Activities

Biosurfactants have also been reported to inhibit microbial adhesion and biofilm formation without exerting antimicrobial activity [69,133,134]. Despite the precise mechanisms of such activity not being fully understood, biosurfactants may affect interactions between microbes and surfaces through several modes of action: (1) modification of the physico-chemical properties (e.g., surface charge, hydrophobicity and surface energy) of the surface, which reduces microbial adhesion [111]; (2) suppression of the expression of biofilm-related genes, which inhibits microbial adhesion [135]; (3) promotion of the solubilization of biofilms encouraging bacterial detachment [136]; and (4) the interference of quorum sensing leading to decreased biofilm formation [70]. Numerous studies have shown that the prior adhesion of BSs to catheter surfaces (surface conditioning) reduced microbial adhesion and colonization [137–139].

In general, bacterial adhesion to a surface is regulated by diverse factors (e.g., growth medium, substrate and cell surface). The most frequently cited theory is the two-step adhesion model in which the adhesion process is divided into two distinct phases: reversible adhesion and irreversible adhesion [11,12,140]. Reversible adhesion describes a dynamic process in which bacteria can easily attach to or detach from a surface due to a combination of surface–cell interactions including van der Waals, electrostatic double-layer, Lewis acid-base, Brownian motion and hydrophobic interactions [64,141]. Walencka et al. [142] reported that BSs can affect cell-to-surface interactions by altering surface tension and charge to overcome the initial electrostatic repulsion barrier. For instance, Meylheuc et al. [143] reported that a stainless-steel surface coated with the BS produced by *Pseudomonas fluorescens* significantly reduced microbial adhesion. The presence of BS in the conditioned surface remarkably reduced the surface energy and enhanced surface hydrophilicity, leading to a decrease in attraction due to a reduction in the van der Waals forces and an increase in electron–donor/electron–acceptor characteristics. Jemil et al. [144] also reported that electrostatic repulsion between negatively charged surfaces (coated with anionic lipopeptides) and the negatively charged microbial surface could aid in inhibiting microbial adhesion. However, following reversible adhesion, microbial attachment gradually becomes stronger with time through a range of interfacial rearrangements (e.g., removal of interfacial water, protein conformational changes and an increase in hydrophobic interactions) and the production of adhesins, eventually form biofilms [145]. Despite numerous studies highlighting the difficulties in eliminating biofilms, BSs have been shown to disrupt or remove biofilms by penetrating and absorbing at the interface between the solid substrate and the biofilm, thereby reducing interfacial tension [134,146].

Antiadhesive and antibiofilm activities have also been reported for marine microbial-derived BSs. Hamza et al. [134] reported a non-toxic glycolipid BS (SLSZ2) derived from a marine epizootic bacterium *Staphylococcus lentus* SZ2 that effectively prevented the adhesion of *Vibrio harveyi* and *Pseudomonas aeruginosa* without showing bactericidal activity. In addition, this BS efficiently inhibited biofilm formation and disrupted the pre-formed biofilms of both strains by ~80%. Another glycolipid BS produced from a marine *Symphylia* sp. also exhibited antiadhesive activity against a range of pathogens (*Candida albicans*, *Pseudomonas aeruginosa* and *Bacillus pumilus*) and could disrupt pre-formed biofilms of these cultures in a concentration-dependent manner [122]. Similarly, a glycolipid BS isolated from the marine actinobacterium *Brevibacterium casei* MSA19 disrupted biofilm formation in *Escherichia coli*, *Pseudomonas aeruginosa* and *Vibrio* spp. under dynamic conditions. Moreover, biofilm disruption activity was consistent against mixed and individual biofilm bacteria at ~30 µg/mL. The lipopeptide BS produced by marine *Bacillus circulans* exhibited promising antiadhesive activity against several potential pathogenic strains, and the BS-coated surface effectively reduced microbial adhesion by up to 89% at a concentration of 0.1 g/L. Moreover, the pre-formed biofilms were removed with efficiencies between 59 and 94% for all the strains tested, demonstrating its potential in biomedical applications [147]. Song et al. [148] reported a lipopeptide BS produced by marine *Bacillus amyloliquefaciens* anti-CA that inhibited biofilm formation and dispersed pre-formed biofilms of *Pseudomonas aeruginosa* PAO1 and *Bacillus cereus*. The obtained data indicated that the BS could suppress the expression of the PslC gene which is associated with exopolysaccharide production in *Pseudomonas aeruginosa* PAO1. Pradhan et al. [149] also reported a lipopeptide BS produced by a marine *Bacillus tequilensis* CH which effectively inhibited pathogenic biofilms (*Escherichia coli* and *Streptococcus mutans*) on both hydrophilic and hydrophobic surfaces at a concentration of 50 µg/mL.

Table 3. Marine microbial-derived BSs with antimicrobial, antiadhesive or antibiofilm activities.

Source	Type	Activity	Reference
Staphylococcus saprophyticus SBPS 15	Glycolipid	Antibacterial activity against *Klebsiella Pneumoniae*, *Escherichia coli*, *Pseudomonas aeruginosa*, *Bacillus subtilis*, *Salmonella paratyphi* and *Staphylococcus aureus* Antifungal activity against *Aspergillus niger*, *Candida albicans* and *Cryptococcus neoformans*	[121]
Serratia marcescens	Glycolipid	Antibacterial activity against *Pseudomonas aeruginosa* and *Bacillus pumilus* Antifungal activity against *Candida albicans* Antiadhesive activity against *Pseudomonas aeruginosa*, *Bacillus pumilus* and *Candida albicans*	[122]
Brevibacterium casei MSA19	Glycolipid	Antibacterial activity against *Escherichia coli*, *Klebsiella pneumoniae*, *Proteus mirabilis*, *Pseudomonas aeruginosa*, *Vibrio parahaemolyticus* and *Vibrio vulnificus* Antibiofilm activity against mixed and individual cultures of *Escherichia coli*, *Pseudomonas aeruginosa* and *Vibrio* spp.	[123]

Table 3. *Cont.*

Source	Type	Activity	Reference
Streptomyces sp. MAB36	Glycolipid	Antibacterial activity against *Bacillus cereus, Enterococcus faecalis, Proteus mirabilis, Pseudomonas aeruginosa, Staphylococcus aureus, Staphylococcus epidermidis, Shigella dysenteriae* and *Shigella boydii* Antifungal activity against *Candida albicans*	[124]
Brachybacterium paraconglomeratum MSA21	Glycolipid	Antibacterial activity against *Bacillus subtilis, Escherichia coli, Enterococcus faecalis, Klebsiella pneumoniae, Micrococcus luteus, Pseudomonas aeruginosa, Proteus mirabilis, Streptococcus* sp., *Staphylococcus aureus* and *Staphylococcus epidermidis* Antifungal activity against *Candida albicans*	[125]
Buttiauxella sp. M44	Glycolipid	Antibacterial activity against *Escherichia coli, Salmonella enterica, Bacillus cereus, Bacillus subtilis* and *Staphylococcus aureus* Antifungal activity against *Candida albicans* and *Aspergillus niger*	[126]
Staphylococcus lentus SZ2	Glycolipid	Antiadhesive activity against *Vibrio harveyi* and *Pseudomonas aeruginosa* Antibiofilm activity against *Vibrio harveyi* and *Pseudomonas aeruginosa*	[134]
Bacillus velezensis H3	Lipopeptide	Antibacterial activity against *Staphyloccocus aureus, Mycobacterium, Klebsiella peneumoniae* and *Pseudomonas aeruginosa* Antifungal activity against *Candida albicans*	[71]
Halobacterium salinarum	Lipopeptide	Antibacterial activity against *Escherichia coli, Bacillus* sps., *Pseudomonas* sp., *Streptococcus* sp. And *Staphylococcus aureus* Antifungal activity against *Aspergillus niger* and *Candida albicans*	[127]
Nocardiopsis alba MSA10	Lipopeptide	Antibacterial activity against *Enterococcus faecalis, Klebsiella pneumoniae, Micrococcus luteus, Proteus mirabilis, Staphylococcus aureus* and *Staphylococcus epidermidis* Antifungal activity against *Candida albicans*	[128]
Aneurinibacillus aneurinilyticus SBP-11	Lipopeptide	Antibacterial activity against *Klebsiella pneumoniae, Escherichia coli, Staphylococcus aureus, Pseudomonas aeruginosa, Bacillus subtilis* and *Vibrio cholerae*	[129]
Bacillus licheniformis NIOT-AMKV06	Lipopeptide	Antibacterial activity against *Enterococcus faecalis, Klebsiella pneumoniae, Micrococcus luteus, Proteus mirabilis, Salmonella typhi, Shigella flexneri, Staphylococcus aureus* and *Vibrio cholera*	[131]
Pontibacter korlensis strain SBK-47	Lipopeptide	Antibacterial activity against *Streptococcus mutans, Micrococcus luteus, Salmonella typhi* and *Klebsiella oxytoca* Antiadhesion potential against *Bacillus subtilis, Staphylococcus aureus, Salmonella typhi* and *Vibrio cholerae*	[130]
Bacillus tequilensis CH	Lipopeptide	Antibiofilm activity against *Escherichia coli* and *Streptococcus mutans*	[149]
Bacillus Amyloliquefaciens anti-CA	Lipopeptide	Antibiofilm activity against *Pseudomonas aeruginosa* and *Bacillus cereus*	[148]
Bacillus circulans	Lipopeptide	Antiadhesive activity against *Escherichia coli, Micrococcus flavus, Serratia marcescens, Salmonella typhimurium, Proteus vulgaris, Citrobacter freundii, Alcaligenes faecalis,* and *Klebsiella aerogenes*	[147]
Aspergillus ustus MSF3	Glycolipoprotein	Antibacterial activity against *Enterococcus faecalis, Escherichia coli, Klebsiella pneumoniae, Micrococcus luteus, Pseudomonas aeruginosa, Proteus mirabilis, Staphylococcus aureus, Staphylococcus epidermidis* and haemolytic *Streptococcus* Antifungal activity against *Candida albicans*	[150]
Streptomyces sp. B3	Mixture of proteins, carbohydrates and lipids	Antibacterial activity against *Escherichia coli* and *Pseudomonas aeruginosa* Antifungal activity against *Candida albicans*	[151]
Oceanobacillus iheyensis BK6	Extracellular polysacchrides	Antibiofilm activity against *Staphylococcus aureus*	[152]

6. Opportunities, Challenges and Future Perspectives

Currently, research on anti-infection materials for urinary catheters is still increasing, and there is a growing demand for catheters with stronger antibiofilm and antiencrustation capabilities. Compared to the conservative strategy of optimizing existing products (e.g., widening the internal lumen [1], replacing bulk silver with silver nanoparticles [4], and redesign of micro/nano-scale surface topography [153]), the exploration of novel anti-infection materials from marine resources has clearly become an exciting potential solution to address some current limitations. Owing to the vast diversity of marine microorganisms, a number of new bioactive molecules with antimicrobial, antiadhesive and antibiofilm activities have been discovered that could be potentially combined with urinary catheters to combat CAUTIs.

The antimicrobial strategy aims to endow urinary catheters with microbicidal or microbiostatic properties to prevent the contact of microbes with the catheter surface or inhibit microbial migration along the catheter, thus preventing biofilm formation and encrustation. For short-term catheters, the use of antibiotics has proven to be the most efficient and cost-effective strategy, whereas the application of conventional antibiotics (e.g., nitrofurazone) has been questioned due to the safety concerns and the presence of antibiotic resistance. Despite attempts having been made to develop new antibiotics to solve this problem, the difficulty in identifying novel and effective compounds has led to a slowdown of research in this field. In recent decades, the isolation of microbes from previously unexplored marine habitats has led to the discovery of a number of novel antimicrobial compounds with new modes of action to combat the current antibiotic resistance threat. Several of these have been proven to possess broad-spectrum antimicrobial activities against a wide range of uropathogens, which could be potentially applied to urinary catheters to eradicate CAUTIs. Technically, these antimicrobial molecules could be directly deposited on the catheter surfaces or applied in coatings. Considering that CAUTIs may be derived from both extraluminal and intraluminal routes, it would be ideal to endow both surfaces with antimicrobial properties, despite extraluminal infections being clinically more common. For example, commercial catheters have been conventionally impregnated with antimicrobials, such as antibiotics, and function via a release model. However, this is only a temporary solution for short-term catheterization, and microbial contamination can resume once the antibiotics are removed. Given that the efficacy of antimicrobial materials is often concentration dependent, a challenge in this type of catheter modification strategy is to achieve and preserve adequate local delivery of the antimicrobials during catheterization in vivo without inducing resistance and patient cytotoxicity. This could be achieved by developing a novel release system with controlled release kinetics instead of directly altering the drug loading. For example, hydrogel coatings, due to their lubricating properties, have been widely applied in urinary catheters. Milo et al. [154] reported a smart infection-responsive hydrogel coating for urinary catheters. The coating is a dual-layered polymeric system consisting of a lower 'reservoir' layer of poly(vinyl alcohol) (PVA) hydrogel (containing bacteriophage), capped by an upper layer of the pH-responsive polymer. The upper layer swells when urinary pH is elevated due to *P. mirabilis* infection, exposing the PVA reservoir layer to urine, resulting in the release of bacteriophage from the coating to prevent the encrustation and blockage of urinary catheters. In this way, the release of antimicrobials could be controlled in a smart way to prevent/retard CAUTIs and associated complications. Researchers will need to further conduct thorough in vitro and in vivo leaching and cytotoxicity studies to determine the optimum operational conditions and identify any problematic side effects.

In long-term catheterization, extensive biofilms containing >5×10^9 viable cells/cm^2 can be found on catheters and can be responsible for the persistence of the infections [155]. Moreover, the biofilms are often composed of multispecies consortia, which have been reported to be more virulent and have a higher tolerance to antibiotics [7]. Therefore, in addition to killing the uropathogens, attempts have also been made to combine catheter surfaces with antiadhesive materials to retard the occurrence of CAUTIs. To date, only

PTFE and hydrogel have entered clinical use, while their efficacy in resisting CAUTI and encrustation is still controversial [4,17,33]. Other antiadhesive materials, such as polyzwitterions, have recently emerged as promising candidates, although their instability in long-term catheterization hinders practical application [1]. In this scenario, research on marine microbes has led to the discovery of novel antiadhesive molecules with greater activity and stability. For instance, marine microbial-derived antiadhesive materials, such as biosurfactants and cyanobacterial extracellular polymers [59,156], can inhibit microbial adhesion via multimechanisms. Currently, several biosurfactants have been reported to influence both cell-to-cell and cell-to-surface interactions that can inhibit microbial adhesion as well as disrupt biofilm formation [67,70,112]. Technically, biosurfactants could be doped in coatings and act on microbial cells via a contact mode. These features may aid in preventing biofilm formation and encrustation as well as extending the lifetime of indwelling urinary catheters. Furthermore, they could be employed in combination with other strategies (e.g., use of antimicrobial materials and micro/nano patterning) to achieve synergistic effects.

In fact, although these marine microbial-derived molecules have shown potential in combating CAUTI-related pathogens and/or biofilms, it should be noted that their clinical effectiveness still needs to be verified in future. Currently, there has been a lack of accomplished research in this area, and this paper provides a prospective proposal for researchers. Currently, the most significant obstacles hindering the development of marine microbial-derived products are supply issues. This is mainly due to difficulties associated with the isolation and growth of producing microorganisms. In addition, for marine microbial-derived biosurfactants, most of these materials are unidentified mixtures of compounds, and the further pharmaceutical development of such mixtures is very challenging. To date, the development of new chemical and physicochemical approaches and tools has led to great advances in the isolation and structure elucidation of novel minor marine secondary metabolites, which could not be isolated/detected in the past [54]. On the other hand, urinary catheters are still considered as low-cost clinical care products, although commercial 'anti-infective' catheters are usually priced two to five times higher than standard catheters. Therefore, in addition to the cost of employing new materials, a cost-effective coating technology should also be addressed.

7. Conclusions

Marine microorganisms can produce metabolites of varied chemical structures displaying antimicrobial, antiadhesive and antibiofilm activities. These compounds present enormous potential for the discovery of new agents to overcome the current challenges associated with CAUTI. Owing to technical limitations in the past, bioactive compounds derived from marine microorganisms have not yet progressed into clinical trials. However, recent advances in oceanographic science and metabolome screening have led to a boost in the discovery of new species and metabolic profiles as well as new molecules with potent anti-infection activities against CAUTI-associated pathogens. Research efforts should be applied to the exploration of marine microbes in the search for new bioactive compounds for the development of novel anti-infection agents.

Author Contributions: S.Z. and X.L. are first co-authors. Conceptualized and writing, S.Z. and X.L.; Revision and editing, G.M.G. and Q.Z.; Supervision and resources, Q.Z. All authors have read and agreed to the published version of the manuscript.

Funding: This work was supported by the UK Engineering and Physical Sciences Research Council (EP/P00301X/1).

Acknowledgments: The authors acknowledge the financial supports from the UK Engineering and Physical Sciences Research Council (EP/P00301X/1).

Conflicts of Interest: The authors declare no conflict of interest.

References

1. Singha, P.; Locklin, J.; Handa, H. A review of the recent advances in antimicrobial coatings for urinary catheters. *Acta Biomater.* **2017**, *50*, 20–40. [CrossRef]
2. Andersen, M.J.; Flores-Mireles, A.L. Urinary catheter coating modifications: The race against catheter-associated infections. *Coatings* **2020**, *10*, 23. [CrossRef]
3. Jacobsen, S.M.; Stickler, D.J.; Mobley, H.L.; Shirtliff, M.E. Complicated catheter-associated urinary tract infections due to *Escherichia coli* and *Proteus mirabilis*. *Clin. Microbiol. Rev.* **2008**, *21*, 26–59. [CrossRef]
4. Zhang, S.; Wang, L.; Liang, X.; Vorstius, J.; Keatch, R.; Corner, G.; Nabi, G.; Davidson, F.; Gadd, G.M.; Zhao, Q. Enhanced antibacterial and antiadhesive activities of silver-PTFE nanocomposite coating for urinary catheters. *ACS Biomater. Sci. Eng.* **2019**, *5*, 2804–2814. [CrossRef]
5. Stickler, D.J. Clinical complications of urinary catheters caused by crystalline biofilms: Something needs to be done. *J. Intern. Med.* **2014**, *276*, 120–129. [CrossRef] [PubMed]
6. Cortese, Y.J.; Wagner, V.E.; Tierney, M.; Devine, D.; Fogarty, A. Review of catheter-associated urinary tract infections and in vitro urinary tract models. *J. Heal. Eng.* **2018**, *14*, 1–16. [CrossRef]
7. Ramstedt, M.; Ribeiro, I.A.C.; Bujdakova, H.; Mergulhao, F.J.M.; Jordao, L.; Thomsen, P.; Alm, M.; Burmolle, M.; Vladkova, T.; Can, F.; et al. Evaluating efficacy of antimicrobial and antifouling materials for urinary tract medical devices: Challenges and recommendations. *Macromol. Biosci.* **2014**, *19*, e1800384. [CrossRef] [PubMed]
8. Saint, S.; Gaies, E.; Fowler, K.E.; Harrod, M.; Krein, S.L. Introducing a catheter-associated urinary tract infection (CAUTI) prevention guide to patient safety (GPS). *Am. J. Infect. Control* **2014**, *42*, 548–550. [CrossRef]
9. Milo, S.; Nzakizwanayo, J.; Hathaway, H.J.; Jones, B.V.; Jenkins, A.T.A. Emerging medical and engineering strategies for the prevention of long-term indwelling catheter blockage. *Proc. Inst. Mech. Eng. Part H* **2019**, *233*, 68–83. [CrossRef] [PubMed]
10. Stickler, D.J. Bacterial biofilms and the encrustation of urethral catheters. *Biofouling* **1996**, *9*, 13. [CrossRef]
11. Dunne, W.M., Jr. Bacterial adhesion: Seen any good biofilms lately? *Clin. Microbiol. Rev.* **2002**, *15*, 155–166. [CrossRef]
12. Donlan, R.M. Biofilms: Microbial Life on Surfaces. *Emerg. Infect. Dis.* **2002**, *8*, 881–890. [CrossRef]
13. Høiby, N.; Bjarnsholt, T.; Givskov, M.; Molin, S.; Ciofu, O. Antibiotic resistance of bacterial biofilms. *Int. J. Antimicrob. Agents* **2010**, *35*, 322–332. [CrossRef]
14. Hooton, T.M.; Bradley, S.F.; Cardenas, D.D.; Colgan, R.; Geerlings, S.E.; Rice, J.C.; Saint, S.; Schaeffer, A.J.; Tambayh, P.A.; Tenke, P.; et al. Diagnosis, prevention, and treatment of catheter-associated urinary tract infection in adults: 2009 International clinical practice guidelines from the Infectious Diseases Society of America. *CID* **2010**, *50*, 625–663. [CrossRef]
15. Yu, K.; Lo, J.C.; Yan, M.; Yang, X.; Brooks, D.E.; Hancock, R.E.; Lange, D.; Kizhakkedathu, J.N. Anti-adhesive antimicrobial peptide coating prevents catheter associated infection in a mouse urinary infection model. *Biomaterials* **2017**, *116*, 69–81. [CrossRef] [PubMed]
16. Stickler, D.; Ganderton, L.; King, J.; Nettleton, J.; Winters, C. *Proteus mirabilis* biofilms and the encrustation of urethral catheters. *Urol. Res.* **1993**, *21*, 407–411. [CrossRef]
17. Zhang, S.; Liang, X.; Gadd, G.M.; Zhao, Q. Superhydrophobic coatings for urinary catheters to delay bacterial biofilm formation and catheter-associated urinary tract infection. *ACS Appl. Bio Mater.* **2020**, *3*, 282–291. [CrossRef]
18. Pelling, H.; Nzakizwanayo, J.; Milo, S.; Denham, E.L.; MacFarlane, W.M.; Bock, L.J.; Sutton, J.M.; Jones, B.V. Bacterial biofilm formation on indwelling urethral catheters. *Lett. Appl. Microbiol.* **2019**, *68*, 277–293. [CrossRef]
19. Efthimiou, I.; Skrepetis, K. *Prevention of Catheter-Associated Urinary Tract Infections. Recent Advances in the Field of Urinary Tract Infections*; IntechOpen: London, UK, 2013; Available online: https://www.intechopen.com/books/recent-advances-in-the-field-of-urinary-tract-infections/prevention-of-catheter-associated-urinary-tract-infections/ (accessed on 20 September 2020).
20. Al-Qahtani, M.; Safan, A.; Jassim, G.; Abadla, S. Efficacy of anti-microbial catheters in preventing catheter associated urinary tract infections in hospitalized patients: A review on recent updates. *J. Infect. Public Health* **2019**, *12*, 760–766. [CrossRef] [PubMed]
21. Guiton, P.S.; Hung, C.S.; Hancock, L.E.; Caparon, M.G.; Hultgren, S.J. Enterococcal biofilm formation and virulence in an optimized murine model of foreign body-associated urinary tract infections. *Infect. Immun.* **2010**, *78*, 4166–4175. [CrossRef]
22. Johnson, J.R.; Johnston, B.; Kuskowski, M.A. In vitro comparison of nitrofurazone- and silver alloy-coated foley catheters for contact-dependent and diffusible inhibition of urinary tract infection-associated microorganisms. *Antimicrob. Agents Chemother.* **2012**, *56*, 4969–4972. [CrossRef]
23. Peng, D.; Li, X.; Liu, P.; Luo, M.; Chen, S.; Su, K.; Zhang, Z.; He, Q.; Qiu, J.; Li, Y. Epidemiology of pathogens and antimicrobial resistance of catheter-associated urinary tract infections in intensivecare units: A systematic review and meta-analysis. *Am. J. Infect. Control* **2018**, *46*, e81–e90. [CrossRef] [PubMed]
24. Walker, J.N.; Flores-Mireles, A.L.; Pinkner, C.L.; Schreiber, H.L.I.; Joens, M.S.; Park, A.M.; Potretzke, A.M.; Bauman, T.M.; Pinkner, J.S.; Fitzpatrick, J.; et al. Catheterization alters bladder ecology to potentiate Staphylococcus aureus infection of the urinary tract. *Proc. Natl. Acad. Sci. USA* **2017**, *114*, E8721–E8730. [CrossRef] [PubMed]
25. Fisher, L.E.; Hook, A.L.; Ashraf, W.; Yousef, A.; Barrett, D.A.; Scurr, D.J.; Chen, X.; Smith, E.F.; Fay, M.; Parmenter, C.D.; et al. Biomaterial modification of urinary catheters with antimicrobials to give long-term broadspectrum antibiofilm activity. *J. Control. Release* **2015**, *202*, 57–64. [CrossRef] [PubMed]
26. Lawrence, E.L.; Turner, I.G. Materials for urinary catheters: A review of their history and development in the UK. *Med. Eng. Phys.* **2005**, *27*, 443–453. [CrossRef]

27. Morris, N.S.; Stickler, D.J.; Winters, C. Which indwelling urethral catheters resist encrustation by *Proteus mirabilis* biofilms? *Br. J. Urol.* **1997**, *80*, 58–63. [CrossRef]
28. Desai, D.G.; Liao, K.S.; Cevallos, M.E.; Trautner, B.W. Silver or nitrofurazone impregnation of urinary catheters has a minimal effect on uropathogen adherence. *J. Urol.* **2010**, *184*, 2565–2571. [CrossRef]
29. Cohen, A.B.; Dagli, M.; Stavropoulos, S.W.J.; Mondschein, J.I.; Soulen, M.C.; Shlansky-Goldberg, R.D.; Solomon, J.A.; Chittams, J.L.; Trerotola, S.O. Silicone and polyurethane tunneled linfusion catheters: A comparison of durability and breakage rates. *J. Vasc. Interv. Radiol.* **2011**, *22*, 638–641. [CrossRef]
30. Kazmierska, K.A.; Thompson, R.; Morris, N.; Long, A.; Ciach, T. In vitro multicompartmental bladder model for assessing blockage of urinary catheters: Effect of hydrogel coating on dynamics of *Proteus mirabilis* growth. *Urology* **2010**, *76*, e515–e520. [CrossRef]
31. Liu, L.; Shi, H.; Yu, H.; Yan, S.; Luan, S. The recent advances in surface antibacterial strategies for biomedical catheters. *Biomater. Sci.* **2020**, *8*, 4095–4108. [CrossRef]
32. Trautner, B.W.; Hull, R.A.; Darouiche, R.O. Prevention of catheter-associated urinary tract infection. *Curr. Opin. Infect. Dis.* **2005**, *18*, 37–41. [CrossRef]
33. Pickard, R.; Lam, T.; MacLennan, G.; Starr, K.; Kilonzo, M.; McPherson, G.; Gillies, K.; McDonald, A.; Walton, K.; Buckley, B.; et al. Antimicrobial catheters for reduction of symptomatic urinary tract infection in adults requiring short-term catheterisation in hospital: A multicentre randomised controlled trial. *Lancet* **2012**, *380*, 1927–1935. [CrossRef]
34. Zhang, S.; Liang, X.; Gadd, G.M.; Zhao, Q. A sol-gel based silver nanoparticle/polytetrafluorethylene (AgNP/PTFE) coating with enhanced antibacterial and anti-corrosive properties. *Appl. Surf. Sci.* **2021**, *535*, 147675. [CrossRef]
35. Wu, K.; Yang, Y.; Zhang, Y.; Deng, J.; Lin, C. Antimicrobial activity and cytocompatibility of silver nanoparticles coated catheters via a biomimetic surface functionalization strategy. *Int. J. Nanomed.* **2015**, *10*, 7241–7252. [CrossRef]
36. Feneley, R.C.L.; Hopley, I.B.; Wells, P.N.T. Urinary catheters: History, current status, adverse events and research agenda. *J. Med. Eng. Technol.* **2015**, *39*, 459–470. [CrossRef]
37. Prestinaci, F.; Pezzotti, P.; Pantosti, A. Antimicrobial resistance: A global multifaceted phenomenon. *Pathog. Glob. Health* **2015**, *109*, 309–318. [CrossRef]
38. Lam, T.B.; Omar, M.I.; Fisher, E.; Gillies, K.; MacLennan, S. Types of indwelling urethral catheters for short-term catheterisation in hospitalised adults. *Cochrane Database Syst. Rev.* **2014**, *23*, CD004013. [CrossRef] [PubMed]
39. Hiraku, Y.; Sekine, A.; Nabeshi, H.; Midorikawa, K.; Murata, M.; Kumagai, Y.; Kawanishi, S. Mechanism of carcinogenesis induced by a veterinary antimicrobial drug, nitrofurazone, via oxidative DNA damage and cell proliferation. *Cancer Lett.* **2004**, *215*, 141–150. [CrossRef] [PubMed]
40. Sankar, S.; Rajalakshmi, T. Application of poly ethylene glycol hydrogel to overcome latex urinary catheter related problems. *Biofactors* **2007**, *30*, 217–225. [CrossRef]
41. Carlsson, S.; Weitzberg, E.; Wiklund, P.; Lundberg, J.O. Intravesical nitric oxide delivery for prevention of catheter-associated urinary tract infections. *Antimicrob. Agents Chemother.* **2005**, *49*, 2352–2355. [CrossRef]
42. Li, X.; Li, P.; Saravanan, R.; Basu, A.; Mishra, B.; Lim, S.H.; Su, X.; Tambyah, P.A.; Leong, S.S. Antimicrobial functionalization of silicone surfaces with engineered short peptides having broad spectrum antimicrobial and salt-resistant properties. *Acta Biomater.* **2014**, *10*, 258–266. [CrossRef] [PubMed]
43. Lehman, S.M.; Donlan, R.M. Bacteriophage-mediated control of a two-species biofilm formed by microorganisms causing catheter-associated urinary tract infections in an in vitro urinary catheter model. *Antimicrob. Agents Chemother.* **2015**, *59*, 1127–1137. [CrossRef] [PubMed]
44. Thallinger, B.; Brandauer, M.; Burger, P.; Sygmund, C.; Ludwig, R.; Ivanova, K.; Kun, J.; Scaini, D.; Burnet, M.; Tzanov, T.; et al. Cellobiose dehydrogenase functionalized urinary catheter as novel antibiofilm system. *J. Biomed. Mater. Res. B Appl. Biomater.* **2016**, *104*, 1448–1456. [CrossRef] [PubMed]
45. Santos, D.K.; Rufino, R.D.; Luna, J.M.; Santos, V.A.; Sarubbo, L.A. Biosurfactants: Multifunctional biomolecules of the 21st century. *Int. J. Mol. Sci.* **2016**, *17*, 401. [CrossRef]
46. Lovell, F.M. The structure of a bromine-rich marine antibiotic. *J. Am. Chem. Soc.* **1966**, *88*, 4510–4511. [CrossRef]
47. Nweze, J.A.; Mbaoji, F.N.; Huang, G.; Li, Y.; Yang, L.; Zhang, Y.; Huang, S.; Pan, L.; Yang, D. Antibiotics development and the potentials of marine-derived compounds to stem the tide of multidrug-resistant pathogenic bacteria, fungi, and protozoa. *Mar. Drugs* **2020**, *18*, 145. [CrossRef] [PubMed]
48. Bernan, V.S.; Greenstein, M.; Carter, G.T. Mining marine microorganisms as a source of new antimicrobials and antifungals. *Curr. Med. Chem. Anti-Infect. Agents* **2004**, *3*, 181–195. [CrossRef]
49. Visbeck, M. Ocean science research is key for a sustainable future. *Nat. Commun.* **2018**, *9*, 690. [CrossRef]
50. Penesyan, A.; Kjelleberg, S.; Ega, S. Development of novel drugs from marine surface associated microorganisms. *Mar. Drugs* **2010**, *8*, 438–459. [CrossRef]
51. Stowe, S.D.; Richards, J.J.; Tucker, A.T.; Thompson, R.; Melander, C.; Cavanagh, J. Anti-biofilm compounds derived from marine sponges. *Mar. Drugs* **2011**, *9*, 2010–2035. [CrossRef]
52. Mi, Y.; Zhang, J.; He, S.; Yan, X. New peptides isolated from marine cyanobacteria, an overview over the past decade. *Mar. Drugs* **2017**, *15*, 132. [CrossRef]

53. Seal, B.S.; Drider, D.; Oakley, B.B.; Brussow, H.; Bikard, D.; Rich, J.O.; Miller, S.; Devillany, E.; Kwan, J.; Bertin, G.; et al. Microbial-derived products as potential new antimicrobials. *Vet. Res.* **2018**, *49*, 66. [CrossRef] [PubMed]
54. Dyshlovoy, S.A.; Honecker, F. Marine compounds and cancer: The first two decades of XXI century. *Mar. Drugs* **2020**, *18*, 20. [CrossRef] [PubMed]
55. Satheesh, S.; Ba-akdah, M.A.; Al-Sofyani, A.A. Natural antifouling compound production by microbes associated with marine macroorganisms—A review. *Electron. J. Biotechn.* **2016**, *21*, 26–35. [CrossRef]
56. Mandakhalikar, K.D.; Chua, R.R.; Tambyah, P.A. New technologies for prevention of catheter associated urinary tract infection. *Curr. Treat. Options. Infect. Dis.* **2016**, *8*, 24–41. [CrossRef]
57. Younis, K.M.; Usup, G.; Ahmad, A. Secondary metabolites produced by marine streptomyces as antibiofilm and quorum-sensing inhibitor of uropathogen *Proteus mirabilis*. *Environ. Sci. Pollut. Res. Int.* **2016**, *23*, 4756–4767. [CrossRef]
58. Wang, J.; Nong, X.H.; Zhang, X.Y.; Xu, X.Y.; Amin, M.; Qi, S.H. Screening of antibiofilm compounds from marine-derived fungi and the effects of Secalonic Acid D on *Staphylococcus aureus* biofilm. *J. Microbiol. Biotechnol.* **2017**, *27*, 1078–1089. [CrossRef]
59. Costa, B.; Mota, R.; Tamagnini, P.; Martins, M.C.L.; Costa, F. Natural cyanobacterial polymer-based coating as a preventive strategy to avoid catheter-associated urinary tract infections. *Mar. Drugs* **2020**, *18*, 279. [CrossRef]
60. Rahman, H.; Austin, B.; Mitchell, W.J.; Morris, P.C.; Jamieson, D.J.; Adams, D.R.; Spragg, A.M.; Schweizer, M. Novel anti-infective compounds from marine bacteria. *Mar. Drugs* **2010**, *8*, 498–518. [CrossRef]
61. Tortorella, E.; Tedesco, P.; Esposito, F.P.; January, G.G.; Fani, R.; Jaspars, M.; De Pascale, D. Antibiotics from deep-sea microorganisms: Current discoveries and perspectives. *Mar. Drugs* **2018**, *16*, 355. [CrossRef]
62. Pereira, F. Have marine natural product drug discovery efforts been productive and how can we improve their efficiency? *Expert. Opin. Drug Discov.* **2019**, *14*, 717–722. [CrossRef]
63. Stickler, D.J.; Morgan, S.D. Observations on the development of the crystalline bacterial biofilms that encrust and block Foley catheters. *J. Hosp. Infect.* **2008**, *69*, 350–360. [CrossRef]
64. Zhang, S.; Liang, X.; Gadd, G.M.; Zhao, Q. Advanced titanium dioxide-polytetrafluoroethylene (TiO2-PTFE) nanocomposite coatings on stainless steel surfaces with antibacterial and anti-corrosion properties. *Appl. Surf. Sci.* **2019**, *490*, 231–241. [CrossRef]
65. Ndlovu, T.; Rautenbach, M.; Vosloo, J.A.; Khan, S.; Khan, W. Characterization and antimicrobial activity of biosurfactant extracts produced by *Bacillus amyloliquefaciens* and *Pseudomonas aeruginosa* isolated from a wastewater treatment plant. *AMB Express* **2017**, *7*, 108. [CrossRef]
66. Harshada, K. Biosurfactant: A potent antimicrobial agent. *J. Microbiol. Exp.* **2014**, *1*, 173–177. [CrossRef]
67. Gudiña, E.J.; Rocha, V.; Teixeira, J.A.; Rodrigues, L.R. Antimicrobial and anti-adhesive properties of biosurfactant produced by *lactobacilli* isolates, biofilm formation and aggregation ability. *J. Gen. Appl. Microbiol.* **2013**, *59*, 425–436.
68. Rienzo, M.A.D.D.; Stevenson, P.; Marchant, R.; Banat, I.M. Antibacterial properties of biosurfactants against selected Gram-positive and Gram-negative bacteria. *FEMS. Microbiol. Lett.* **2016**, *363*, fnv224. [CrossRef]
69. Rodrigues, L.; Banat, I.M.; Teixeira, J.; Oliveira, R. Biosurfactants: Potential applications in medicine. *J. Antimicrob. Chemother.* **2006**, *57*, 609–618. [CrossRef]
70. Paraszkiewicz, K.; Moryl, M.; Płaza, G.; Bhagat, D.; Satpute, S.K.; Bernat, P. Surfactants of microbial origin as antibiofilm agents. *Int. J. Environ. Heal. Res.* **2019**, *11*, 1–20. [CrossRef]
71. Liu, X.; Ren, B.; Chen, M.; Wang, H.; Kokare, C.R.; Zhou, X.; Wang, J.; Dai, H.; Song, F.; Liu, M.; et al. Production and characterization of a group of bioemulsifiers from the marine *Bacillus velezensis* strain H3. *Appl. Microbiol. Biotechnol.* **2010**, *87*, 1881–1893. [CrossRef]
72. Bonmatin, J.M.; Laprevote, O.; Peypoux, F. Diversity among microbial cyclic lipopeptides: Iturins and surfactins. Activity-Structure relationships to design new bioactive agents. *Comb. Chem. High. Throughput Screen.* **2003**, *6*, 541–556. [CrossRef]
73. Busscher, H.J.; Van Hoogmoed, C.G.; Geertsema-Doornbusch, G.I.; Van Der Kuijl-Booij, M.; Van Der Mei, H.C. *Streptococcus thermophilus* and its biosurfactants inhibit adhesion by *Candida* spp. on silicone rubber. *Appl. Environ. Microbiol.* **1997**, *63*, 3810–3817. [CrossRef]
74. Kasanah, N.; Hamann, M.T. Development of antibiotics and the future of marine microorganisms to stem the tide of antibiotic resistance. *Curr. Opin. Investig. Drugs* **2004**, *5*, 827–837.
75. Kapoor, G.; Saigal, S.; Elongavan, A. Action and resistance mechanisms of antibiotics: A guide for clinicians. *J. Anaesthesiol. Clin. Pharmacol.* **2017**, *33*, 300–305. [CrossRef]
76. Rourke, A.O.; Beyhan, S.; Choi, Y.; Morales, P.; Chan, A.P.; Espinoza, J.L.; Dupont, C.L.; Meyer, K.J.; Spoering, A.; Lewis, K.; et al. Mechanism-of-action classification of antibiotics by global transcriptome profiling. *Antimicrob. Agents Chemother.* **2020**, *64*, e01207–e01219.
77. Davies, J.; Davies, D. Origins and evolution of antibiotic resistance. *Microbiol. Mol. Biol. Rev.* **2010**, *74*, 417–433. [CrossRef]
78. Sun, D.; Jeannot, K.; Xiao, Y.; Knapp, C.W. Editorial: Horizontal gene transfer mediated bacterial antibiotic resistance. *Front. Microbiol.* **2019**, *10*, 1933. [CrossRef]
79. Rabin, N.; Zheng, Y.; Opoku-Temeng, C.; Du, Y.; Bonsu, E.; Sintim, H.O. Agents that inhibit bacterial biofilm formation. *Future Med. Chem.* **2015**, *7*, 647–671. [CrossRef]
80. Liang, Y.; Xie, X.; Chen, L.; Yan, S.; Ye, X.; Anjum, K.; Huang, H.; Lian, X.; Zhang, Z. Bioactive polycyclic quinones from marine *Streptomyces* sp. 182SMLY. *Mar. Drugs* **2016**, *14*, 10. [CrossRef]

81. Ramesh, C.; Vinithkumar, N.V.; Kirubagaran, R. Marine pigmented bacteria: A prospective source of antibacterial compounds. *J. Nat. Sci. Biol. Med.* **2019**, *10*, 104–113. [CrossRef]
82. Wiese, J.; Imhoff, J.F. Marine bacteria and fungi as promising source for new antibiotics. *Drug Dev. Res.* **2019**, *80*, 24–27. [CrossRef]
83. Hughes, C.C.; Fenical, W. Antibacterials from the sea. *Chemistry* **2010**, *16*, 12512–12525. [CrossRef] [PubMed]
84. Schumacher, R.W.; Talmage, S.C.; Miller, S.A.; Sarris, K.E.; Davidson, B.S.; Goldberg, A. Isolation and structure determination of an antimicrobial ester from a marine sediment-derived bacterium. *J. Nat. Prod.* **2003**, *66*, 1291–1293. [CrossRef]
85. Habbu, P.; Warad, V.; Shastri, R.; Madagundi, S.; Kulkarni, V.H. Antimicrobial metabolites from marine microorganisms. *Chin. J. Nat. Med.* **2016**, *14*, 101–116. [CrossRef]
86. Manivasagan, P.; Venkatesan, J.; Sivakumar, K.; Kim, S.K. Pharmaceutically active secondary metabolites of marine actinobacteria. *Microbiol. Res.* **2014**, *169*, 262–278. [CrossRef]
87. Stincone, P.; Brandelli, A. Marine bacteria as source of antimicrobial compounds. *Crit. Rev. Biotechnol.* **2020**, *40*, 306–319. [CrossRef] [PubMed]
88. Tareq, F.S.; Kim, J.H.; Lee, M.A.; Lee, H.; Lee, Y.; Lee, J.S.; Shin, H.J. Ieodoglucomides A and B from a marine derived bacterium *Bacillus licheniformis*. *Org. Lett.* **2012**, *14*, 1464–1467. [CrossRef]
89. Tareq, F.S.; Kim, J.H.; Lee, M.A.; Lee, H.S.; Lee, J.S.; Lee, Y.J.; Shin, H.J.V. Antimicrobial gageomacrolactins characterized from the fermentation of the marine-derived bacterium *Bacillus subtilis* under optimum growth conditions. *J. Agric. Food Chem.* **2013**, *61*, 3428–3434. [CrossRef] [PubMed]
90. Tareq, F.S.; Lee, M.A.; Lee, H.S.; Lee, Y.J.; Lee, J.S.; Hasan, C.M.; Islam, M.T.; Shin, H.J. Gageotetrins A–C, noncytotoxic antimicrobial linear lipopeptides from a marine bacterium *Bacillus subtilis*. *Org. Lett.* **2014**, *16*, 928–931. [PubMed]
91. Tareq, F.S.; Lee, M.A.; Lee, H.S.; Lee, Y.J.; Lee, J.S.; Hasan, C.M.; Islam, M.T.; Shin, H.J. Non-cytotoxic antifungal agents: Isolation and structures of gageopeptides A–D from a *Bacillus* strain 109GGC020. *J. Agric. Food. Chem.* **2014**, *62*, 5565–5572.
92. Podilapu, A.R.; Emmadi, M.; Kulkarni, S.S. Expeditious synthesis of ieodoglucomides A and B from the marine-derived bacterium *Bacillus licheniformis*. *Eur. J. Org. Chem.* **2018**, *2018*, 3230–3235. [CrossRef]
93. Uzair, B.; Menaa, F.; Khan, B.A.; Mohammad, F.V.; Ahmad, V.U.; Djeribi, R.; Menaa, B. Isolation, purification, structural elucidation and antimicrobial activities of kocumarin, a novel antibiotic isolated from actinobacterium *Kocuria marina* CMG S2 associated with the brown seaweed *Pelvetia canaliculata*. *Microbiol. Res.* **2018**, *206*, 186–197. [CrossRef]
94. Mondol, M.A.M.; Shin, H.J. Antibacterial and antiyeast compounds from marine-derived bacteria. *Mar. Drugs* **2014**, *12*, 2913–2921. [CrossRef]
95. Yang, S.C.; Lin, C.H.; Sung, C.T.; Fang, J.Y. Antibacterial activities of bacteriocins: Application in foods and pharmaceuticals. *Front. Microbiol.* **2014**, *5*, 241.
96. Elayaraja, S.; Annamalai, N.; Mayavu, P.; Balasubramanian, T. Production, purification and characterization of bacteriocin from *Lactobacillus murinus* AU06 and its broad antibacterial spectrum. *Asian. Pac. J. Trop. Biomed.* **2014**, *4*, S305–S311. [CrossRef] [PubMed]
97. Lucas-Elío, P.; Gómez, D.; Solano, F.; Sanchez-Amat, A. The antimicrobial activity of marinocine, synthesized by *marinomonas mediterranea*, is due to hydrogen peroxide generated by its lysine oxidase activity. *J. Bacteriol.* **2006**, *188*, 2493–2501. [CrossRef]
98. Raju, R.; Khalil, Z.G.; Piggott, A.M.; Blumenthal, A.; Gardiner, D.L.; Skinner-Adams, T.S.; Capon, R.J. Mollemycin A: An antimalarial and antibacterial glyco-hexadepsipeptide-polyketide from an Australian marine-derived *Streptomyces* sp. (CMB-M0244). *Org. Lett.* **2014**, *16*, 1716–1719. [CrossRef]
99. Murphy, A.C.; Gao, S.S.; Han, L.C.; Carobene, S.; Fukuda, D.; Song, Z.; Hothersall, J.; Cox, R.J.; Crosby, J.; Crump, M.P.; et al. Biosynthesis of thiomarinol A and related metabolites of *Pseudoalteromonas* sp. SANK 73390. *Chem. Sci.* **2014**, *5*, 397–402. [CrossRef]
100. Braña, A.F.; Sarmiento-Vizcaíno, A.; Pérez-Victoria, I.; Otero, L.; Fernández, J.; Palacios, J.J.; Martín, J.; Cruz, M.D.L.; Díaz, C.; Vicente, F.; et al. Branimycins B and C, antibiotics produced by the abyssal Actinobacterium *Pseudonocardia carboxydivorans* M-227. *J. Nat. Prod.* **2017**, *80*, 569–573. [CrossRef]
101. Govindarajan, G.; Satheeja, S.V.; Jebakumar, S.R. Antimicrobial potential of phylogenetically unique actinomycete, *Streptomyces* sp. JRG-04 from marine origin. *Biologicals* **2014**, *42*, 305–311. [CrossRef] [PubMed]
102. Mangamuri, U.; Muvva, V.; Poda, S.; Naragani, K.; Munaganti, R.K.; Chitturi, B.; Yenamandra, V. Bioactive metabolites produced by *Streptomyces Cheonanensis* VUK-A from Coringa mangrove sediments: Isolation, structure elucidation and bioactivity. *3 Biotech* **2016**, *6*, 63. [CrossRef] [PubMed]
103. Bae, M.; Kim, H.; Moon, K.; Nam, S.; Shin, J.; Oh, K.; Oh, D. Mohangamides A and B, new dilactone-tethered pseudo-dimeric peptides inhibiting *Candida albicans* isocitrate lyase. *Org. Lett.* **2015**, *17*, 712–715. [CrossRef] [PubMed]
104. Subramenium, G.A.; Swetha, T.K.; Iyer, P.M.; Balamurugan, K.; Pandian, S.K. 5-hydroxymethyl-2-furaldehyde from marine bacterium *Bacillus subtilis* inhibits biofilm and virulence of *Candida albicans*. *Microbiol. Res.* **2018**, *207*, 19–32. [CrossRef] [PubMed]
105. Anjum, K.; Sadiq, I.; Chen, L.; Kaleem, S.; Li, X.; Zhang, Z.; Lian, X. Novel antifungal janthinopolyenemycins A and B from a co-culture of marine-associated *Janthinobacterium* spp. ZZ145 and ZZ148. *Tetrahedron Lett.* **2018**, *59*, 3490–3494. [CrossRef]
106. Wu, B.; Oesker, V.; Wiese, J.; Schmaljohann, R.; Imhoff, J.F. Two new antibiotic pyridones produced by a marine fungus, *Trichoderma* sp. strain MF106. *Mar. Drugs* **2014**, *12*, 1208–1219. [CrossRef]

107. Haga, A.; Tamoto, H.; Ishino, M.; Kimura, E.; Sugita, T.; Kinoshita, K.; Takahashi, K.; Shiro, M.; Koyama, K. Pyridone alkaloids from a marine-derived fungus, *Stagonosporopsis cucurbitacearum*, and their activities against azole-resistant *Candida albicans*. *J. Nat. Prod.* **2013**, *76*, 750–754. [CrossRef]
108. Yin, Q.; Liang, J.; Zhang, W.; Zhang, L.; Hu, Z.L.; Zhang, Y.; Xu, Y. Butenolide, a marine-derived broad-spectrum antibiofilm agent against both Gram-positive and Gram-negative pathogenic bacteria. *Mar. Biotechnol.* **2019**, *21*, 88–98. [CrossRef]
109. Böhringer, N.; Fisc, K.M.; Schillo, D.; Bara, R.; Hertzer, C.; Grein, F.; Eisenbarth, J.H.; Kaligis, F.; Schneider, T.; Wägele, H.; et al. Antimicrobial potential of bacteria associated with marine sea slugs from North Sulawesi, *Indonesia*. *Front. Microbiol.* **2017**, *8*, 1092. [CrossRef]
110. Rosa, C.F.C.; Freire, D.M.G.; Ferraz, E.C. Biosurfactant microfoam: Application in the removal of pollutants from soil. *J. Environ. Chem. Eng.* **2015**, *3*, 89–94. [CrossRef]
111. Giri, S.S.; Ryu, E.C.; Sukumaran, V.; Park, S.C. Antioxidant, antibacterial, and anti-adhesive activities of biosurfactants isolated from *Bacillus* strains. *Microbial. Pathog.* **2019**, *132*, 66–72. [CrossRef]
112. Kubicki, S.; Bollinger, A.; Katzke, N.; Jaeger, K.E.; Loeschcke, A.; Thies, S. Marine Biosurfactants: Biosynthesis, structural diversity and biotechnological applications. *Mar. Drugs* **2019**, *17*, 408. [CrossRef]
113. Sun, W.; Wang, Y.; Zhang, W.; Ying, H.; Wang, P. Novel surfactant peptide for removal of biofilms. *Coll. Surf. B. Biointerfaces* **2018**, *172*, 180–186. [CrossRef] [PubMed]
114. Fenibo, E.O.; Ijoma, G.N.; Selvarajan, R.; Chikere, C.B. Microbial surfactants: The next generation multifunctional biomolecules for applications in the petroleum industry and its associated environmental remediation. *Microorganisms* **2019**, *7*, 581. [CrossRef] [PubMed]
115. Gudiña, E.J.; Teixeira, J.A.; Rodrigues, L.R. Biosurfactants produced by marine microorganisms with therapeutic applications. *Mar. Drugs.* **2016**, *14*, 38. [CrossRef]
116. Naughton, P.J.; Marchant, R.; Naughton, V.; Banat, I.M. Microbial biosurfactants: Current trends and applications in agricultural and biomedical industries. *J. Appl. Microbiol.* **2019**, *127*, 12–28. [CrossRef] [PubMed]
117. Rodrigues, A.I.; Gudiña, E.J.; Teixeira, J.A.; Rodrigues, L.R. Sodium chloride effect on the aggregation behaviour of rhamnolipids and their antifungal activity. *Sci. Rep.* **2017**, *7*, 12907. [CrossRef]
118. Sen, S.; Borah, S.N.; Bora, A.; Deka, S. Production, characterization, and antifungal activity of a biosurfactant produced by *Rhodotorula babjevae* YS3. *Microb. Cell Factories* **2017**, *16*, 1–14. [CrossRef] [PubMed]
119. Desai, J.D.; Banat, I.M. Microbial production of surfactants and their commercial potential. *Microbiol. Mol. Biol. Rev.* **1997**, *61*, 47–64. [CrossRef]
120. Banat, I.M.; Franzetti, A.; Gandolfi, I.; Bestetti, G.; Martinotti, M.G.; Fracchia, L.; Smyth, T.J.; Marchant, R. Microbial biosurfactants production, applications and future potential. *Appl. Microbiol. Biotechnol.* **2010**, *87*, 427–444. [CrossRef]
121. Mani, P.; Dineshkumar, G.; Jayaseelan, T.; Deepalakshmi, K.; Kumar, C.G.; Balan, S.S. Antimicrobial activities of a promising glycolipid biosurfactant from a novel marine *Staphylococcus saprophyticus* SBPS 15. *3 Biotech* **2016**, *6*, 163. [CrossRef]
122. Dusane, D.H.; Pawar, V.S.; Nancharaiah, Y.V.; Venugopalan, V.P.; Kumar, A.R.; Zinjarde, S.S. Anti-biofilm potential of a glycolipid surfactant produced by a tropical marine strain of *Serratia marcescens*. *Biofouling* **2011**, *27*, 645–654. [CrossRef] [PubMed]
123. Kiran, G.S.; Sabarathnam, B.; Selvin, J. Biofilm disruption potential of a glycolipid biosurfactant from marine *Brevibacterium casei*. *FEMS. Immunol. Med. Microbiol.* **2010**, *59*, 432–438. [CrossRef]
124. Manivasagan, P.; Sivasankar, P.; Venkatesan, J.; Sivakumar, K.; Kim, S. Optimization, production and characterization of glycolipid biosurfactant from the marine actinobacterium, *Streptomyces* sp. MAB36. *Bioprocess Biosyst. Eng.* **2014**, *37*, 783–797. [CrossRef]
125. Kiran, G.S.; Sabarathnam, B.; Thajuddin, N.; Selvin, J. Production of glycolipid biosurfactant from spongeassociated marine actinobacterium *Brachybacterium paraconglomeratum* MSA21. *J. Surfactants. Deterg.* **2014**, *17*, 531–542. [CrossRef]
126. Marzban, A.; Ebrahimipour, G.; Danesh, A. Bioactivity of a novel glycolipid produced by a *Halophilic Buttiauxella* sp. and improving submerged fermentation using a response surface method. *Molecules* **2016**, *21*, 1256. [CrossRef] [PubMed]
127. Sumaiya, M.; Devi, C.A.; Leela, K. A study on biosurfactant production from marine bacteria. *Int. J. Sci. Res.* **2017**, *7*, 139–145.
128. Gandhimathi, R.; Kiran, G.S.; Hema, T.A.; Selvin, J.; Raviji, T.R.; Shanmughapriya, S. Production and characterization of lipopeptide biosurfactant by a sponge-associated marine actinomycetes *Nocardiopsis alba* MSA10. *Bioprocess Biosyst. Eng.* **2009**, *32*, 825–835. [CrossRef]
129. Balan, S.S.; Kumar, C.G.; Jayalakshmi, S. Aneurinifactin, a new lipopeptide biosurfactant produced by a marine *Aneurinibacillus aneurinilyticus* SBP-11 isolated from Gulf of Mannar: Purification, characterization and its biological evaluation. *Microbiol. Res.* **2017**, *194*, 1–9. [CrossRef] [PubMed]
130. Balan, S.S.; Kumar, C.G.; Jayalakshmi, S. Pontifactin, a new lipopeptide biosurfactant produced by a marine *Pontibacter korlensis* strain SBK-47: Purification, characterization and its biological evaluation. *Process. Biochem.* **2016**, *51*, 2198–2207. [CrossRef]
131. Lawrance, A.; Balakrishnan, M.; Joseph, T.C.; Sukumaran, D.P.; Valsalan, V.N.; Gopal, D.; Ramalingam, K. Functional and molecular characterization of a lipopeptide surfactant from the marine sponge-associated eubacteria *Bacillus licheniformis* NIOT-AMKV06 of Andaman and Nicobar Islands, India. *Mar. Pollut. Bull.* **2014**, *82*, 76–85. [CrossRef]
132. Anestopoulos, I.; Kiousi, D.E.; Klavaris, A.; Maijo, M.; Serpico, A.; Suarez, A.; Sanchez, G.; Salek, K.; Chasapi, S.A.; Zompra, A.A.; et al. Marine-derived surface active agents: Health-promoting properties and blue biotechnology-based applications. *Biomolecules* **2020**, *10*, 885. [CrossRef]

133. Tahmourespour, A.; Salehi, R.; Kermanshahi, R.K. *Lactobacillus Acidophilus*-derived biosurfactant effect on GTFB and GTFC expression level in *Streptococcus Mutans* biofilm cells. *Braz. J. Microbiol.* **2011**, *42*, 330–339. [CrossRef]
134. Hamza, F.; Satpute, S.; Banpurkar, A.; Kumar, A.R.; Zinjarde, S. Biosurfactant from a marine bacterium disrupts biofilms of pathogenic bacteria in a tropical aquaculture system. *FEMS Microbiol. Ecol.* **2017**, *93*, 140. [CrossRef]
135. Ohadi, M.; Forootanfar, H.; Dehghannoudeh, G.; Eslaminejad, T.; Ameri, A.; Shakibaie, M.; Adeli-Sardou, M. Antimicrobial, anti-biofilm, and anti-proliferative activities of lipopeptide biosurfactant produced by *Acinetobacter junii* B6. *Microb. Pathog.* **2020**, *138*, 103806. [CrossRef] [PubMed]
136. Silva, S.S.E.; Carvalho, J.W.P.; Aires, C.P.; Nitschke, M. Disruption of *Staphylococcus aureus* biofilms using rhamnolipid biosurfactants. *J. Dairy. Sci.* **2017**, *100*, 7864–7873. [CrossRef] [PubMed]
137. Mireles, J.R.; Toguchi, A.; Harshey, R.M. *Salmonella enterica* serovar typhimurium swarming mutants with altered biofilm-forming abilities: Surfactin inhibits biofilm formation. *J. Bacteriol.* **2001**, *183*, 5848–5854. [CrossRef]
138. Janek, T.; Krasowska, A.; Czyżnikowska, Ż.; Łukaszewicz, M. Trehalose lipid biosurfactant reduces adhesion of microbial pathogens to polystyrene and silicone surfaces: An experimental and computational approach. *Front. Microbiol.* **2018**, *9*, 2441. [CrossRef] [PubMed]
139. Falagas, M.E.; Makris, G.C. Probiotic bacteria and biosurfactants for nosocomial infection control: A hypothesis. *J. Hosp. Infect.* **2009**, *71*, 301–306. [CrossRef]
140. Hermansson, M. The DLVO theory in microbial adhesion. *Colloids Surf. B.* **1999**, *14*, 105–119. [CrossRef]
141. Katsikogianni, M.; Missirlis, Y.F. Concise review of mechanisms of bacterial adhesion to biomaterials and of techniques used in estimating bacteria-material interactions. *Eur. Cells. Mater.* **2004**, *8*, 37–57. [CrossRef] [PubMed]
142. Walencka, E.; Rozalska, S.; Sadowska, B.; Rozalska, B. The influence of *Lactobacillus acidophilus*-derived surfactants on *staphylococcal* adhesion and biofilm formation. *Folia Microbiol.* **2008**, *53*, 61–66. [CrossRef]
143. Meylheuc, T.; Oss, C.J.V.; Bellon-Fontaine, M.N. Adsorption of biosurfactant on solid surfaces and consequences regarding the bioadhesion of *Listeria monocytogenes* LO28. *J. Appl. Microbiol.* **2001**, *91*, 822–832. [CrossRef]
144. Jemil, N.; Ayed, H.B.; Manresa, A.; Nasri, M.; Hmidet, N. Antioxidant properties, antimicrobial and anti-adhesive activities of DCS1 lipopeptides from *Bacillus methylotrophicus* DCS1. *BMC Microbiol.* **2017**, *17*, 144. [CrossRef] [PubMed]
145. Kimkes, T.E.P.; Heinemann, M. How bacteria recognise and respond to surface contact. *FEMS Microbiol. Rev.* **2020**, *44*, 106–122. [CrossRef]
146. Gomes, M.Z.d.V.; Nitschke, M. Evaluation of rhamnolipid and surfactin to reduce the adhesion and remove biofilms of individual and mixed cultures of food pathogenic bacteria. *Food Control* **2012**, *25*, 441–447. [CrossRef]
147. Das, P.; Mukherjee, S.; Sen, R. Antiadhesive action of a marine microbial surfactant. *Colloids Surf. B Biointerfaces* **2009**, *71*, 183–186. [CrossRef]
148. Song, B.; Wang, Y.; Wang, G.; Liu, G.L.; Li, W.; Yan, F. The lipopeptide 6-2 produced by *Bacillus amyloliquefaciens* anti-CA has potent activity against the biofilm-forming organisms. *Mar. Pollut. Bull.* **2016**, *108*, 62. [CrossRef] [PubMed]
149. Pradhan, A.K.; Pradhan, N.; Mall, G.; Panda, H.T.; Sukla, L.B.; Panda, P.K.; Mishra, B.K. Application of lipopeptide biosurfactant isolated from a halophile: *Bacillus tequilensis* CH for inhibition of biofilm. *Appl. Biochem. Biotechnol.* **2013**, *171*, 1362–1375. [CrossRef]
150. Kiran, G.S.; Hema, T.A.; Gandhimathi, R.; Selvin, J.; Thomas, T.A.; Ravji, T.R.; Natarajaseenivasan, K. Optimization and production of a biosurfactant from the sponge-associated marine fungus *Aspergillus ustus* MSF3. *Colloids Surf. B. Biointerfaces* **2009**, *73*, 250–256. [CrossRef]
151. Khopade, A.; Ren, B.; Liu, X.Y.; Mahadik, K.; Zhang, L.; Kokare, C. Production and characterization of biosurfactant from marine *Streptomyces* species B3. *J. Colloid Interface Sci.* **2012**, *367*, 311–318. [CrossRef]
152. Kavita, K.; Singh, V.K.; Mishra, A.; Jha, B. Characterisation and anti-biofilm activity of extracellular polymeric substances from Oceanobacillus iheyensis. *Carbohydr. Polym.* **2014**, *101*, 29–35. [CrossRef]
153. Gu, H.; Lee, S.W.; Carnicelli, J.; Zhang, T.; Ren, D. Magnetically driven active topography for long-term biofilm control. *Nat. Commun.* **2020**, *11*, 2211. [CrossRef] [PubMed]
154. Milo, S.; Hathaway, H.; Nzakizwanayo, J.; Alves, D.R.; Esteban, P.P.; Jonesc, B.V.; Jenkins, A.T.A. Prevention of encrustation and blockage of urinary catheters by *Proteus mirabilis* via pH-triggered release of bacteriophage. *J. Mater. Chem. B* **2017**, *5*, 5403–5411. [CrossRef] [PubMed]
155. Jordan, R.P.C.; Nicolle, L.E. *Biofilms in Infection Prevention and Control*; Academic Press: Cambridge, MA, USA, 2014; pp. 287–309.
156. Costa, B.; Mota, R.; Parreira, P.; Tamagnini, P.; Martins, M.C.L.; Costa, F. Broad-spectrum anti-adhesive coating based on an extracellular polymer from a marine cyanobacterium. *Mar. Drugs* **2019**, *17*, 243. [CrossRef] [PubMed]

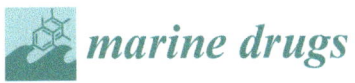

Review

Research Strategies to Develop Environmentally Friendly Marine Antifouling Coatings

Yunqing Gu [1], Lingzhi Yu [1], Jiegang Mou [1,*], Denghao Wu [1], Maosen Xu [1], Peijian Zhou [1] and Yun Ren [2]

1. College of Metrology &Measurement Engineering, China Jiliang University, Hangzhou 310018, China; guyunqing@cjlu.edu.cn (Y.G.); s1902080449@cjlu.edu.cn (L.Y.); wdh@cjlu.edu.cn (D.W.); msxu@zjut.edu.cn (M.X.); 19a0205122@cjlu.edu.cn (P.Z.)
2. Zhijiang College, Zhejiang University of Technology, Shaoxing 312030, China; renyun_ry@hotmail.com
* Correspondence: mjg@cjlu.edu.cn

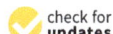

Received: 22 June 2020; Accepted: 16 July 2020; Published: 18 July 2020

Abstract: There are a large number of fouling organisms in the ocean, which easily attach to the surface of ships, oil platforms and breeding facilities, corrode the surface of equipment, accelerate the aging of equipment, affect the stability and safety of marine facilities and cause serious economic losses. Antifouling coating is an effective method to prevent marine biological fouling. Traditional organic tin and copper oxide coatings are toxic and will contaminate seawater and destroy marine ecology and have been banned or restricted. Environmentally friendly antifouling coatings have become a research hotspot. Among them, the use of natural biological products with antifouling activity as antifouling agents is an important research direction. In addition, some fouling release coatings without antifoulants, biomimetic coatings, photocatalytic coatings and other novel antifouling coatings have also developed rapidly. On the basis of revealing the mechanism of marine biofouling, this paper reviews the latest research strategies to develop environmentally friendly marine antifouling coatings. The composition, antifouling characteristics, antifouling mechanism and effects of various coatings were analyzed emphatically. Finally, the development prospects and future development directions of marine antifouling coatings are forecasted.

Keywords: antifouling mechanism; antifouling coating; antifoulant; environmentally friendly; polymer

1. Introduction

Marine fouling organisms refer to the general term for all kinds of marine organisms attached to the surface of marine facilities and causing damage to human marine economy [1]. Marine fouling organisms not only endanger the development of the marine economy, but also hinder human exploitation of the ocean. At present, more than 4000 marine fouling organisms have been discovered [2], such as microorganisms mainly including bacteria, diatoms and Ulva spores, etc.; large fouling organisms mainly include barnacles, bryozoans, mussels and algae.

Various fouling organisms easily attach to ships, oil platforms and breeding facilities in the ocean [3]. Barnacles and other invertebrates are firmly attached to the hull surface by secreting a biological adhesive. As the barnacle grows, its edges will destroy the anticorrosion layer on the hull surface, thereby accelerating the hull corrosion [4]. As shown in Figure 1 [5], when the hull surface is attached, fouling organisms will corrode the hull surface and increase the roughness of the hull surface, thereby reducing the speed of the ship [6–8], increasing fuel consumption and greenhouse gas emissions [9,10]. In recent years, with the rapid development of offshore industries such as submarine oil and marine power generation, the damage of marine fouling organisms to man-made facilities has become more severe. For example, when an offshore oil platform is attached, it will increase the weight of the facility and weaken its ability to resist tsunami and storm risks. In addition, fouling organisms can block drainage pipes, jeopardizing the safety and service life of marine facilities. Some marine fouling organisms enter the non-native land by attaching to the bottom of the ship, thereby causing biological invasion and causing great harm to the global marine ecology [11]. Every year, a lot of money is invested in ship surface cleaning and maintenance of marine facilities. With the continuous development of the human marine economy, the economic losses caused by marine fouling organisms are getting larger and larger, thus, effective and economic prevention methods are getting more and more attention.

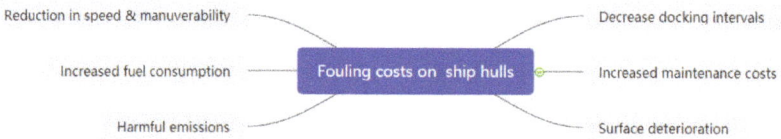

Figure 1. Hull attached to fouling organisms [5].

The key to managing biological attachment is to block biological attachment from the source. Applying antifouling coating is currently the easiest and most widely used antifouling method. Traditional antifouling coating often use poisonous drugs to poison fouling organisms, the main components of which are organic tin [12] and cuprous oxide. However, the accumulation of metal elements in metal compounds in fish and shellfish will cause biological variation and death and pollute seawater, and thus harm the marine ecological environment. Taking into account the greater harm of organic tin to the marine environment [13], organic tin coatings have been banned worldwide. Although cuprous oxide is less toxic, as it continues to accumulate, its impact on marine ecology will become greater and greater. Therefore, the development of efficient and environmentally friendly marine antifouling coatings has become a research hotspot [14].

There are two main research directions for new antifouling coatings. One direction is to develop non-toxic and environmentally friendly antifoulants that replace metal compounds, that is, to find antifouling active substances from the ocean. An antifoulant developed by marine natural products can effectively reduce the harm to the environment, which is also one of the hot issues in current research [2,15]. In addition, some terrestrial biological products have also attracted attention. The purification or modification of natural products through chemical methods can obtain antifoulants with extremely strong antifouling capabilities. The second direction focuses on fouling release coatings, which will modify the surface characteristics of the material, making it difficult for fouling organisms to adhere or make them easier to remove after attachment. Due to the complex diversity of the marine environment, it is becoming more and more difficult for a single mechanism of antifouling coating to meet the requirements of use, and some composite antifouling coatings that combine multiple antifouling principles have also appeared. With the development and application of nanotechnology and polymer materials, the antifouling ability of antifouling coatings has been further improved [16].

This article first reveals the fouling mechanism of marine fouling organisms. On this basis, it mainly summarizes the development status of environmentally friendly antifouling coatings in three aspects from antifoulant type antifouling coatings, fouling release antifouling coatings and other important antifouling coatings. Our analysis reveals the antifouling mechanism of various antifouling coatings, and reviews the advantages and disadvantages of the new coating. Finally, the development trend of marine antifouling coatings is forecasted.

2. Formation Mechanism of Fouling

In order to better solve the problem of marine biological fouling, it is necessary to understand how the attachment of marine fouling organisms to the surface of objects occurs. Marine biological fouling is a process where biological communities accumulate on the surface of materials. The process is complex. As shown in Figure 2, biological fouling can be divided into three stages: conditioned film, micro-fouling and macro-fouling.

(1) Conditioned film [17]: When a clean surface is placed in seawater, a layer of organic matter, including polysaccharides, lipids and protein molecules, will accumulate within minutes. The physical adsorption of these molecules on the surface of the material causes the accumulation of organic molecules to form a thin film, which is usually called the conditioned film. This adsorption is reversible, relying only on weak non-covalent bond forces, such as van der Waals forces, electrostatic forces and hydrogen bonding.

(2) Micro-fouling [18,19]: After the conditioned film is formed, bacteria and diatoms and other microorganisms will adhere to the conditioned film within 24 h, and floating bacteria will gather on the surface. These attached bacteria and algae will secrete new extracellular polymers (EPS) in order to further improve their fixation ability with the material surface or conditioned film, thereby forming a biofilm composed of water, organic matter, microorganisms and extracellular metabolites. This process is irreversible, and this process is called micro-fouling.

(3) Macro-fouling [20]: The formation of micro-fouling can further aggravate the generation of biological fouling. Biofilms provide abundant food and nutrition for the attachment of larvae of multicellular species and large marine organisms. Barnacles, shellfish and other large fouling organisms adhere to and grow within a few days, and complex biomes slowly form, and large-scale fouling will form in a few months. This is called macro-fouling. This process can be completed within 1–2 months and organisms can be attached to the surface for several years.

However, this model cannot apply to all marine fouling organisms. The actual fouling of the ocean is sometimes not in this order. For example, the cyprids of barnacle *Amphibalanus amphitrite* can adhere to the surface of materials without biofilm.

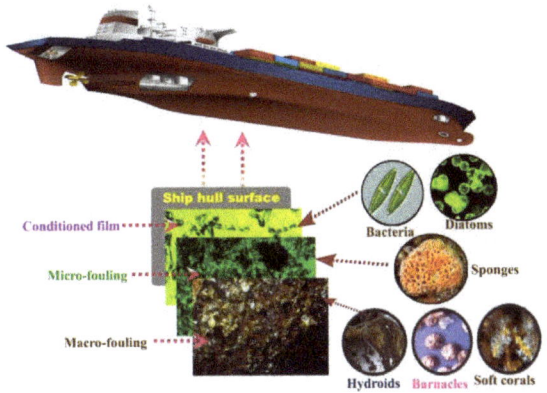

Figure 2. Hull surface fouling process and main fouling organisms [5].

3. Marine Antifouling Coating

Thus far, the application of antifouling coating is the most effective means of antifouling. Self-polishing copolymer-based coatings containing TBT had high efficiency in preventing the settlement and growth of marine fouling organisms, thus they were once used widely. However, they were globally banned in 2008 due to their persistent toxicity to non-target organisms. It is time to develop environmentally friendly systems to prevent marine biofouling. Table 1 summarizes the current popular research directions of environmentally friendly marine antifouling coating.

Table 1. Main research directions of marine antifouling coatings.

Type	Components	Mechanism	Characteristic	Referent
Coatings with antifoulant	Chemical antifoulant.	Poisoning or inhibiting biological growth.	Currently widely used; There are hidden environmental hazards.	[12–16]
	Natural product antifoulant.	Inhibiting settlement and adhesion of marine organisms.	Difficult or expensive to obtain; It is hard to retain activity.	[21–49]
Fouling release coatings	Silicone; Organic fluorine.	Low surface energy makes organisms difficult to attach.	Commercially available; Vulnerable; Low efficiency at static.	[50–54]
Biomimetic coatings	Micro-structured surfaces.	Increase the difficulty of attaching fouling organisms.	Poor effect; It is hard to be applied.	[55–68]
Other	Photocatalytic Antifouling Coating.	Photocatalysis enhances surface oxidizability and reducibility.	Have almost no effect at night and in deep sea.	[69–71]
	Nano-composite coating.	Strong sterilization ability; Hydrophobic.	Enhance the compatibility of other ingredients.	[72–74]

3.1. Natural Product Antifoulant

Cuprous oxide antifouling coatings have been used widely in today's marine ship. However, it also has potential environmental risks. Because the copper element in the cuprous oxide coating is enriched in the ocean, it causes a lot of death of seaweed and destroys the ecological balance, and will eventually be restricted or banned. In order to prevent the antifouling coating from harming the ecological environment, the researchers tried to find useful substances from nature to replace copper-based coatings. At present, the research of new antifoulants mainly focuses on the extraction and optimization of natural products. Many natural substances extracted from animals and plants have a good antifouling effect [21]. Compounds such as terpenoids, steroids, carotenoids, phenolics, furanones, alkaloids, peptides and lactones extracted from the ocean all have antifouling activity [22,23]. Irritation substances extracted from terrestrial plants such as oleander and pepper are also important sources of antifoulants.

3.1.1. Marine Products with Antifouling Activity

Some marine organisms produce certain metabolites that inhibit fouling biological activity, which helps to develop pollution-free antifoulants composed of natural products [24]. In the past few years, some marine biological products with anti-pollution function have been discovered [25,26]. For example, Zhang et al. [27] discovered subergorgic acid (SA) from *Subergorgia suberosa*, which proves that it is non-toxic and has a strong inhibitory effect on attachments. In addition, Zhang et al. [28] conducted an in-depth study on the structure-activity relationship of SA and found that both ketone carbonyl and the double bond are necessary elements with antifouling activity. The experimental scheme is shown in Figure 3. Firstly, the esterification product 1 was readily obtained from SA using CH_3I and K_2CO_3; secondly, $NaBH_4$ or $LiAIH_4$ was used to reduce ketone carbonyl to hydroxyl group; thirdly, LiOH(3eq)/TFH/H_2O was used, trying to remove the methyl to give 3; finally, a strong oxidant 30%H_2O_2/TFA was used to modify the double bond of SA into two hydroxyl groups to obtain product 4. Products 1 and 2 still have antifouling activity, while products 3 and 4 have no antifouling activity, thus, ketone carbonyl and double bond groups are necessary elements for antifouling effect. On this basis, benzyl esters and methylene chains with proven antifouling activity were added to SA to form new SA derivatives. According to the methods depicted in Figure 3b, with dry DMF as solvent and

K$_2$CO$_3$ as base, SA can smoothly react with various benzyl halides and quantitatively obtain the desired benzyl ester. As shown in Figure 3c, using SA and dibromoalkanes of various lengths as starting materials, compounds 15–20 were easily synthesized in good yields. The antifouling test results show that the antifouling effect of all benzyl esters of SA is basically the same or stronger than that of SA containing unsubstituted benzyl rings. The results also show that the antifouling effect of SA derivatives containing methylene chains is not as good as that of SA, and the influence of the length of methylene chains on the antifouling effect of SA derivatives depends on the functional group at the opposite position of the methylene chain. The impact of this type of antifouling agent on non-target marine life needs further testing. However, the antifouling active functional groups proved in its experiments have certain value for the research of antifouling compounds.

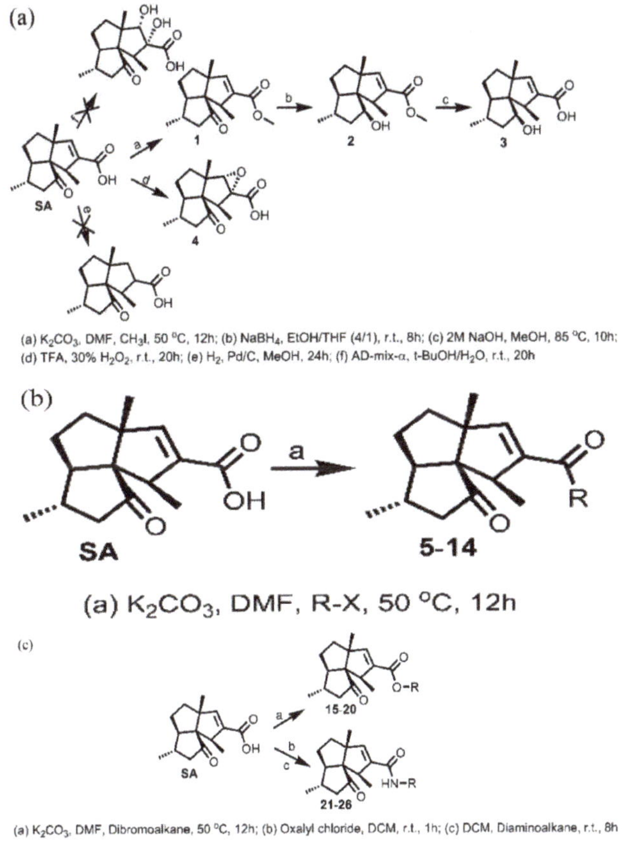

Figure 3. Research and preparation of subergorgic acid (SA) compounds. (**a**) Identification of bioactive functional groups of SA. (**b**) Synthesis of benzyl esters of SA. (**c**) Synthesis of SA derivatives containing methylene chain of various lengths [28].

In nature, marine organisms have evolved many biological strategies to interact with microorganisms to protect themselves from pathogens or from being parasitized. [29]. In particular, sponges and their associated microbiota produce compounds that interfere with quorum sensing (QS) mechanisms [30,31]. Quorum sensing is a synchronization mechanism within a bacterial population. The bacteria use QS to communicate, regulate their behavior and assess their population density. The use of marine biological secretions to interfere with bacterial QS can effectively inhibit the formation of bacterial biofilms, making it difficult for other organisms to attach [32]. Tintillier et al. [33] studied the marine sponge *Pseudoceratina sp. 2081* and isolated four new tetrabromotyrosine derivatives exhibiting antifouling and quorum sensing inhibition (QSi) properties. Structures of the isolated bromotyrosine metabolites is showed in Figure 4. They tested the antifouling activity of 6 kinds of extracts. Among the six compounds tested, the most active were 1, 3 and 5. The mode of action of those compounds are not based on toxicity. They operate through a targeted mode of action on bacteria and microalgae, as they only affect adherence and not growth.

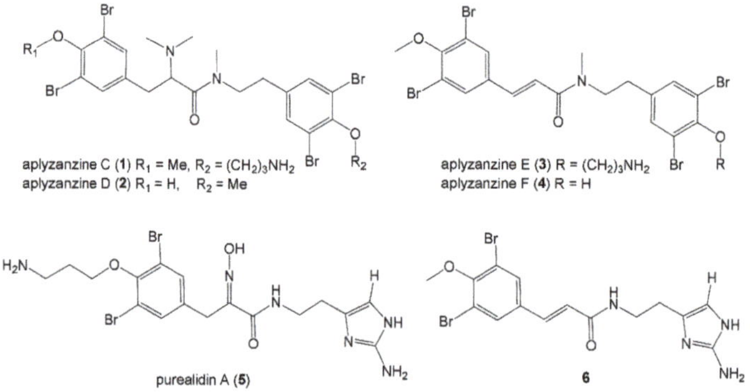

Figure 4. Structures of the isolated bromotyrosine metabolites [33].

Indole derivatives found in bryozoans and ascidians have been shown to have antifouling effects [34]. However, due to the uncontrollable release rate of indole derivatives in antifouling coatings, the effect of antifouling coatings with added indole derivatives is poor. Feng et al. [35] prepared acrylate resins suspending the indole derivative structure in their side chain by the free-radical polymerization. Its preparation method and antifouling principle are shown in Figure 5. The prepared indole derivatives have good antibacterial and algae inhibiting effects. The self-polishing rate of the acrylate resin polymerized with indole derivatives is reduced, thereby obtaining a long-term self-polishing effect. The dynamic simulation measurements and static immersion measurements of the coating were performed to study in the marine environment. The results show that acrylate resin containing indole derivatives has long-lasting efficacy in biological control and the acrylate resins suspending the indole derivative structure in their side chain can make fouling organisms difficult to grow. In addition, indole derivatives inhibit the marine algae growth by interfering with the equilibrium of calcium ions in algal cells and decreasing the abundance of cellular Ca^{2+} [36]. Under the action of seawater, the acrylic resin continuously renews its surface through the hydrolysis of ester groups. This self-polishing property makes attached organisms easily fall off the surface, exposing new indole derivative structures. Therefore, the combination of these two functions of the resins can significantly improve their antifouling properties. Since indole derivatives are easily degraded by microorganisms, they will not cause a great impact on the ecological environment.

Most marine fouling organisms secrete bio-gum to enhance surface adhesion. Bio-glue is a protein, and many biological enzymes in nature can degrade proteins. The essence of biological enzyme is protein, which is easy to decompose, causes no pollution and will not damage the marine ecology, thus, the biological enzyme with antifouling function is an ideal antifoulant. Wang et al. [37] isolated a marine proteolytic bacterial strain of *Bacillus velezensis* from sea mud and found that the protease produced by it had obvious inhibitory effects on barnacles, diatoms and mussels. This method uses bacteria to obtain proteases, which has the possibility of mass production. However, because marine fouling organisms secrete complex binders, polysaccharides and even lipids, it is difficult to control marine fouling by a single protease. Therefore, in the application research of enzyme-based environmental protection antifouling materials, it is necessary to use a combination of several enzymes to control marine antifouling.

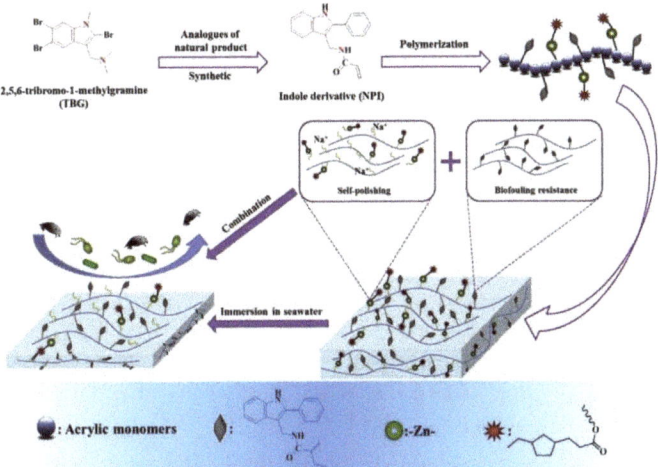

Figure 5. Preparation process and working mechanism of acrylate resin with indole derivatives [35].

Currently, these marine biological antifoulant usually cannot obtain a sufficient amount from the ocean, and are difficult to chemically synthesize at low cost, thus, to a certain extent, it is still difficult to commercially mass-produce. However, it is important to develop a more perfect antifoulant by studying its antifouling mechanism through chemical methods and exploring the functions of various groups.

3.1.2. Terrestrial Products with Antifouling Activity

Terrestrial organisms are also a valuable source of natural antifoulants. Compared with marine life, many terrestrial plants are easy to produce commercially because of their wide distribution or large-scale cultivation [38]. Liu et al. [39] isolated four cardenolides from *Nerium oleander L.* and evaluated their antifouling activity and toxicity to non-target organisms. The result showed that all of the tested compounds showed a strong inhibitory activity against barnacle settlement, with very low or moderate toxicity to non-target organisms. Their antifouling effect far exceeds that of TBT, Irgarol and copper. However, before it is widely used, its degradability and toxicity to non-target organisms need further study.

Chalcone is a compound commonly found in natural products. Celery was once the main source of chalcone, and now it is mainly synthesized by chemical means. Almeida et al. [40] studied the synthesis methods of 16 kinds of chalcone derivatives and studied the antifouling properties and ecotoxicity of chalcone through biological experiments. The results show that chalcone can effectively prevent the settlement of mussel larvae and inhibit the accumulation of other fouling microorganisms. In addition, they proved that these compounds have low ecotoxicity and clarified their great potential in the field of marine antifouling. Sathicq et al. [41] evaluated the synthetic furan-based chalcone antifouling coatings. They used furan rings instead of B rings to make a variety of different furylchalcones antifouling coatings, and conducted field experiments. Experimental results show that: using furylchalcones as an antifouling coating is an effective means of preventing marine fouling organisms; the synthesis of furylchalcone is simple and efficient, which is beneficial to reduce economic costs; furylchalcone is degradable, having little impact on the marine environment. Despite this, the mechanism of action of chalcone derivatives as antifoulant is not yet clear, thus, it is necessary to thoroughly understand the toxicity of furanyl chalcone in non-target marine organisms before applying it to the marine environment.

Camphor extracted from the trunk of camphor tree is a terpene natural organic compound, which can also be synthesized in large quantities by chemical means [42]. It is often used to repel insects and mosquitoes in daily life. In theory, it is a potential compound with antifouling capabilities [43]. Borneol extracted from herbs such as lavender and chamomile is a crystalline cyclic alcohol. Borneol-based polymer, isobornyl methacrylate (IBOMA) has been proven to have a strong activity against bacterial infections and can be used to prepare antibacterial coatings [44]. Hu et al. [45] synthesized an environmentally friendly antifouling coating based on antibacterial polymer (IBOMA) and natural antifouling agent (camphor). The prepared coating can slowly degrade in sea water and release borneol. Borneol itself has antibacterial properties [46], and at the same time, it provides a self-renewing surface to prevent dirt from sticking. In addition, camphor was released, providing a special antibiosis and antifouling surface with sterilized polymers to play a synergistic antifouling effect. Due to the hydrolysis of acrylic silicone resin and the increase in carboxylate content after immersion, the hydrophobicity of the coating surface quickly becomes dehydrated. The experiment proves that the produced coating can be controlled and slowly released, and has a continuous effect. Marine testing has shown the great potential of the coating, but the coating still needs a longer time to evaluate.

Capsaicin extracted from chili is a spicy vanillin amide alkaloid with antibacterial effects and is also regarded as a natural non-toxic antifoulant [47]. Wang et al. [48] conducted extensive research on capsaicin and its derivatives and reported six capsaicin derivatives for the first time, proving that capsaicin and its derivatives have excellent antifouling properties. Liu et al. [49] used capsaicin as an antifoulant and used high-density polyethylene (HDPE) as a substrate to make an antifouling coating by flame spray. Capsaicin, HDPE and coating preparation methods are shown in Figure 6. Compared with the raw materials, the morphology and grain size of capsaicin in the coating have changed significantly, and the coating has significant antibacterial and antifouling capabilities. In addition, capsaicin can be extracted from capsicum relatively easily, thus, this antifouling technology has low cost and high feasibility, and is suitable for widespread promotion.

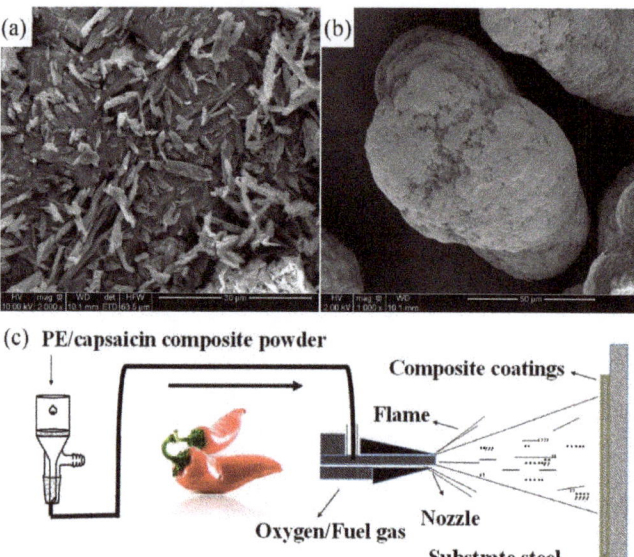

Figure 6. Capsaicin coating raw materials and preparation method. (**a**) FESEM image of the starting capsaicin powder; (**b**) FESEM image of the starting high-density polyethylene (HDPE) powder; (**c**) the fabrication route for the HDPE–capsaicin antifouling coatings [49].

Biological antifoulants come from a wide range of sources, and the effect is quite excellent. However, the method of extracting it from organisms is still difficult to use on a large scale. Even though some biologically active substances can be artificially synthesized, it is far less convenient than metal compounds. In addition, natural product antifouling agents may have ecotoxicity, that is, they might be toxic to non-target organisms. Therefore, for the research of natural antifouling agents, we should not only pay attention to their antifouling properties, but also explore their ecotoxicity.

3.2. Fouling Release Coatings

The fouling release coatings (FRC) itself does not contain antifoulants, mainly to use the dual characteristics of fouling organisms that are difficult to attach to the surface of low surface energy materials or easy to desorb on the surface to prevent or reduce the attachment of marine fouling organism. Compared with traditional self-polishing antifouling coatings (SPC), FRC uses its own physical properties to hinder the attachment of fouling organisms, and will not release antifouling agents into the ocean, thereby not causing pollution to the marine environment.

Biological attachment behavior has a direct relationship with the surface characteristics of materials. Different surfaces have different or even opposite effects on biological adhesion. Low surface energy coatings mainly inhibit the attachment of fouling organisms by physical means, that is, the use of the characteristics that fouling organisms are difficult to attach to the surface of low surface energy materials to prevent or reduce the attachment of marine fouling organisms. Research shows that when the surface energy is less than 25 mJ/m^2, that is, the contact angle between the coating and the liquid is greater than 98°, and it can effectively reduce the adhesion of fouling organism [50]. At present, this type of antifouling coating mainly includes two major categories of silicone and organic fluorine.

3.2.1. Organic Fluorine

In fluorine-containing polymers, due to the strong electronegativity of fluorine atoms, low polarizability and high C-F bond energy (460 kJ/mol), these materials are given high chemical stability and oleophobic and hydrophobic properties [51]. Arukalam et al. [52] prepared a perfluorodecyltrichlorosilane-based poly (dimethylsiloxane)-ZnO (FDTS-based PDMS-ZnO) nanocomposite coatings with surface energies within 20–30 mN/m for possible antifouling and anti-corrosion applications. ZnO is that the coating has antibacterial ability and changes the roughness of the coating surface, thereby improving its anti-adhesion ability. FDTS can modify the surface energy of the coating to keep its surface energy within 20–30 mN/m. Electrochemical impedance spectroscopy (EIS) test shows that the coating has excellent corrosion resistance. These characteristics mean that this coating has a good application prospect in the field of marine antifouling. Xu et al. [53] prepared a polymer with pendant branched poly (ethylene glycol) (PEO) and poly (2,2,2-trifluoroethyl methacrylate) (PFMA) structural units. The structure is shown in Figure 7. The b-PFMA-PEO asymmetric molecular brush with its side chains densely distributed with the same repeat unit is used to prepare a fluorine-containing synergistic nonfouling/fouling-release surface. A spin-cast thin film of the b-PFMA-PEO asymmetric molecular brush exhibits a synergistic antifouling property, in which PEO side chains endow the surface with a nonfouling characteristic, whereas PFMA side chains display the fouling-release functionality because of their low surface energy. Compared with the bare surface, the protein adsorption of the surface of the coating containing asymmetric molecular brushes is reduced by 45–75%, and the cell adhesion is reduced by 70–90%, showing considerable antifouling performance.

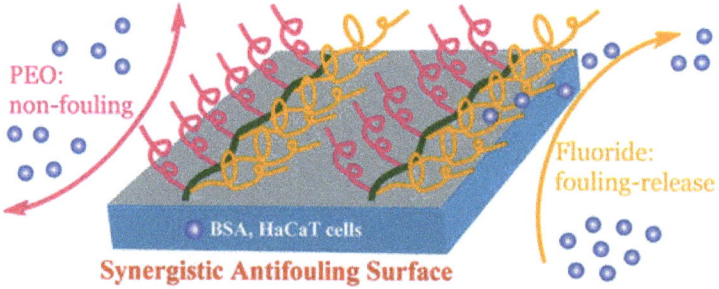

Figure 7. The structure of synergistic antifouling surface [53].

3.2.2. Silicone

Due to the high price and difficulty in preparation, fluoropolymers currently have few commercial products, and silicone polymer antifouling coatings have become a research and development hotspot. The silicone polymer has good desorption ability, and can easily make marine fouling organisms fall off by brushing or flowing. For example, PDMS has a combination of low surface energy and low elastic modulus, and it has gradually become the base of most antifouling coatings. Selim et al. [54] prepared a super-hydrophobic PDMS-Ag@SiO$_2$ core-shell nanocomposite antifouling coating using the modified Stöber methods. The formation process of the coating is shown in Figure 8. The Ag@SiO$_2$ core-shell nanofiller was inserted into the surface of the PDMS material by the solution casting method, and a strong coating was formed according to the hydrazination curing mechanism. The water contact angle (WCA) of the coating was determined to be 156°, and the surface free energy was 11.15 mJ/m^2. Biological tests prove that the coating has significant inhibitory effects on different bacterial strains, yeasts and fungi.

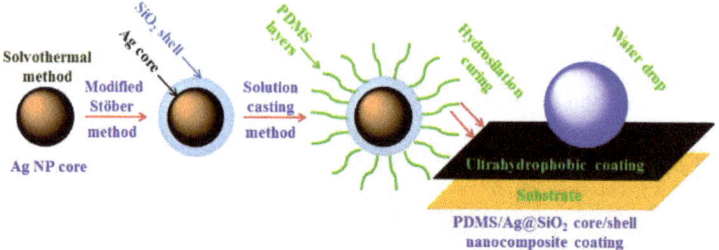

Figure 8. Schematic diagram of Ag@SiO$_2$ core-shell nanosphere structure [54].

Low surface energy coatings do not require the use of antifoulant and they generally have a smooth surface, which is of great significance for reducing the navigation resistance of the vessels and reducing fuel consumption. The obvious disadvantage of low surface energy coatings is the poor adhesion on the hull surface. In practical applications, intermediate coatings must be used to enhance the adhesion of the coatings, which complicates the coating application process and increases the cost of use. Compared with other types of coatings, low surface energy coatings are more easily destroyed. In addition, most low surface energy coatings have poor desorption ability to strong adherent organisms such as diatoms.

3.3. Biomimetic Antifouling Coating

Biomimetic antifouling coating, also known as microstructured surface antifouling coating, its mechanism of action is to destroy the physical attachment of marine organic matter by preparing a surface similar to the microstructure contained in the biological epidermis. For example, the skin or surface of sharks, shells, etc. [55,56] all have different structures of microstructures. This microstructured surface plays an important role in preventing or inhibiting the pollution of barnacles, algae and bacteria. The current main methods of making microstructured surfaces include laser etching [57], photolithography [58], three-dimensional (3D) printing [59], etc.

The shark skin surface structure has been extensively studied due to its drag reduction [60,61] and antifouling properties, and its various microstructures have been proven [62,63]. For example, in order to further study the antifouling effect of bionic shark skin, Pu et al. [64] prepared the biomimetic shark skin using the polydimethylsiloxane (PDMS)-embedded elastomeric stamping (PEES) method. PDMS itself is a low surface energy antifouling material, which has a certain antifouling ability, but it is prone to bioaccumulation in static or low flow state. The surface microstructure of shark skin is constructed on PDMS material, and the coating still has a low surface energy and exhibits extremely strong hydrophobicity. Air is hidden in the surface microstructure to form a thin layer of air, which can effectively reduce the interaction between the surface and protein molecules. Therefore, it is difficult for the protein to adhere to the surface and inhibit the attachment of some fouling organisms. The structure of shark skin and biomimetic shark skin is shown in Figure 9. Marine field tests show that the hydrophobicity of the PDMS material itself and the surface microstructure can effectively prevent the attachment of marine fouling organisms.

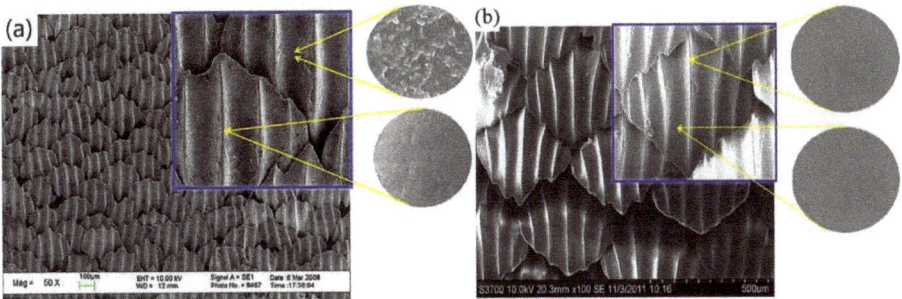

Figure 9. SEM images of shark skin and biomimetic shark skin: (**a**) the riblet structures of shark surface; (**b**) the surface of biomimetic shark skin prepared [64].

In marine environment, *Laminaria japonica* still has excellent antifouling ability in a relatively static state compared to those parade creatures. Zhao et al. [65] reported the synergistic effect between surface topography and chemical modification, and used sodium alginate and guanidine-hexamethylenediamine-PEI to replicate the surface microstructure on the surface of PDMS replicas by a layer-by-layer assembly method. The production process is shown in Figure 10. The water contact angle of PDMS with a microstructured surface is reduced to 35.3°, which is more hydrophilic. After the algae test and the bacteria test, the surface has extremely strong antifouling performance, and the antibacterial ability is up to 96.2 ± 1.3%.

Lotus leaf surface is one of the most famous superhydrophobic surfaces and displays excellent anti-biofouling performances [66,67]. Jiang et al. [68] investigate the super-repellency of the lotus leaf towards the bacterial medium, together with its mechanical bactericidal activity against the attached bacteria, and for the first time reveal the synergistic antibacterial effects of its bacterial repellency and physical rupture by nanotubes. They designed and developed a hierarchically structured superhydrophobic surface integrated with regularly spaced micro-pillar arrays and packed nanoneedles. This surface can remarkably prolong its efficiency under much harsh conditions with respect to the conventional superhydrophobic surfaces, without causing any potential antimicrobial resistance. Schematic illustration of fabrication procedure of lotus leaf-like structures is shown in Figure 11, and the microscale structure of the surface is showed in Figure 12. The surface static water contact angle exceeds 170°, and the rolling angle is less than 1°. The surface's anti-adhesion efficiency for *E. coli* can reach more than 99%. A small amount of adhered bacteria can be completely killed, effectively overcoming the disadvantages of bacteria adhesion accumulation on the surface of a single structure sterilization.

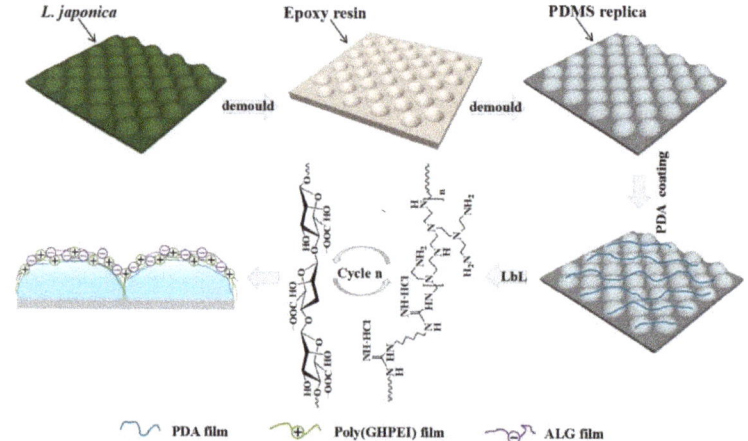

Figure 10. Schematic diagram of material preparation process [65].

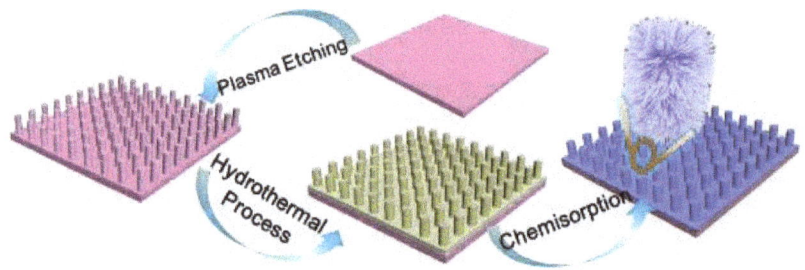

Figure 11. Schematic illustration of fabrication procedure of lotus leaf-like structures [68].

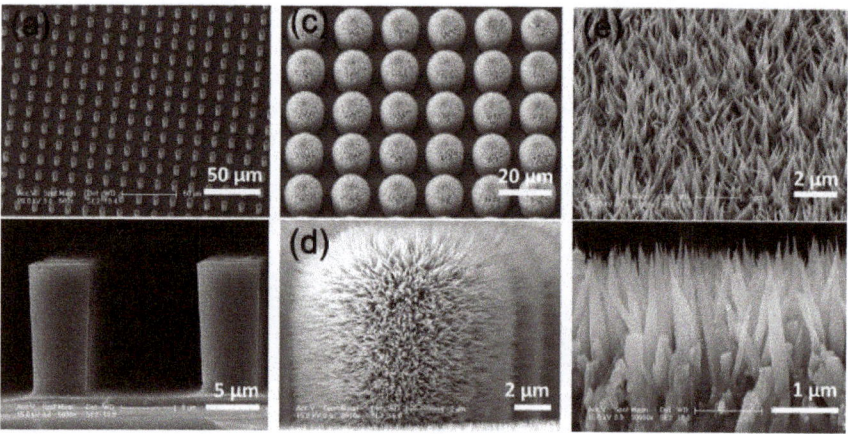

Figure 12. Microscale structure of different scales on the patterned surface [68].

The biomimetic antifouling coating contains no antifoulant and will not release compounds into the sea water. It is an eco-friendly antifouling coating. However, the construction of surface microstructures is more complicated, it is difficult to repair after damage and it is less effective in real marine environments. With the rapid development of Micro-Electro-Mechanical System (MEMS) and laser repair technologies, bionic antifouling coatings are still a promising development direction.

3.4. Photocatalytic Antifouling Coating

The use of photocatalytic to enhance the antifouling ability of the hull has attracted the attention of many scholars [69]. When some nanocomposites are exposed to sunlight, their surfaces exhibit strong oxidizing and reducing properties. Considering both economic and ecological aspects, this method has no pollution and low cost. TiO_2 nanocrystals are widely used materials that modify coating surfaces to provide considerable mechanical reinforcement and surface wettability. Selim et al. [70] conducted an in-depth study on photocatalytic antifouling coatings, and prepared a PDMS/TiO_2 hybrid nanocomposite. Its preparation method and action mechanism are shown in Figure 13. When sunlight illuminates TiO_2 nanoparticles, it will excite carriers such as electrons and holes. The photogenerated electrons are transferred from the valence band to the conduction band, while the holes remain in the valence band. The electrons in the conduction band can be reduced to superoxide anion radicals, and the holes with strong oxidizing ability can oxidize water to produce hydroxyl groups. Hydroxyl groups still have strong oxidizing properties, which can attack the unsaturated bonds of organic substances or extract H atoms of organic substances to generate new free radicals. The chain reaction is excited and the bacteria are decomposed. In addition, the modified material exhibits strong hydrophilicity, which will produce a thin water film on the surface to block the adhesion of fouling organisms.

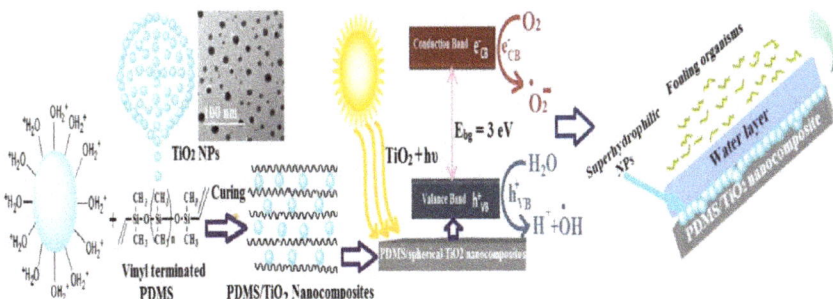

Figure 13. Preparation and catalytic principle of silicone/TiO_2 nanocomposite [70].

However, because the band gap of TiO_2 nanoparticles is 4% of sunlight, they can only absorb ultraviolet rays. Therefore, it is necessary to further improve the visible light absorption effect of the material. Zhang et al. [71] synthesized a new visible light-sensitive $InVO_4$/$AgVO_3$ photocatalyst with a PN node structure through ion exchange and in-situ growth process. Its mechanism of action is shown in Figure 14. When the bacteria come into contact with the catalyst, the H^+ and O^{2-} ions catalyzed by the surface of $InVO_4$/$AgVO_3$ will destroy these cell walls and cell membranes, resulting in severe cell rupture, cell effluent and DNA molecule destruction. About 99.9999% of *Pseudomonas aeruginosa* (*P. aeruginosa*), *Escherichia coli* (*E. coli*) and *Staphylococcus aureus* (*S. aureus*) were killed over 0.5 $InVO_4$/$AgVO_3$ at 30 min.

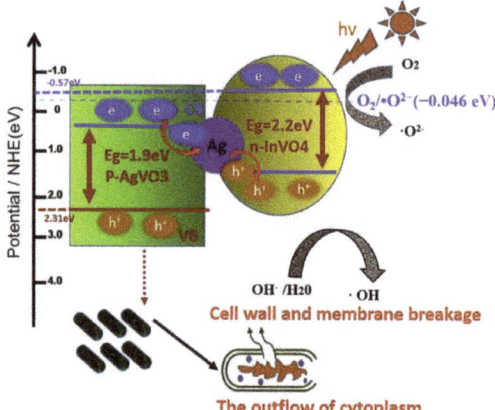

Figure 14. Mechanism of InVO$_4$/AgVO$_3$ under light [71].

3.5. Nano-Composite Antifouling Coating

Due to the diversity of the working environment and the increased use requirements, it is difficult to achieve a better antifouling effect with a single performance antifouling coating. Composite antifouling coatings have become the mainstream of current antifouling coatings research [72]. Tian et al. [73] prepared a series of composite antifouling coatings consisting of silicone elastomer and nanocomposite hydrogel. They use AgNPs as cross-linking agents to improve the compatibility of hydrogels and PDMS, combine different antifouling mechanisms together, and improve the antifouling performance of hybrid coatings. The preparation principle of the coating is shown in Figure 15. Silicone and hydrogel work together to improve the desorption ability of the coating. Nanoparticles AgNPs are not only used to enhance the compatibility of silicone and hydrogel, but also make the coating have a bactericidal effect. After soaking in seawater for two years, the surface of the coating has no barnacles nor other scaling phenomena, further verifying its antifouling ability.

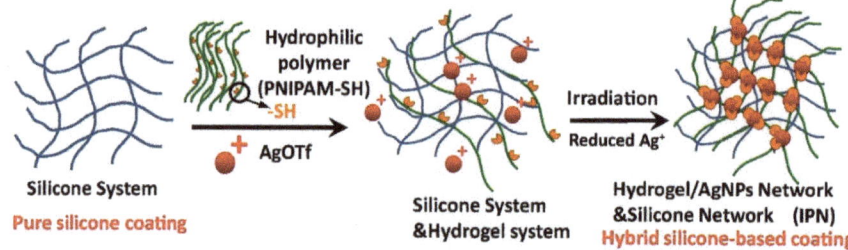

Figure 15. Schematic illustration of the formation of the pure silicone film and the hybrid coatings [73].

Selim et al. [74] prepared a superhydrophobic coating of silicone/β-MnO$_2$ nanorod composite for marine antifouling. They studied how the self-cleaning and antifouling features were affected by controlling the β-MnO$_2$ nanorod preparation and distribution in the silicone matrix. The preparation method of β-MnO$_2$ and the construction method of the coating are shown in Figure 16. PDMS, as the substrate of the coating, is itself a low surface energy coating. By using β-MnO$_2$ nanorods to construct a rough structure on the surface of PDMS, the coating is made superhydrophobic. The composite coating prevents fouling organisms from adhering through super-hydrophobicity and low surface energy. In addition, β-MnO$_2$ nanomaterials also enhance the stability of the coating to temperature and PH.

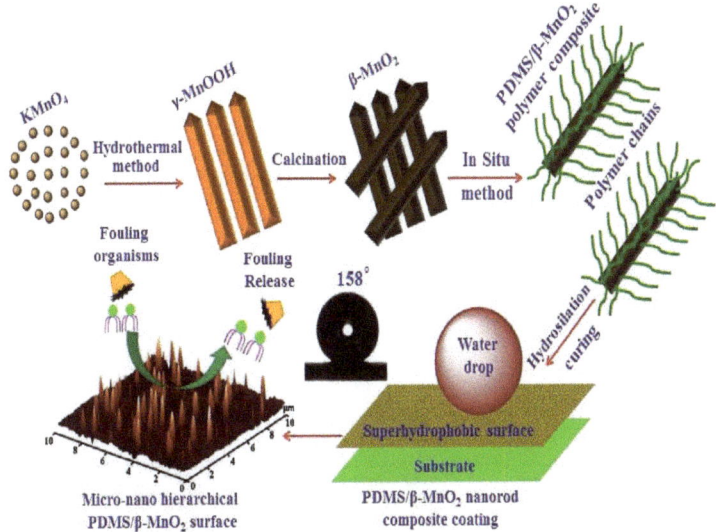

Figure 16. The preparation method of β-MnO₂ and the construction method of the coating [74].

3.6. Other Antifouling Coatings

In addition to the several coatings introduced above, some novel research results have emerged in recent years. These novel coatings have novel ideas and are expected to become new hot spots in antifouling coatings.

3.6.1. Microcapsules Coating

Li et al. [75] prepared a form of environment-friendly microcapsules through mini-emulsion polymerization as show in Figure 17. They used zinc acrylate resin to wrap the synthetic microcapsules into a coating, and investigated the slow release efficiency and antifouling effect of the coating. The microcapsules had a poly(urea-formaldehyde) (PUF) shell and a mixed core of silicone oil and capsaicin. Dimethyl silicone oil has low surface tension, good water repellency, good lubricity and has the characteristics of pollution resistance, antifouling, anti-adhesion and so on. Capsaicin extracted from natural peppers does not destroy the biological chain, and can be used as a marine antifouling agent to kill plant spores and animal larvae attached to the outer surface of ships. It has broad application prospects in the field of antifouling materials. PUF microcapsules can combine multiple ingredients to delay the release rate of silicone oil and capsaicin, and extend the service life of the coating. Since the surface of the microcapsule antifouling paint has a micro-nano raised structure and the internal material can be slowly released, it has good hydrophobicity and antifouling properties. The release rate of the antifouling agents from the coating is determined by their slow release from the microcapsules to the surrounding coating matrix, and the encapsulated biocide is protected from degradation. This research has certain guiding significance for the development of long-term antifouling coatings.

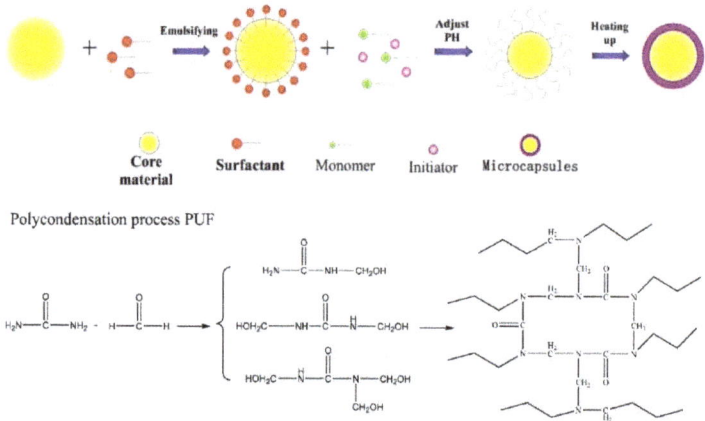

Figure 17. Mechanism of urea-formaldehyde microcapsule formation [75].

3.6.2. Dynamic Surface Antifouling

Xie et al. [76] first proposed the concept of Dynamic Surface Antifouling (DSA). The dynamic surface refers to a changing surface that continuously renews itself in seawater and thus decreases the adhesion of biofouling. Based on this strategy, they developed a series of biodegradable and reproducible polymer dynamic surface coatings, which have excellent antifouling properties and mechanical properties. The dynamic surface can shorten the contact time between the organisms and the surface, and make the interaction between them close to non-adhesion, thereby reducing the interaction force between the surface and the fouling organisms, making the fouling organisms difficult to attach. For degradable polymers, the surface renewal is a spontaneous process where water flow is not necessary. They developed degradable self-polishing copolymers (DSPC), made of poly (ester-co-silyl methacrylate) [77]. They inserted ester bonds into the backbone of a silyl acrylate copolymer for the first time by copolymerizing 2-methylene-1, 3-dioxepane (MDO), tributylsilyl methacrylate (TBSM) and methyl methacrylate (MMA) via radical ring opening polymerization (RROP). The degradable main chains can significantly improve the erosion of the TBSM based copolymer and avoid swelling. Consequently, the coating has excellent antifouling properties during static immersion in seawater. In addition, this type of coating can be used as a carrier and release control system for antifouling agents.

3.6.3. Oil-Infused Polymers

Oil-infused 'slippery' polymer surfaces and engineered surface textures have been separately shown to reduce settlement or adhesion strength of marine biofouling organisms. Kommeren et al. [78] created liquid-infused surfaces embossed with surface structures. They used a photo-embossing process to create perfluorinated oil-infused fluorinated meth (acrylate) coatings with tuneable surface topography. Figure 18 showed the changed in coating surface morphology with the addition of oil-infused. Oil-infused polymers are made by exposing bulk polymeric materials such as fluoropolymer or PDMS to an excess of a chemically-matched oil, such as silicone or perfluorinated oils. The polymers absorb the oil, leaving a thin liquid layer on the material surface and a reservoir of oil in the bulk polymer. This allows oil to diffuse to the interface and replenish the surface liquid layer as it becomes depleted. The antifouling coating of this strategy can effectively resist bacterial adhesion under static and flowing conditions. The performance of the coating can be adjusted by controlling the surface fluctuations, thus, the coating can adapt to a variety of use environments.

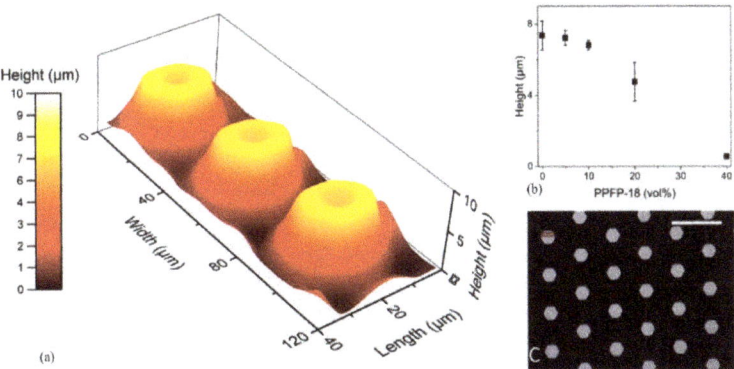

Figure 18. Microstructure of the coating surface. (**a**) A three-dimensional (3D) height profile of the photo-embossed features in a polymerized coating without the addition of perfluorinated oil. (**b**) Measured feature height. (**c**) Micrograph of coating surface. [78].

3.6.4. Sol-Gel Coating

Sol-gel derived functional coatings are commercially available for many practical applications and are emerging as suitable non-toxic alternatives to biocidal antifouling coatings. The sol-gel process provides the capacity to include inorganic and organic components at the nanometric scale. The surface energy of sol-gel is low and through modification can change the hydrophobicity and hydrophilicity of its surface. Richards et al. [79] studied several novel transparent sol-gel materials and determined their effectiveness as antifouling coatings for potential application to marine deployed sensors, camera lenses, solar panels or other related technologies. They developed a range of sol-gel coating with increasing water surface wettability and roughness. The surface energy of antifouling coatings was altered by modification of surface chemistry, while surface topology was roughened by the incorporation of amorphous fumed silica within the sol-gel. A future application of this work would be to incorporate sol gel coatings on the optical windows of sensors to reduce early stage fouling.

3.6.5. Coating Based on a Synergistic Strategy

Xie et al. [80] designed a new type of antifouling costing with a longer period of validity based on a synergistic antifouling strategy. As shown in Figure 19, the antifouling paint is made of polyacrylates, tert-butyldimethylsilyl methacrylate (TBSM), eugenol methacrylate (EM) and poly(vinylpyrrolidone) (PVP). EM can add eugenol groups to the coating covalently, so that the coating has the function of contact inhibition. PVP can enhance the hydrophilicity of the coating to block biological adhesion. Eugenol can be gradually released into the sea water to expel marine life. Methyl methacrylate (MMA) ethyl acrylate (EA) and n-butyl acrylate (BA) are used in the coating to enhance the mechanical properties and adhesion of the coating, thereby improving the durability of the coating. TBSM can make the coating have a stable hydrolysis rate, so that eugenol can be released stably. Antifouling tests show that the coating can effectively prevent protein adsorption, bacterial adhesion and diatom adhesion. The actual marine environment test shows that the validity period of the coating is at least 8 months. This research has created conditions for the development of environmentally friendly, efficient and long-lasting antifouling paints.

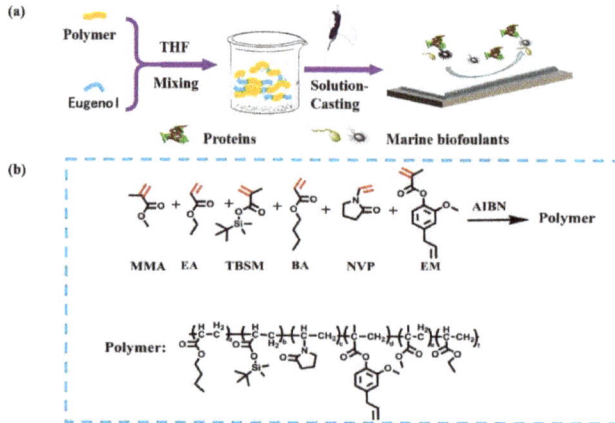

Figure 19. Preparation of synergistic antifouling coating [80]. (**a**) Schematic diagram of coating preparation. (**b**) Synthesis of key copolymer PAPS-EM.

4. Concluding Remarks

Every year, marine fouling organisms cause huge economic losses, and antifouling coating is currently the most direct and effective means of prevention. It is important to develop stable, durable and environmentally friendly antifouling coatings. The current antifouling coatings are difficult to cover in terms of stability, toxicity and cost of use, which seriously hinders its popularization and use. In the future, the research and use of marine antifouling coating will surely develop in the direction of being highly efficient, non-toxic, non-polluting and degradable.

Antifouling coating containing antifoulant mostly outperform coatings without antifoulant. It is imperative to develop new and highly effective antifoulant to replace cuprous oxide, which is currently widely used. Obtaining natural antifouling substances from nature, especially extracting antifouling active substances from marine organisms, is the most ideal source of antifoulants. Through in-depth research on the antifouling mechanism of natural antifouling active substances, the development of highly effective and non-polluting antifouling agents is an important direction of the development of antifoulants. In addition, releasable coatings are environmentally friendly and have potential development prospects. The fouling release coating is mostly suitable for ships with high speed and fast travel, and it is less effective for ships that are moored for a long time or traveling at low speed.

Coatings that rely on a single antifouling mechanism cannot achieve the desired antifouling effect, and future trend will need to integrate multiple methods. Composite coatings that integrate multiple antifouling mechanisms will surely become a research hotspot, especially some nano-composite and modified coatings. With the use of nanotechnology, marine antifouling technology has been greatly improved. When the material reaches the nanometer level, its performance will change qualitatively, and the surface performance of the coating or the release efficiency of the antifoulant will be significantly improved. In addition, combining antifoulant with fouling release coatings is also an important development direction.

Author Contributions: Conceptualization and design, Y.G., L.Y. and J.M.; Writing—manuscript preparation, Y.G., L.Y. and D.W.; Writing—review and editing, L.Y., M.X., P.Z. and Y.R. All authors have read and agreed to the published version of the manuscript.

Funding: This research was funded by the Zhejiang Provincial Natural Science Foundation of China (LY19E050003) and by the National Natural Science Foundation of China (51779226).

Conflicts of Interest: The authors declare no conflict of interest.

References

1. Schultz, M.P.; Bendick, J.A.; Holm, E.R.; Hertel, W.M. Economic impact of biofouling on a naval surface ship. *Biofouling* **2011**, *27*, 87–98. [CrossRef] [PubMed]
2. Satheesh, S.; Ba-akdah, M.A.; Al-Sofyani, A.A. Natural antifouling compound production by microbes associated with marine macroorganisms—A review. *Electron. J. Biotechnol.* **2016**, *21*, 26–35. [CrossRef]
3. Dafforn, K.A.; Lewis, J.A.; Johnston, E.L. Antifouling strategies: History and regulation, ecological impacts and mitigation. *Mar. Pollut. Bull.* **2011**, *62*, 453–465. [CrossRef] [PubMed]
4. Lejars, M.; Margaillan, A.; Bressy, C. Fouling release coatings: A nontoxic alternative to biocidal antifouling coatings. *Chem. Rev.* **2012**, *112*, 4347–4390. [CrossRef]
5. Selim, M.S.; Shenashen, M.A.; El-Safty, S.A.; Higazy, S.A.; Selim, M.M.; Isago, H.; Elmarakbi, A. Recent progress in marine foul-release polymeric nanocomposite coatings. *Prog. Mater. Sci.* **2017**, *87*, 1–32. [CrossRef]
6. Schultz, M.P. Effects of coating roughness and biofouling on ship resistance and powering. *Biofouling* **2007**, *23*, 331–341. [CrossRef]
7. Gu, Y.Q.; Yu, S.W.; Mou, J.G.; Wu, D.H.; Zheng, S.H. Research progress on the collaborative drag reduction effect of polymers and surfactants. *Materials* **2020**, *13*, 444. [CrossRef] [PubMed]
8. Gu, Y.Q.; Mou, J.G.; Dai, D.S.; Zheng, S.H.; Jiang, L.F.; Wu, D.H.; Ren, Y.; Liu, F.Q. Characteristics on drag reduction of bionic jet surface based on earthworm's back orifice jet. *Acta Phys. Sin.* **2015**, *64*, 024701.
9. Dupraz, V.; Stachowski-Haberkorn, H.S.; Ménard, D.; Limon, G.; Akcha, F.; Budzinski, H.; Cedergreen, N. Combined effects of antifouling biocides on the growth of three marine microalgal species. *Chemosphere* **2018**, *209*, 801–814. [CrossRef]
10. Feng, D.Q.; He, J.; Chen, S.Y.; Su, P.; Ke, C.H.; Wang, W. The plant alkaloid camptothecin as a novel antifouling compound for marine paints: Laboratory bioassays and field trials. *Mar. Biotechnol.* **2018**, *20*, 623–638. [CrossRef]
11. Miralles, L.; Ardura, A.; Arias, A.; Borrell, Y.J.; Clusa, L.; Dopico, E.; de Rojas, A.H.; Lopez, B.; Munoz-Colmenero, M.; Roca, A.; et al. Barcodes of marine invertebrates from north Iberian ports: Native diversity and resistance to biological invasions. *Mar. Pollut. Bull.* **2016**, *112*, 183–188. [CrossRef]
12. Maia, F.; Silva, A.P.; Fernandes, S.; Cunha, A.; Almeida, A.; Tedim, J.; Zheludkevich, M.L.; Ferreira, M.G.S. Incorporation of biocides in nanocapsules for protective coatings used in maritime applications. *Chem. Eng. J.* **2015**, *270*, 150–157. [CrossRef]
13. Ytreberg, E.; Bighiu, M.A.; Lundgren, L.; Eklund, B. XRF measurements of tin, copper and zinc in antifouling paints coated on leisure boats. *Environ. Pollut.* **2016**, *213*, 594–599. [CrossRef] [PubMed]
14. Selim, M.S.; El-Safty, S.A.; El-Sockary, M.A.; Hashem, A.I.; Elenien, O.M.A.; El-Saeed, A.M.; Fatthallah, N.A. Modeling of spherical silver nanoparticles in silicone-based nanocomposites for marine antifouling. *RSC Adv.* **2015**, *5*, 63175–63185. [CrossRef]
15. Qian, P.Y.; Li, Z.R.; Xu, Y.; Fusetani, N. Mini-review: Marine natural products and their synthetic analogs as antifouling compounds: 2009–2014. *Biofouling* **2015**, *31*, 101–122. [CrossRef]
16. Sun, Z.Z.; Yang, L.; Zhang, D.; Bian, F.G.; Song, W.L. High-performance biocompatible nano-biocomposite artificial muscles based on a renewable ionic electrolyte made of cellulose dissolved in ionic liquid. *Nanotechnology* **2019**, *30*, 285503. [CrossRef] [PubMed]
17. Yebra, D.M.; Kiil, S.; Weinell, C.E.; Dam-Johansen, K. Presence and effects of marine microbial biofilms on biocide-based antifouling paints. *Biofouling* **2006**, *22*, 33–41. [CrossRef]
18. Rosenhahn, A.; Schilp, S.; Kreuzer, H.J.; Grunze, M. The role of "inert" surface chemistry in marine biofouling prevention. *Phys. Chem. Chem. Phys.* **2010**, *12*, 4275–4286. [CrossRef] [PubMed]
19. Magin, C.M.; Cooper, S.P.; Brennan, A.B. Non-toxic antifouling strategies. *Mater. Today* **2010**, *13*, 36–44. [CrossRef]
20. Callow, J.A.; Callow, M.E. Trends in the development of environmentally friendly fouling-resistant marine coatings. *Nat. Commun.* **2011**, *2*, 244. [CrossRef] [PubMed]
21. Wang, Q.C.; Uzunoglu, E.; Wu, Y.; Libera, M. Self-assembled poly (ethylene glycol)-co-acrylic acid microgels to inhibit bacterial colonization of synthetic surfaces. *ACS Appl. Mater. Interfaces* **2012**, *4*, 2498–2506. [CrossRef] [PubMed]

22. Almeida, J.R.; Vasconcelos, V. Natural antifouling compounds: Effectiveness in preventing invertebrate settlement and adhesion. *Biotechnol. Adv.* **2015**, *33*, 343–357. [CrossRef] [PubMed]
23. Chen, C.L.; Maki, J.S.; Rittschof, D.; Teo, S.L.M. Early marine bacterial biofilm on a copper-based antifouling paint. *Int. Biodeterior. Biodegrad.* **2013**, *83*, 71–76. [CrossRef]
24. Qian, P.Y.; Wong, Y.H.; Zhang, Y. Changes in the proteome and phosphoproteome expression in the bryozoan *Bugula neritina* larvae in response to the antifouling agent butenolide. *Proteomics* **2010**, *10*, 3435–3446. [CrossRef] [PubMed]
25. Zhang, Y.F.; Zhang, H.M.; He, L.S.; Liu, C.D.; Xu, Y.; Qian, P.Y. Butenolide inhibits marine fouling by altering the primary metabolism of three target organisms. *ACS Chem. Biol.* **2012**, *7*, 1049–1058. [CrossRef]
26. Li, Y.X.; Zhang, F.Y.; Xu, Y.; Matsumura, K.; Han, Z.; Liu, L.L.; Lin, W.H.; Jia, Y.X.; Qian, P.Y. Structural optimization and evaluation of butenolides as potent antifouling agents: Modification of the side chain affects the biological activities of compounds. *Biofouling* **2012**, *28*, 857–864. [CrossRef]
27. Zhang, J.; Liang, Y.; Liao, X.J.; Deng, Z.; Xu, S.H. Isolation of a new butenolide from the South China Sea gorgonian coral *Subergorgia suberosa*. *Nat. Prod. Res.* **2014**, *28*, 150–155. [CrossRef]
28. Zhang, J.; Ling, W.; Yang, Z.Q.; Liang, Y.; Zhang, L.Y.; Guo, C.; Wang, K.L.; Zhong, B.L.; Xu, S.H.; Xu, Y. Isolation and structure-activity relationship of subergorgic acid and synthesis of its derivatives as antifouling agent. *Mar. Drugs* **2019**, *17*, 101. [CrossRef]
29. Puglisi, M.P.; Sneed, J.M.; Sharp, K.H.; Ritson-Williams, R.; Paul, V.J. Marine chemical ecology in benthic environments. *Nat. Prod. Rep.* **2019**, *31*, 1510–1553. [CrossRef]
30. Borges, A.; Simoes, M. Quorum sensing inhibition by marine bacteria. *Mar. Drugs* **2019**, *17*, 427. [CrossRef]
31. Saurav, K.; Borbone, N.; Burgsdorf, I.; Teta, R.; Caso, A.; Bar-Shalom, R.; Esposito, G.; Britstein, M.; Steindler, L.; Costantino, V. Identification of quorum sensing activators and inhibitors in the marine sponge sarcotragus spinosulus. *Mar. Drugs* **2020**, *18*, 127. [CrossRef] [PubMed]
32. Toupoint, N.; Mohit, V.; Linossier, I.; Bourgougnon, N.; Myrand, B.; Olivier, F.; Lovejoy, C.; Tremblay, R. Effect of biofilm age on settlement of mytilus edulis. *Biofouling* **2012**, *28*, 985–1001. [CrossRef] [PubMed]
33. Tintillier, F.; Moriou, C.; Petek, S.; Fauchon, M.; Hellio, C.; Saulnier, D.; Ekins, M.; Hooper, J.N.A.; AI-Mourabit, A.; Debitus, C. Quorum sensing inhibitory and antifouling activities of new bromotyrosine metabolites from the polynesian sponge *pseudoceratina* n. sp. *Mar. Drugs* **2020**, *18*, 272. [CrossRef]
34. Penez, N.; Culioli, G.; Perez, T.; Briand, J.F.; Thomas, O.P.; Blache, Y. Antifouling properties of simple indole and purine alkaloids from the Mediterranean gorgonian paramuricea clavata. *J. Nat. Prod.* **2011**, *74*, 2304–2308. [CrossRef] [PubMed]
35. Feng, K.; Ni, C.H.; Yu, L.M.; Zhou, W.J.; Li, X. Synthesis and evaluation of acrylate resins suspending indole derivative structure in the side chain for marine antifouling. *Colloids Surf. B Biointerfaces* **2019**, *184*, 110518. [CrossRef] [PubMed]
36. Chen, L.G.; Qian, P.Y. Review on molecular mechanisms of antifouling compounds: An update since 2012. *Mar. Drugs* **2017**, *15*, 264. [CrossRef]
37. Wang, L.; Yu, L.M.; Lin, C.G. Extraction of protease produced by sea mud bacteria and evaluation of antifouling performance. *J. Ocean Univ. China* **2019**, *18*, 1139–1146. [CrossRef]
38. Perez, M.; Sanchez, M.; Stupak, M.; Garcia, M.; de Almeida, M.T.R.; Oberti, J.C.; Palermo, J.A.; Blustein, G. Antifouling activity of celastroids isolated from maytenus species, natural and sustainable alternatives for marine coatings. *Ind. Eng. Chem. Res.* **2014**, *53*, 7655–7659. [CrossRef]
39. Liu, H.; Chen, S.Y.; Guo, J.Y.; Su, P.; Qiu, Y.K.; Ke, C.H.; Feng, D.Q. Effective natural antifouling compounds from the plant *Nerium oleander* and testing. *Int. Biodeterior. Biodegrad.* **2018**, *127*, 170–177. [CrossRef]
40. Almeida, J.R.; Moreira, J.; Pereira, D.; Pereira, S.; Antunes, J.; Palmeira, A.; Vasconcelos, V.; Pinto, M.; Correia-da-Silva, M.; Cidade, H. Potential of synthetic chalcone derivatives to prevent marine biofouling. *Sci. Total Environ.* **2018**, *643*, 98–106. [CrossRef]
41. Sathicq, A.; Paola, A.; Perez, M.; Dallesandro, O.; Garcia, M.; Roldan, J.P.; Romanelli, G.; Blustein, G. Furylchalcones as new potential marine antifoulants. *Int. Biodeterior. Biodegrad.* **2019**, *143*, 104730. [CrossRef]
42. Chaturvedi, T.; Kumar, A.; Verma, R.S.; Padalia, R.C.; Sundaresan, V.; Chauhan, A.; Saikia, D.; Singh, V.R. Chemical composition, genetic diversity, antibacterial, antifungal and antioxidant activities of camphor-basil (Ocimum kilimandscharicum Guerke). *Ind. Crops Prod.* **2018**, *118*, 246–258. [CrossRef]
43. Akella, V.S.; Singh, D.K.; Mandre, S.; Bandi, M.M. Dynamics of a camphoric acid boat at the air–water interface. *Phys. Lett. A* **2018**, *382*, 1176–1180. [CrossRef]

44. Wang, X.; Jing, S.Y.; Liu, Y.Y.; Liu, S.J.; Tan, Y.B. Diblock copolymer containing bioinspired borneol and dopamine moieties: Synthesis and antibacterial coating applications. *Polymer* **2017**, *116*, 314–323. [CrossRef]
45. Hu, J.K.; Sun, B.K.; Zhang, H.C.; Lu, A.; Zhang, H.Q.; Zhang, H.L. Terpolymer resin containing bioinspired borneol and controlled release of camphor: Synthesis and antifouling coating application. *Nature* **2020**, *10*, 10375.
46. Santos, S.E.; Ribeiro, F.P.; Menezes, P.M.; Duarte-Fiho, L.A.; Quintans, J.S.; Quintans-Junior, L.J.; Silva, F.S.; Ribeiro, L.A. New insights on relaxant effects of-borneol monoterpene in rat aortic rings. *Fundam. Clin. Pharmacol.* **2019**, *33*, 148–158. [CrossRef] [PubMed]
47. Qian, P.Y.; Xu, Y.; Fusetani, N. Natural products as antifouling compounds: Recent progress and future perspectives. *Biofouling* **2010**, *26*, 223–234. [CrossRef]
48. Wang, X.; Yu, L.M.; Liu, Y.J.; Jiang, X.H. Synthesis and fouling resistance of capsaicin derivatives containing amide groups. *Sci. Total Environ.* **2020**, *710*, 136361. [CrossRef]
49. Liu, Y.; Shao, X.Q.; Huang, J.; Li, H. Flame sprayed environmentally friendly high density polyethylene (HDPE)-capsaicin composite coatings for marine antifouling applications. *Mater. Lett.* **2019**, *238*, 46–50. [CrossRef]
50. David, R.; Neumann, A.W. Contact angle patterns on low-energy surfaces. *Adv. Colloid Interface Sci.* **2014**, *206*, 46–56. [CrossRef]
51. Gao, Z.Q.; Jiang, S.M.; Zhang, Q.F.; Li, X.G. Advances in research of marine antifouling fluorine resin coatings with low surface energy. *Electropating Finish.* **2017**, *36*, 273–279.
52. Arukalam, I.O.; Oguzie, E.E.; Li, Y. Fabrication of FDTS-modified PDMS-ZnO nanocomposite hydrophobic coating with anti-fouling capability for corrosion protection of Q235 steel. *J. Colloid Interface Sci.* **2016**, *484*, 220–228. [CrossRef]
53. Xu, B.B.; Liu, Y.J.; Sun, X.W.; Hu, J.H.; Shi, P.; Huang, X.Y. Semifluorinated synergistic nonfouling/fouling-release surface. *ACS Appl. Mater. Interfaces* **2017**, *9*, 16517–16523. [CrossRef] [PubMed]
54. Selim, M.S.; Yang, H.; Wang, F.Q.; Li, X.; Huang, Y.; Fatthallah, N.A. Silicone/Ag@SiO$_2$ core-shell nanocomposite as a self-cleaning antifouling coating material. *RSC Adv.* **2018**, *8*, 9910–9921. [CrossRef]
55. Carman, M.L.; Estes, T.G.; Feinberg, A.W.; Schumacher, J.F.; Wikerson, W.; Wilson, L.H.; Callow, M.E.; Callow, J.A.; Brennan, A.B. Engineered antifouling microtopographies-correlating wettability with cell attachment. *Biofouling* **2006**, *22*, 11–21. [CrossRef]
56. Scardino, A.J.; Guenther, J.; de Nys, R. Attachment point theory revisited: The fouling response to a microtextured matrix. *Biofouling* **2008**, *24*, 45–53. [CrossRef]
57. Bixler, G.D.; Bhushan, B. Shark skin inspired low-drag micro-structured surfaces in closed channel flow. *J. Colloid Interface Sci.* **2013**, *393*, 384–396. [CrossRef] [PubMed]
58. Schumacher, J.F.; Carman, M.L.; Estes, T.G.; Feinberg, A.W.; Wilson, L.H.; Callow, M.E.; Callow, J.A.; Finlay, J.A.; Brennan, A.B. Engineered antifouling microtopographies-effect of feature size, geometry, and roughness on settlement of zoospores of the green alga Ulva. *Biofouling* **2007**, *23*, 55–62. [CrossRef] [PubMed]
59. Wen, L.; Weaver, J.C.; Lauder, G.V. Biomimetic shark skin: Design, fabrication and hydrodynamic function. *J. Exp. Biol.* **2014**, *217*, 1656–1666. [CrossRef]
60. Gu, Y.Q.; Zhao, G.; Zheng, J.X.; Li, Z.Y.; Liu, W.B.; Muhammad, F.K. Experimental and numerical investigation on drag reduction of non-smooth bionic jet surface. *Ocean. Eng.* **2014**, *81*, 50–57. [CrossRef]
61. Gu, Y.Q.; Yu, S.W.; Mou, J.G.; Fan, T.X.; Zheng, S.H.; Zhao, G. Experimental study of drag reduction characteristics related to the multifactor coupling of a bionic jet surface. *J. Hydrodyn.* **2019**, *31*, 186–194. [CrossRef]
62. Luo, Y.H.; Zhang, D.Y. Investigation on fabricating continuous vivid sharkskin surface by bio-replicated rolling method. *Appl. Surf. Sci.* **2013**, *282*, 370–375.
63. Gu, Y.Q.; Fan, T.X.; Mou, J.G.; Wu, D.H.; Zheng, S.H.; Wang, E. Characteristics and mechanism investigation on drag reduction of oblique riblets. *J. Cent. South Univ.* **2017**, *24*, 1379–1386. [CrossRef]
64. Pu, X.; Li, G.J.; Huang, H.L. Preparation, anti-biofouling and drag-reduction properties of a biomimetic shark skin surface. *Biol. Open* **2016**, *5*, 389–396. [CrossRef] [PubMed]
65. Zhao, L.M.; Chen, R.R.; Lou, L.G.; Jing, X.Y.; Liu, Q.; Liu, J.Y.; Yu, J.; Liu, P.L.; Wang, J. Layer-by-Layer-Assembled antifouling films with surface microtopography inspired by Laminaria japonica. *Appl. Surf. Sci.* **2020**, *511*, 145564. [CrossRef]

66. Zhang, P.C.; Lin, L.; Zang, D.M.; Guo, X.L.; Liu, M.J. Designing Bioinspired Anti-Biofouling Surfaces based on a Superwettability Strategy. *Small* **2016**, *13*, 1503334. [CrossRef] [PubMed]
67. Darmanin, T.; Guittard, F. Superhydrophobic and superoleophobic properties in nature. *Mater. Today* **2015**, *18*, 273–285. [CrossRef]
68. Jiang, R.J.; Hao, L.W.; Song, L.J.; Tian, L.M.; Fan, Y.; Zhao, J.; Liu, C.Z.; Ming, W.H.; Ren, L.Q. Lotus-leaf-inspired hierarchical structured surface with non-fouling and mechanical bactericidal performances. *Chem. Eng. J.* **2020**, *398*, 125609. [CrossRef]
69. Sun, Z.Z.; Li, Z.X.; Li, W.Z.; Bian, F.G. Mesoporous cellulose/TiO_2/SiO_2/TiN-based nanocomposite hydrogels for efficient solar steam evaporation: Low thermal conductivity and high light-heat conversion. *Cellulose* **2020**, *27*, 481–491. [CrossRef]
70. Selim, M.S.; El-Safty, S.A.; El-Sockary, M.A.; Hashem, A.I.; Elenien, O.M.A.; EL-Saeed, A.M.; Fatthallah, N.A. Smart photo-induced silicone/TiO_2 nanocomposites with dominant [110] exposed surfaces for self-cleaning foul-release coatings of ship hulls. *Mater. Des.* **2016**, *101*, 218–225. [CrossRef]
71. Zhang, X.; Zhang, J.; Yu, J.Q.; Zhang, Y.; Cui, Z.X.; Sun, Y.; Hou, B.R. Fabrication of $InVO_4$/$AgVO_3$ heterojunctions with enhanced photocatalytic antifouling efficiency under visible-light. *Appl. Catal.* **2018**, *220*, 57–66. [CrossRef]
72. Gu, Y.Q.; Xia, K.; Wu, D.H.; Mou, J.G.; Zheng, S.H. Technical characteristics and wear-resistant mechanism of Nano coatings: A review. *Coatings* **2020**, *10*, 233. [CrossRef]
73. Tian, S.; Jiang, D.Y.; Pu, J.B.; Sun, X.F.; Li, Z.M.; Wu, B.; Zheng, W.R.; Liu, W.Q.; Liu, Z.X. A new hybrid silicone-based antifouling coating with nanocomposite hydrogel for durable antifouling properties. *Chem. Eng. J.* **2019**, *370*, 1–9. [CrossRef]
74. Selim, M.S.; Yang, H.; El-Safty, A.S.; Fatthallah, N.A.; Shenashen, M.A.; Wang, F.Q.; Huang, Y. Superhydrophobic coating of silicone/β–MnO_2 nanorod composite for marine antifouling. *Colloids Surf.* **2019**, *570*, 518–530. [CrossRef]
75. Li, Y.; Wang, G.Q.; Guo, Z.H.; Wang, P.Q.; Wang, A.M. Preparation of microcapsules coating and the study of their bionic anti-fouling performance. *Materials* **2020**, *13*, 1669. [CrossRef] [PubMed]
76. Xie, Q.Y.; Pan, J.S.; Ma, C.F.; Zhang, G.Z. Dynamic surface antifouling: Mechanism and systems. *Soft Matter* **2019**, *15*, 1087–1107. [CrossRef] [PubMed]
77. Zhou, X.; Xie, Q.Y.; Ma, C.F.; Chen, Z.J.; Zhang, G.Z. Inhibition of marine biofouling by use of degradable and hydrolyzable silyl acrylate copolymer. *Ind. Eng. Chem. Res.* **2015**, *54*, 9559–9565. [CrossRef]
78. Kommeren, S.; Guerin, A.J.; Dale, M.L.; Ferguson, J.; Lyall, G.; Reynolds, K.J.; Clare, A.S.; Bastiaansen, C.W.M.; Sullivan, T. Antifouling and fouling-release performance of photo-embossed fluorogel elastomers. *J. Mar. Sci. Eng.* **2019**, *7*, 419. [CrossRef]
79. Richards, C.; Briciu-Burghina, C.; Jacobs, M.R.; Barrett, A.; Regan, F. Assessment of antifouling potential of novel transparent sol gel coatings for application in the marine environment. *Molecules* **2019**, *24*, 2983. [CrossRef]
80. Xie, C.H.; Guo, H.S.; Zhao, W.Q.; Zhang, L. Environmentally friendly marine antifouling coating based on a synergistic strategy. *Langmuir* **2020**, *36*, 2396–2402. [CrossRef]

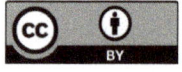 © 2020 by the authors. Licensee MDPI, Basel, Switzerland. This article is an open access article distributed under the terms and conditions of the Creative Commons Attribution (CC BY) license (http://creativecommons.org/licenses/by/4.0/).

MDPI
St. Alban-Anlage 66
4052 Basel
Switzerland
Tel. +41 61 683 77 34
Fax +41 61 302 89 18
www.mdpi.com

Marine Drugs Editorial Office
E-mail: marinedrugs@mdpi.com
www.mdpi.com/journal/marinedrugs

www.ingramcontent.com/pod-product-compliance
Lightning Source LLC
LaVergne TN
LVHW070620100526
838202LV00012B/689